T35774

tical
Guide to
Sports Injuries

Acquisitions editor: Melanie Tait
Development editor: Myriam Brearley
Production controller: Chris Jarvis
Desk editor: Jane Campbell
Cover designer: Alan Studholme

A Practical Guide to Sports Injuries

Malcolm T. F. Read

MA MB Bchir MRCGP DRCOG
DM-SMed FISM

*Consultant in Orthopaedic and Sports
Medicine, London, UK*

BUTTERWORTH
HEINEMANN

OXFORD AUCKLAND BOSTON JOHANNESBURG MELBOURNE NEW DELHI

Butterworth-Heinemann
Linacre House, Jordan Hill, Oxford OX2 8DP
225 Wildwood Avenue, Woburn, MA 01801-2041
A division of Reed Educational and Professional Publishing Ltd

ℛ A member of the Reed Elsevier plc group

First published 2000

British Library Cataloguing in Publication Data
Read, Malcolm
    A practical guide to sports injuries
    1. Sports injuries   2. Sports injuries – Treatment   3. Sports injuries – Diagnosis
    I. Title
    617.1'027

Library of Congress Cataloguing in Publication Data
Read, Malcolm
    A practical guide to sports injuries/Malcolm Read.
    p. cm.
    Includes bibliographical references and index.
    ISBN 0 7506 3251 8
    1. Sports injuries.   I. Title.
    RD97.R427
    617.1'027–dc21

ISBN 0 7506 3251 8

Every effort has been made to contact Copyright holders requesting permission to reproduce their illustra-
tions in this book. Any omissions will be rectified in subsequent printings if notice is given to the
Publisher.

Typeset by David Gregson Associates, Beccles, Suffolk
Printed and bound in Great Britain by Martins the Printers Ltd, Berwick upon Tweed

Contents

Foreword

This book is full of practical advice and observation based on Malcolm Read's years of experience as a sports and exercise medicine doctor. I learned most of my sports medicine from Malcolm Read in the 1980s, and within these pages can see all that knowledge, advice and practical experience easily presented. There are clear pictorial summaries at the beginning of every chapter, and you can use this book as an easy reference. There are also regular caveats which represent the important potential banana skins to look out for, and useful tiops to give to your patients.

As the title suggests, this is a practical guide, and is not full of abstract theory or extensive references. It is full of personal observations, treatments and practical measures of how to deal with real-life sports injuries and musculo-skeletal problems. It is based on the author's many years of experience, and represents the forefront of practice in sports and exercise medicine. There is useful and honest comment on the limitations of treatments which should provide an invaluable guide to practice as well as an entertaining and informative read.

Richard Budgett
British Olympic Medical Officer
Olympic Gold Medalist

Acknowledgement

My heartfelt thanks go to my wife Rosemary, who has interpreted illegible train-vibrated scrawl and typed and retyped this manuscript over many long evenings, and to Dr Hugh Foster for his advice during the editing. To Stephanie Pain, our daughter, and Alan Pain my thanks for the action photographs.

Introduction

This book is not a textbook of sports medicine but a practical guide to the problems that can face a doctor or physiotherapist with a sports team or in a sports clinic.

General

The book can be used by selecting the *anatomical area* concerned, e.g. the knee, where a list of *differential diagnoses* is presented depending upon the locality of the problem, e.g. medial knee pain. The book is designed for practical reference with localized areas of pain highlighted. In some areas, such as the knee, this is then divided into elements of the history that group them together, such as swollen or non-swollen, and medial or lateral areas of pain reference. These are then further subdivided as follows.

Findings
Findings include the history, and signs and symptoms that are specific to the problem. Many sports injuries have a primary injury which may have a pure complete diagnostic picture, but many have a combination of injuries – a lateral epicondylitis and a radio-humeral joint arthropathy. The findings only deal with the elements under discussion, not the combinations, although the reader is referred on to the relevant chapter to complete the diagnostic whole. Perhaps the most important principle of orthopaedic medicine is to realize that many patients develop a trick move to protect the primary injury – when this trick move becomes over-strained then pain appears elsewhere and may in fact be the presenting feature. Thus a knee may be protected by 'rolling round' the hip, producing a trochanteric bursitis, or the hamstring insertion becomes flared, whilst protecting a weak knee.

Cause
The mechanism of the injury and the tissues damaged are suggested as no treatment is complete, and the injury will reoccur, if the cause has not been dealt with.

Investigations
These do not include investigations to exclude the differentials unless they are watershed investigations. It is not cost-effective to carry out investigations if the clinical diagnosis is clear and the patient is improving, so these are defined as 'none clinically required'. As MRI improves, so its role may develop further; as of now MRI is not as reliable as CT for cortical bone, but is certainly better for soft tissue injuries, but by no means perfect. Whether MRI or SPECT scanning can pick up early bone lesions may depend upon whether the lesion is medullary or cortical. Bone scanning is a good watershed investigation – if it is 'hot' (an increased uptake of technetium-99), then concentrate the investigation on the bone – if not, treat as a soft tissue problem. This may make the difference to immobilizing or exercising the affected part. X-ray may still be the best and cheapest investigation for myositis ossificans, calcific tendinitis, loose bodies and joint instability.

Treatment
Treatment is not covered in detail but in principle. Details of the pulse rate and fluctuations of ultrasound or the wavelength of laser are for other books, as are the techniques and doses of injections. The aim of treatment in sports injuries, indeed all locomotor problems, is to return the patient to locomotor efficiency and a series of

rehabilitation ladders are included that may be used to guide recovery. Patients left to themselves will rest until pain-free and then return to full activity, break down again, rest and return to full activity ad nauseam, until advised properly. The body responds to incremental loads and these loads must be within the injury tolerance or the injury will reoccur. The ladder principles develop a rehabilitation rate that is dependent upon the individual's progress, not some arbitrary healing rate. These are expanded in the chapter on Rehabilitation (see Chapter 20). *Proprioceptive training*, balance and coordination cannot be trained by 30 minutes of physiotherapy twice a week, but require regular exercises that can be done every hour over the day, including for amateurs, the working day. Thus, for example, balancing on one leg whilst cleaning teeth or adding a half knee bend whilst answering the telephone, plus walking up stairs without using the calf will all aid a weak uncoordinated knee more effectively than 20 minutes on a wobble board twice a week. *Cross-training* is the ideal way to maintain cardiovascular fitness using other exercise programmes to maintain fitness whilst resting the injured part and these regimens are referred to in the chapter on Rehabilitation. Rhythm which controls technique by not allowing a trick move must be encouraged. Athletes are goal achievers who will cheat to reach their goals by using other techniques that will function at lower skills or speed, but will break down at high speed or higher skill levels. It is better to progress correctly, even if more slowly. All athletes, if left to themselves, will practise what they are good at – injury can sometimes be the best time to work on poor skills – use injury lay-off as a friend not an enemy.

Caveats

These are problem areas where it is easy to overlook a totally different diagnosis or complications and remind the reader to think wider and further.

Sports

This section deals with those sports that have technical problems that either cause the injury or require a particular type of rehabilitation or training technique. Reference will be to a right-handed player.

Comments

Comments are made as observations and thoughts of the author reflecting nearly three decades of experience, but without scientific evidence to back them up.

Rehabilitation

This includes cross-training advice to maintain aerobic fitness, standard advice on incremental training and rehabilitation ladders that can be given to the patient for guidance on training with an injury. Some ladders are for technical problems, e.g. tennis elbow, and others, e.g. for the knee, will have two or more ladders that can be used. Patients who jump the ladder steps often produce a recurrence of the injury and a new problem developing during rehabilitation suggests that the old injury is being protected by a trick movement, which is now also suffering injury. This trick movement must be recognized and corrected before it becomes 'patterned' into the rehabilitation. Be pedantic about skill, not rapidity, of return to competition.

Team doctor

The section on team doctoring is to introduce those who go with teams or advise on exercise about some of the physiological, and dope and sex testing problems that might be encountered. Not every variant or problem can be covered, but a working idea of what might be expected if the reader were to travel with a team is presented. Large textbooks are written on the physiology of exercise, and this chapter is to afford a brief insight and understanding of the problems that affect your exercising patient.

Glossary

Some specialist letters refer only to eponyms and many of these and other technical terms are explained in more detail in this chapter. Eponyms have been used in the diagnostic section so that this section can be used as a quick reference for those familiar with the terms. Others who may be less familiar with a particular diagnostic technique are referred on to the Glossary and this chapter will give the reader a brief idea of the 'how, what and why' of the test.

1

Head injuries

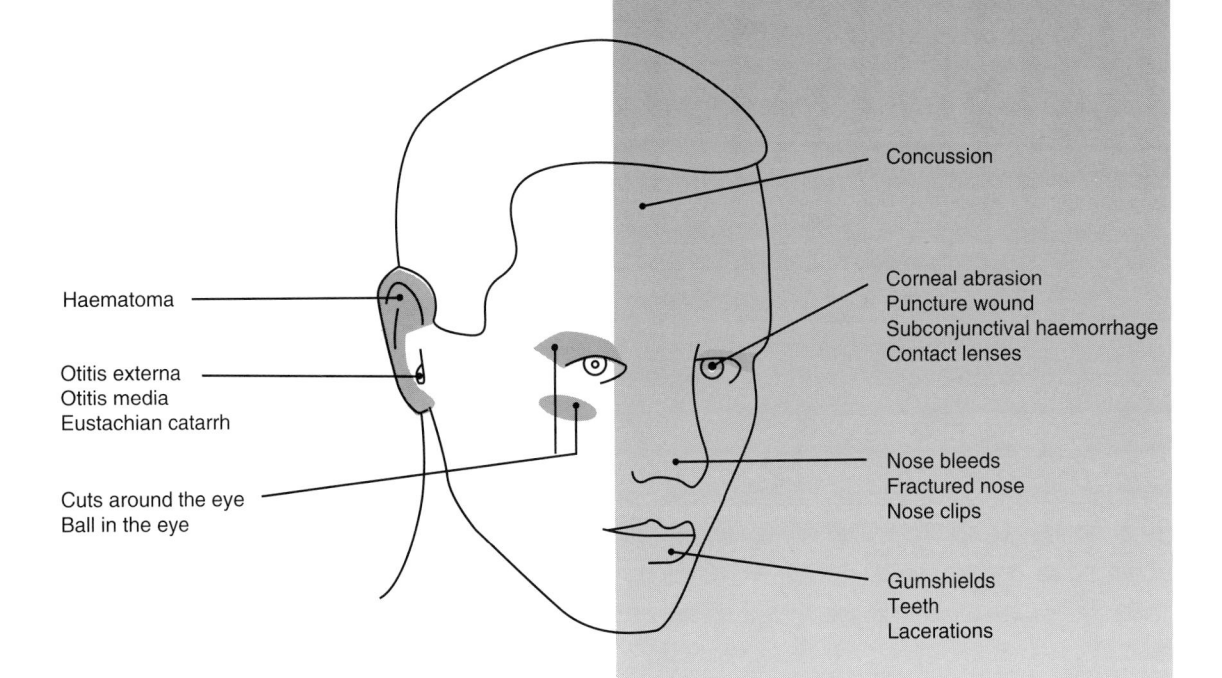

Concussion

Corneal abrasion
Puncture wound
Subconjunctival haemorrhage
Contact lenses

Haematoma

Nose bleeds
Fractured nose
Nose clips

Otitis externa
Otitis media
Eustachian catarrh

Gumshields
Teeth
Lacerations

Cuts around the eye
Ball in the eye

It is important to learn and maintain advanced life-saving techniques. This book is a guide and not a substitute for books or courses directed to that end.

Concussion

Thorough preparation at the venue is important. Know the whereabouts of the stretchers, preferably a scoop stretcher, and semi-rigid lock-on cervical collars. Know the whereabouts of the resuscitation equipment, either from the venue or attending paramedics at the site, and that it is working. Know the telephone number of the nearest hospital competent to handle emergencies and preferably inform the management of that hospital that there is an event in the vicinity.

Airway or neck protection

The airway is vital and its restoration must take precedence even in the presence of spinal injury.

Signs of concussion – if:

(a) There has been even the shortest time of unresponsiveness.
(b) The player was confused as to where he was, what to do or which way to play.
(c) Unsteady – get them to walk heel to toe – or unable to hold the ball.
(d) Giddiness, double vision or vomiting.
(e) Has been unconscious or has spasms or convulsions.
(f) Is unable to remember the time, day, month and year, the name of the other team, and what the score is, plus how long the game has been going.
(g) This amnesia may begin 30 seconds or so after the trauma.

Action to be taken

(a) A concussed player should be removed from the pitch.
(b) If the player has been stunned or dazed less than 1 minute but no other pathological signs are found then return to the field of play but observe for any deterioration.
(c) Any athlete who has been unconscious should be removed from the pitch, preferably on a stretcher, for further examination, having first removed the gumshield and cleared the airway [1].

Off the pitch check

AVPU
A   Alertness
V   Responds to verbal commands
P   Responds to pain
U   Unconscious

Transfer to hospital

(a) Unconscious longer than 5 minutes – note the Glasgow Coma Score and send a record with the patient (tape the chart to the inside of your medical case so you can remember it).
(b) Increasing headache, nausea or vomiting.
(c) Unequal pupils.
(d) Changing neurological signs.
(e) Convulsion.
(f) Rising blood pressure or falling pulse, head down position may aggravate the blood pressure.
(g) Treat with continuous oxygen.

Check

(a) Lacerations – remember a small skin wound can hide a fracture.
(b) Scalp tenderness.
(c) Haematoma for possible underlying fracture.
(d) Blood or cerebrospinal fluid from ears or nose.
(e) Subconjunctival haemorrhage.

All of which require further investigation.

Instructions to friends or relative of an athlete sent home

Advise them that any deterioration in consciousness or drowsiness, onset of headache, double vision or vomiting require immediate medical attention.

Return to competition or training

Should not occur until the athlete has passed a full neurological examination, has no headache and no headache after exercise [2], probably at about 1 week in non-contact sports. Some sports have an arbitrary time to match fitness, e.g. rugby 3 weeks, and boxing 28 days first time, 84 days second time and 1 year third time.

Caveat – Although contact sports can be expected at times to cause problems, a major source of head injuries comes from youngsters swinging golf clubs and being too close to other players and thus hitting them with the club. All coaches and players should be aware.

Protective helmets

No helmet can prevent all head and neck injuries a player might receive. The helmet does not prevent the contra coup injury [2], but is effective against lacerations and haematoma. The hard outer shell dissipates incidental blows but the crumpling of the polystyrene inner shell absorbs most of the energy. Any crash helmet that has been subject to damage should be changed as the integrity of the inner shell cannot be guaranteed.

Eyes

Prevention is better than cure! Snow blindness has occurred in those removing sun glasses to take photographs and water may reflect the sun's rays to cause similar problems. Polarized dark glasses may be made to visual acuity and may also permit changeable prescription lenses to be slipped underneath. Cages or helmets at cricket or American football and motorcycle helmets protect the face and eyes from trauma, and sparring helmets functionally deepen the orbit. However, specially designed squash and badminton eye guards are often ignored, although both the squash ball and shuttlecock 'fit' the orbit and a 'blow out' fracture of the orbit can cause total loss of an eye. Emphasis in these games, beside eye protection, is the calling of 'lets' and 'penalty points', especially for those players with less skill, who tend to hit the ball regardless of the opponent's position of danger.

Medical 'eye injury kit'

(a) Small mirror.
(b) Pencil torch.
(c) Ophthalmoscope.
(d) Sterile washout fluid.
(e) Local anaesthetic eye drops.

(f) Fluorescein.
(g) Antibiotic drops or ointment – check expiry dates regularly.
(h) Eye patches – micropore or clear tape.
(i) Visual acuity chart.
(j) Contact lens fluid.

Cuts around the eye

Allow 3–4 weeks for adequate healing.
(a) Acute. Remove from the field of play, 1 : 1000 adrenaline swabs, steristrips or Embucrylate and/or suturing. Cover the wound.
(b) Subacute. Subcuticular suturing and enzyme creams.

Caveat – Eyelids or medial epicanthic folds, which may involve the tear duct, require specialist referral.

Corneal abrasion

Amethocaine, fluorescein, antibiotic cream or drops. Close the eyelid and cover for 24–48 hours. Remove loose foreign bodies.

Caveat – Embedded foreign body, penetrating injury, hyphaemia (blood in anterior chamber) or dendritic ulcer – refer for ophthalmic opinion.

Puncture wound of the eye

Note any history of penetrating wound, hyphaemia, pear-shaped iris, enlarged or poorly reacting pupil, cloudy vision and impaired visual acuity. Refer for ophthalmic opinion.

Caveat – A late sequelae may be a sympathetic response in the other eye.

Ball in the eye

(a) Large. (Cricket ball plus in size). Then a check for hyphaemia and orbital fractures, especially the inferior orbit, must be made. Note diplopia may also occur as a late sequela when the inferior rectus muscle is tied into the healing inferior orbital fracture. If in doubt, refer for ophthalmic opinion.

(b) Small. A small ball in the eye will fit the orbit and may be catastrophic, causing a blow out fracture of the orbit and loss of an eye [3]. Check for hyphaemia and posterior chamber bleed when the fundus and retina are not visible. If in doubt, refer for ophthalmic opinion.

Subconjunctival haemorrhage

If the haemorrhage appears segmental in the posterior aspect it is probably of no consequence, but if the posterior aspect cannot be visualized then consider trauma to the eye, a fractured skull and cerebral contusion, and refer for a further opinion. If visual problems or possible penetrating injury have occurred, refer for ophthalmic opinion.

Contact lenses

These should be soft and a spare pair should be available, as they are usually displaced around the eye but are occasionally lost outside the eye.

Glasses

These should be (plastic) polycarbonate, have sprung ear clips and have a nose bridge that holds the glasses away from the face to prevent misting up.

Eyes at risk from trauma

In the case of only one functioning eye, check for previous retinal detachment or Marfan's syndrome.

Unfortunately laser surgery does not alter the risk of possible retinal detachment in severe myopia.

Vision

Increasing amounts of work are being done on training vision in sport and particularly the non-dominant eye. Defective vision may be remediable and a full assessment is advised [4].

Ears

Prevention is better than cure. Scrum caps or taping prevent damage to the pinna and ear muffs should prevent acoustic trauma.

Haematoma of the pinna (cauliflower ear)

(a) Acute. Aspirate and compression bandage. The aspiration must be aseptic and will probably require repeating on several occasions.

(b) Chronic. No treatment, but cosmetic surgery can be advised when the playing days are over. Perichondral tears should be well aligned, sutured and covered by antibiotics. This may require referral to a plastic surgeon.

Otitis externa

In particular, can occur following swimming; however, soft moulded ear plugs may help or may cause the problem during insertion. Dry the ears but do not use cotton wool buds on sticks which excoriate the external auditory meatus. Warm olive oil drops pre-swimming and 5% acetic acid in isopropyl alcohol drops after swimming may help. Swab for *Staphylococcus* or *Candida* if troublesome and treat as required.

Otitis media

May play sports if non-toxic but diving, especially scuba, should be avoided. Swimming should cease with a perforation, but ENT surgeons may vary as to whether the presence of grommets should prevent swimming.

Eustachian and sinus catarrh

Acutely may be relieved by menthol inhalations and dope test-negative nasal decongestants, but great care should be taken to avoid medicines with ephedrine, pseudoephedrine or phenyl propranalamine, or any other banned substance. The allergic element may be controlled with steroid insufflation, cromoglyconates and non-sedative antihistamines but parenteral steroids are banned. Surprisingly, once scuba divers learn to repressurize their ears, diving is said to help the condition.

Mouth

Gumshields should be cast made to allow maximum compression thickness over the teeth cusps but allow the least interference with the palate for easy mouth breathing. They should be worn in all sports where potential impact may occur, including squash, where blows from the racket can occur but education as to their advantage may be required [5, 6]. Displaced teeth should be replaced and splinted. Avulsed teeth and crown fragments should be kept but handled only by the crown. In an alert patient replace within 60 minutes, but if not fully alert store in a sterile solution (saline) and get to a dentist within 2 hours. X-ray for missing teeth or fragments if not found. Lacerations in the tongue and mucosa often heal well without sutures.

Nose

Nose bleeds
Sit the patient and tip the head forwards, compress externally over Little's area, preferably for 5 minutes by a person other than the patient. 1 : 1000 adrenaline packs may be used but continued bleeding or posterior nasal cavity bleed – refer to ENT department.

Caveat – The presence of cerebrospinal fluid equates to a cranial fracture.

Fractured nose
(a) Undisplaced. May be treated by managing the bleeding and soft tissue injury.
(b) Displaced. Should be reduced, especially in the young, as a fracture may reduce the size of the nasal passage and increase the likelihood of sinusitis.

Caveat – A septal haematoma will present with increasing pain, fever and an appearance of local, red swollen, septum which requires evacuation and aspiration.

Nose clips
(a) Sprung to close the external nares for synchronized swimming.
(b) Strips to open the nares do nothing to increase respiration during exercise as this is dominantly by mouth breathing, but during the recovery phase allows more nose breathing and thus a feeling of more controlled and easy respiration.

Further reading

1. National Health and Medical Research Council (1995) *Head and Neck Injuries in Football*. Australian Government Publishing Service, Canberra.
2. Ryan, A. J. (1991) Protecting the sportsman's brain (concussion in sport). *Br. J. Sports Med.* **25**, 81–86.
3. Jones, N. P. (1994) Orbital blowout fractures in sport. *Br. J. Sports Med.* **28**, 272–275.
4. Loran, D. F. and MacEwan, C. J. (1995) *Sports Vision*. Butterworth-Heinemann, Oxford.
5. Chapman, P. J. (1990) Orofacial injuries and international rugby players' attitudes to mouth guards. *Br. J. Sports Med.* **24**, 156–158.
6. Jennings, D. C. (1990) Injuries sustained by users and non users of gum shields in local rugby union. *Br. J. Sports Med.* **24**, 159–165.

Bruckner, P. and Khan, K. (1993) *Clinical Sports Medicine*. McGraw-Hill, New York.
Reid, R. (1992) *Sports Injury Assessment and Rehabilitation*. Churchill Livingstone, Edinburgh.

2

Back

Part 1
Functional anatomy

The disk

Each disc has a central nucleus pulposus, a surrounding annulus fibrosis and the limiting cartilage end plates.

Nucleus pulposus

The nucleus pulposus is a soft hydrophilic substance contained within the centre of the disc.

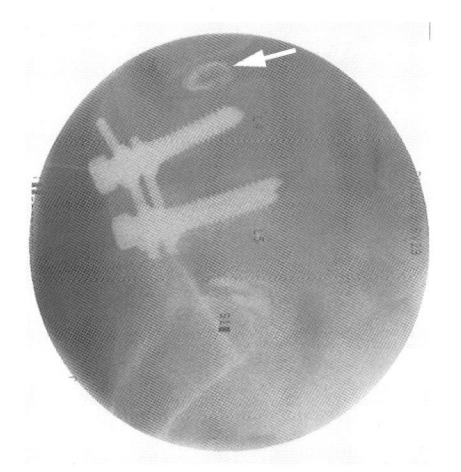

Figure 2.1 The discogram clearly outlines a normal nucleus pulposus at L3/4. L4/5 vertebrae are surgically stabilized.

The nucleus pulposus can move within the confines of the annulus fibrosis. See Fig. 2.1.

Annulus fibrosis

The posterior lateral region is less orderly, and is the area that is weakest during ageing thus predisposing to nucleus pulposus herniations towards the spinal canal.

Cartilage end plate

This represents the anatomical limit of the disc. The annular epiphyses of the vertebral body develop in the marginal part of this thin end plate. Stress changes across this area in the teenager produce pain and diagnostic X-ray changes of Scheuermann's. See Fig. 2.2.

Ligaments

The anterior longitudinal ligament supports the anterior aspect of the vertebral bodies including the discs. The posterior longitudinal ligament is attached to the posterior aspect of the vertebral bodies but creates the anterior wall of the spinal canal. It is not as strong as the anterior ligament.

The ligamentum flavum forms the posterior aspect of the spinal canal. It is an elastic ligament that helps the upright posture and the return of the spinal column to its erect position after bending.

The supraspinous ligament runs over the tips of the spines and connects with the interspinous ligament that joins the spinous processes – they are strongest at the lumbar level.

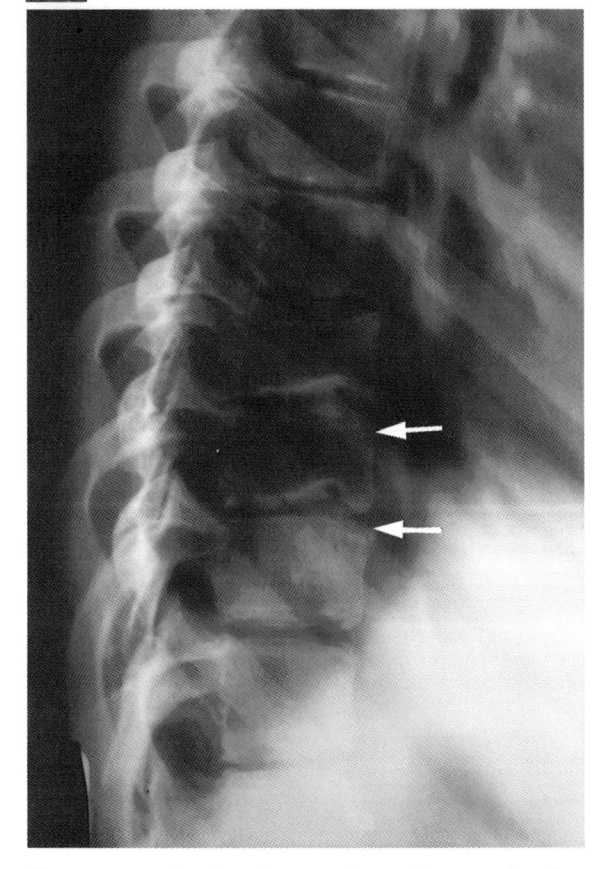

Figure 2.2 The dorsal spine shows the irregular disc spaces and end plates of Scheuermann's.

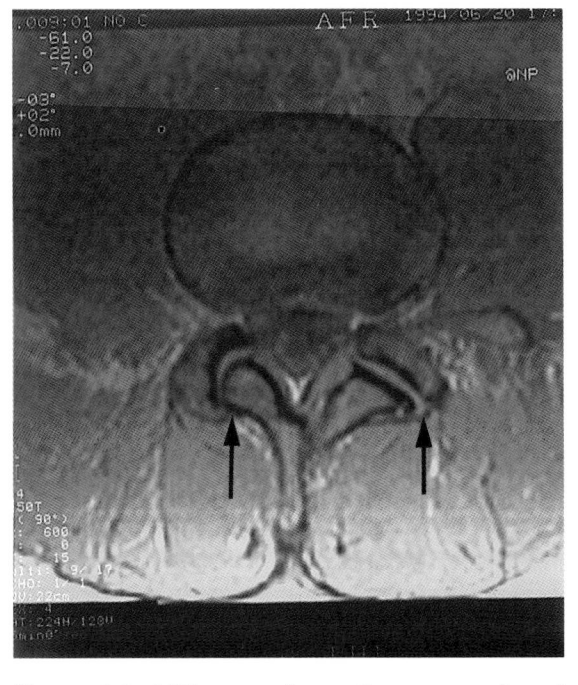

Figure 2.3 MRI scan shows the zygoapophyseal (facet) joints. These illustrated are abnormally asymmetric and as such may produce an unstable movement pattern.

Facet joints

The vertebral arches are united by the synovial zygoapophyseal joints whose shape will control the range of movement between the concomitant vertebrae. The thoracic vertebrae favour lateral bending and rotation, whilst the lumbar facets favour flexion, extension and lateral bending at the higher lumbar levels. See Fig. 2.3.

Innervation

The innervation of the disc, posterior longitudinal ligament, periosteum, venous sinuses and spinal dura is from the sinu vertebral nerve, and contains spinal and sympathetic branches; it may also provide fibres to the facet joints. (This nerve is divided by cryo- or radiorhizotomy to treat chronic facetal pain.)

Function

The major function of the vertebral column is to support and protect the spinal cord from physical trauma. The spinal cord ends at the level between L1/2 and below this are the out-going nerves bound in meningeal coverings to S2, the cauda equina. A filum terminale connects the meninges to their eventual insertion.

The ligaments can support the vertebral column so that less muscle energy is required to maintain its erect posture. During movement the large mass of posterior vertebral muscles are primarily responsible for intrinsic stability; however, with increased dynamic loading both intra-abdominal and intrathoracic pressure increases, acting like a pneumatic cushion (tyre) to support the anterior aspect of the vertebral column – a principle used in functional muscle control of the back.

In the lumbar spine the movements of flexion, extension and side flexion compress the disc on one edge and stretch the other, and this movement pushes the nucleus pulposus towards the stretched surface, so that in flexion the nucleus pulposus will move posteriorly. See Fig. 2.4.

Flexion of the spine is limited by the elasticity of the ligamentum flavum, the inter- and supra-spinous ligaments, the posterior part of the disc, and the posterior longitudinal ligament, whereas extension is limited by the anterior longitudinal ligament, the anterior part of the disc, and the close packing of the facet joints and spinous pro-cesses against one another.

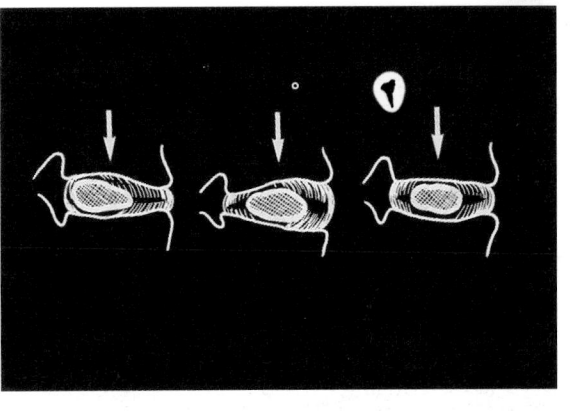

Figure 2.4 The nucleus pulposus moves in relation to back position.

Referred pain

Damage to the lumbar spine may cause localized pain, or referred pain to the groin, buttock, thigh, shin, calf, ankle or foot, with no accompanying local back pain. It is therefore essential to include examination of the back when assessing a patient who presents with pain in the lower limbs.

Leg pain
Clues in the history that pain is nerve or dura:

(a) Night pain, waking the patient from sleep as opposed to whilst turning in bed.
(b) 'Pins and needles' and numbness.
(c) Worse on coughing or blowing the nose.
(d) Worse with extension, L5 S1 collar stud, L2/3/4 disc and lateral canal entrapment.
(e) Radiation of pain into the foot is usually nerve, not facet or sacro-iliac joint.
(f) Burning, hypersensitive, water flowing in arm or leg; however, burning, eternal pain in a stocking distribution = possible reflex sympathetic dystrophy.
(g) Intensity of pain description – there may be few clinical findings but the desire of the patient to convince you just how intense the pain is may be diagnostic of dural pain.

Bone pain

All the usual causes of bone pain must be considered when seeing people with sports injuries. Patients with tumours and infections of the spine give a history of a continuous pain that may or may not be affected by biomechanical movement, unlike locomotor problems, which are affected by normal biomechanical patterns and can be pain-free at times. In young patients, it is important to consider the possibility of ankylosing spondylitis and the other spondylarthropathies.

Non-mechanical back pain

The possibility of a non-mechanical cause of back pain should be considered with a presentation of:

(a) Night pain.
(b) Unremitting pain.
(c) Pain not made worse by movement.
(d) Lost weight.
(e) Unwell.
(f) Temperature raised.
(g) Generally achy.
(h) Other joints painful.
(i) Flitting joint pains.
(j) Dysuria.
(k) Iritis.
(l) Conjunctivitis.
(m) Urethral discharge.
(n) Skin problems – rash, psoriasis.
(o) Known primary carcinoma.
(p) Hypo/hyperthyroidism.
(q) Family history of spondylarthropathy.

Mechanical back pain

There is no black and white definition of mechanical back problems, and the pointers to diagnosis and management are obtained from the patient's history, examination, and investigations which include MRI, CT and disc probes. Common biomechanical problems include:

(a) Disc herniation or discal pressure on the annulus.
(b) Facet joint arthrosis or arthritis.
(c) Pars interarticularis fractures (spondylolysis and its unstable bilateral form spondylolisthesis).
(d) Wedge collapse fractures of the vertebral body.
(e) Scheuermann's vertebral ring epiphysitis.
(f) Sacro-iliac dysfunction.
(g) Ligamentous strain.
(h) Interspinous impingement.

Coccygeal pain

A fall on the base of the spine may damage the sacro-coccygeal ligaments. Sitting and full flexion are painful. A ring cushion and occasionally posterior mobilization of the coccyx may help, as will steroid injections of the sacro-coccygeal ligaments.

General management

The history
Listening to the history will lead both to the possible diagnosis and also to the best modes of treatment. Biomechanical, non-traumatic, lumbar back lesions may be divided into: flexion-orientated, extension-orientated or mixed. It must always be remembered that, when one area is displaced, there will be some degree of stretch of the adjacent ligaments and alteration in the mechanics of the joints, and therefore a disc displacement will have its main component of flexion-orientated pain, but there will be some consequent displacement of the facet joints and stretch of the surrounding ligaments with secondary spasm of the muscles.

Localized muscle injuries
Localized muscle injuries do occur in the back but there is almost always a history of trauma and, without this, an underlying lesion should always be suspected.

Nerve root damage
There may be signs of a nerve root palsy with reduced motor signs. The degree of sensory disturbances, except perineal, do not alter the treatment and need not be tested as the distribution of their symptoms is a sufficient guide to the root level – MRI being an accurate diagnostic indicator of disc and root level. Nerve root involvement is suggested by: 'pins and needles', numbness, hyperaesthesia, night pain, and a desperation in the patient to convince you it really hurts. The distribution of the symptoms suggests the level, e.g. back of leg to calf, shin or foot, L4/5 S1; front thigh, knee, L2/3/4; groin, T12 L1; perineal or perianal, S3/4. The signs of nerve involvement are: positive dural stress tests, brachial nerve tensioning tests, straight leg raising reduced, Lasegue's, slump and Valsalva tests positive, and femoral stretch test positive (see *Glossary*).

Weakness from nerve root palsy

> **Caveat** – If more than two roots are involved, query diabetes, nerve disease or space-occupying lesion.

Cervical nerve root
Signs and symptoms include:

C1 Rare, pain parietal, weak painful limited neck rotation, no disc; think cancer.
C2 No disc, occipito-facial pain; think facet joint or cancer.
C3 Numb cheek, rare weaker scapular elevation.

C4   Numb point of shoulder, weak scapular elevation – uncommon.

C5   Weak deltoid, supraspinatus, biceps, infraspinatus, biceps and brachioradialis jerk diminished.

C6   Weak extensor carpi radialis, brachialis, biceps, subscapularis and biceps jerk diminished.

C7   Weak latissimus dorsi, triceps, common flexors of wrist and triceps jerk diminished.

Lumbar spine nerve root

Signs and symptoms include:

L1/2   Weak psoas.

L3/4   Weak quadriceps and diminished or absent knee jerk.

L4   Weak tibialis anterior and diminished or absent knee jerk.

L5   Weak extensor halucis, extensor digitorum longus, extensor digitorum brevis, peroneals. Peroneal weakness can present with either L4 or 5 root involvement.

S1   Weak calf, hamstring and diminished or absent ankle jerk.

S1/2   Weak gluteals.

S3/4   Anal sphincter or urinary loss of control or sensation.

> **Caveat** – S3/4 root involvement requires emergency surgery.

Rectal and vaginal examination

Intra-pelvic lesions occur and any suggestion of intra-pelvic or rectal causes should be accompanied by the relevant examination.

Rest

In the acute stage of a disc lesion the patient may be too sensitive to move around and is best rested. Certainly the patient who is better in the morning knows they get better with rest and should be actively persuaded to take time off to rest – it will hasten the healing. Sometimes moving a patient by car for traction or physiotherapy undoes the good of rest and they are better being rested rather than travelling to treatment.

Those not made worse by extension should have periods lying prone and then try gradually increasing the lumbar lordosis with pillows under their chest. An exacerbation or peripheralization of leg pain must stop this exercise. L2/3.3/4 discs are often helped by pillows under the knees or, when lying prone, a pillow under the hips. Hard mattresses encourage extension, soft mattresses encourage flexion, thus the mattress should fit the problem. Once the acute sensitivity has settled then activity should be encouraged.

Posture

Probably 80% of management of painful backs is the correct adjustment of posture for the individual, and correct posture may cure and prevent recurrences of many back conditions. Not every back responds to the same postural correction. Thus a flexion-orientated problem will need extensions to improve and prevent disc creep (see Chapter 5). Facet joints and L5 S1 collar stud discs (Fig. 2.5) will require pelvic tilting to flatten the lordosis. However, the L5 S1 collar stud disc may require pelvic tilting to start with; and, as the disc regresses and loses its collar stud formation it will then require extension manoeuvres, typical of an annular disc. A thoraco-lumbar kyphosis may have a compensatory low lumbar lordosis so that the adjustment of posture in this case will be extension at the thoraco-lumbar junction, but pelvic tilt at the lumbo-sacral junction. Too much postural advice is given in general terms without taking into account the variations within and between backs. Some backs may have to be used in a neutral position, neither emphasizing extension nor flexion.

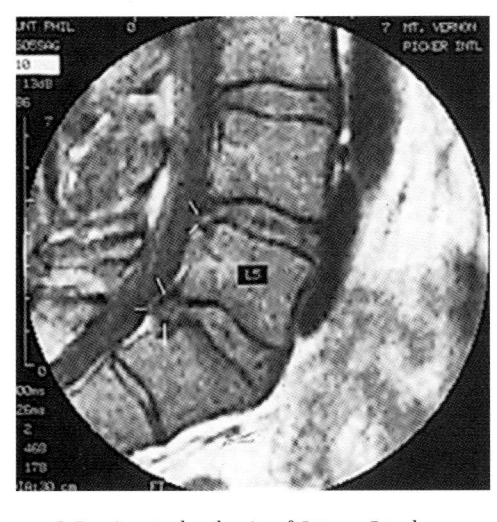

Figure 2.5   A retrolysthesis of L5 on S1 shows on X-ray by a bulging of the disc space into the body of L5. A 'collar stud' prolapse of the disc is seen on MRI and extension will nip this 'collar stud' (arrow).

Correcting the posture

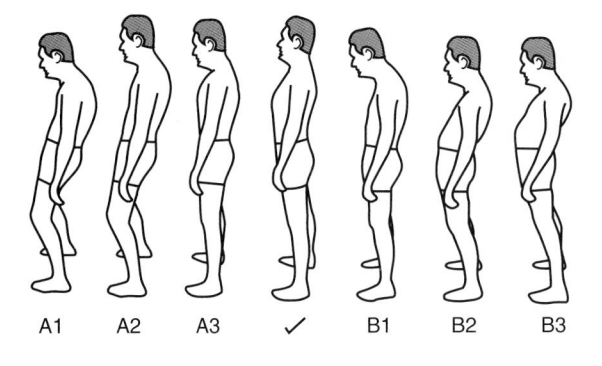

A1   A2   A3   ✓   B1   B2   B3

Group A: Rounded back (A1, A2 and A3)

The pain is worse bending over, sitting, driving and getting out of a chair when the back feels a little stuck and is eased by leaning backwards. Feels better when lying face down and arching backward. More lumbar lordosis is required. Let the weight come forward towards the balls of the feet when standing.

A1   Straighten knees, placing weight on balls of the feet to allow increased lordosis. Straighten dorsal spine, standing tall. Draw back head on shoulders.

A2   Allow lordosis, but flatten stomach muscles. Stand tall through upper spine, straighten head and shoulders.

A3   Too straight; let lordosis occur and reduce pelvic tilt – stand with weight on the balls of the feet.

The neutral position

The neutral position has tolerance and is the ideal posture. Stand with the weight balanced over the middle of the feet, with slight lordosis, stomach muscles gently tightened and dorsal spine straightened. Draw chin and head back, not up. Do not just draw shoulders back like a sergeant major.

Group B: Hollowed (sway) back (B1, B2 and B3)

Applies to those whose pain is worse standing relaxed with a lumbar lordosis, leaning backward and lying face down. It is eased by half sitting on a desk or stool. Less lumbar lordosis required, more flattening of the pelvis. Stand with the weight back, towards the heels.

B1   Stand taller through dorsal spine; straighten rounded back and straighten head and neck.

B2   Flatten stomach to support back.

B3   Tilt pelvis forward to flatten lower back, shift weight towards the heels.

Aids to posture

To increase extension:

(a)   Sleep on a hard mattress/floor/futon.

(b)   When working sit on a low chair with a high desk. Raise computer screen.

(c)   Sit with one knee drawn under the chair or pointing to the ground.

(d)   Use 'wedge' cushion on chair, 'kneel on' chairs or tilt the front of the chair downwards. Use a cushion in the small of the back or a lumbar roll. Try a towel around the waist at night.

(e)   Drive sitting upright with bent arms.

(f)   Stand with centre of gravity towards the balls of feet. Sit and stand tall.

(g)   If slumping in an easy chair, slump with lumbar spine in extension

(h)   When leaning over a solid object stand with legs wide apart to lose height and lean pelvis into object, and maintain the forward lean with an extended spine.

(i) Lock back in extension whilst bending or lifting and splint with abdominal muscles.

To decrease extension:

(a) Sleep on a soft mattress.

(b) Instead of standing obtain some flexion by propping or half sitting on the edge of a table. Use a bar stool even at the kitchen sink. Use a shooting stick.

(c) Stand with one foot resting on an object raised 6–8 inches, i.e. foot rail in a pub.

(d) Stand with the centre of gravity towards the heels.

(e) Use back in neutral position when bending or lifting.

See *Correcting the posture*, p. 13.

Bending

The nucleus pulposus moves posteriorly during flexion of the spine, so when compression of the disc is increased, as in lifting, then the forces on the posterior aspect of the annulus may cause prolapse. Lifting or bending with a slight lordosis helps to prevent this prolapse. Many diagrams show people lifting with a straight back and knees bent but with the bottom tucked in, this position is difficult to hold whilst lifting. When one watches weightlifters and people bending over, working in the fields, these people stand with legs wide apart and stick their bottom out whilst maintaining a neutral back and tense abdomen to lift.

Training

(a) Weights. The back must be locked into neutral, preferably extension, even when sitting. The moment this position cannot be held, stop the exercise. If you have to throw your back into the exercise, then the muscles you are training have fatigued sufficiently for you to recruit other muscles, so you are no

WRONG   RIGHT

longer training the target muscles. If you cannot hold extension, then the weight is too heavy or you are in the wrong technical position for the exercise.

(b) Sit-ups. Neutral back abdominals (Figs 2.6–2.8). Sit-ups with a twist manipulate the spine and should be avoided.

(c) Rowing. Upright rowing risks losing lumbar neutral or extension. The rowing ergo should provide the same effect if used with a hard pull and does not risk the back as much. Lock the back in neutral or extension, do not over reach or 'lay back' too far.

(d) Gymnastics. Walkovers should not be done by hyperextending at L5 S1 but rather spreading the spinal extension up and through the whole lumbar spine

(e) Swimming. Produces extension and thus is excellent for flexion-orientated problems but poor for extension-orientated problems, although back stroke can be tolerated. Running in a floatation jacket may be tolerated.

(f) Cycling. Good for extension-orientated problems but sit upright and raise the handle bars for flexion-orientated problems.

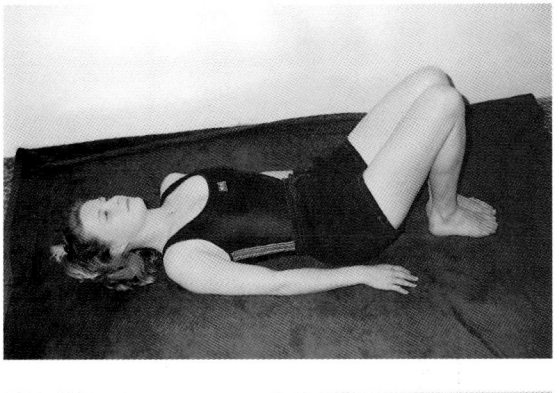

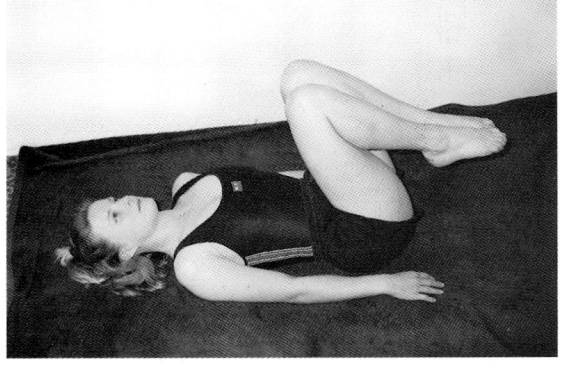

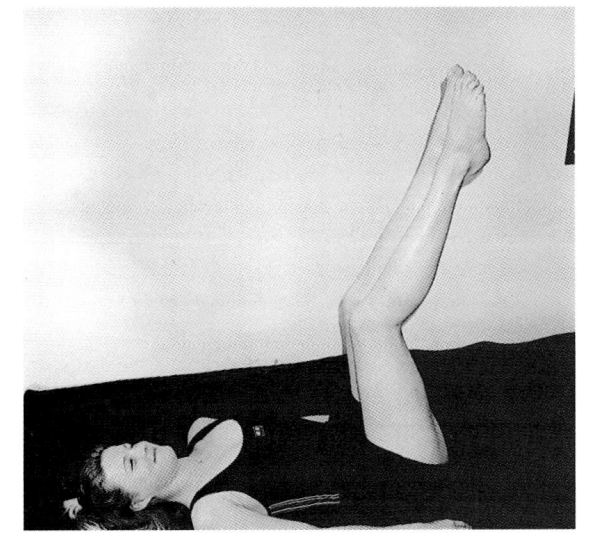

Figure 2.6 Exercise for lower abdominals. (a) Lie supine. (b) Bend the knees to flatten the back and support it on the couch. (c) Straighten the knees so there is no tension on the back and then lower the legs until the back starts to extend, re-flex the hips until the back is neutral again, then hold, either for a count of 7 or as long as one can.

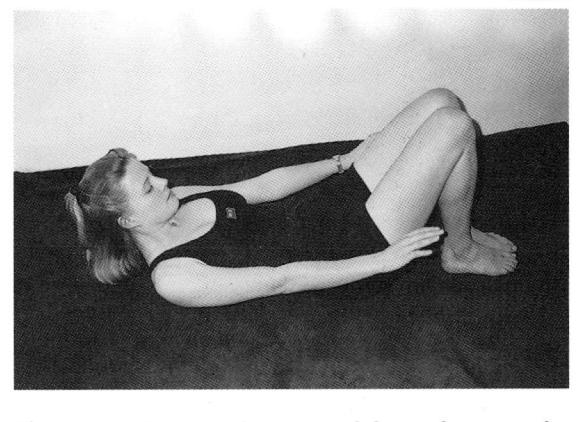

Figure 2.7 Exercise for upper abdominals. Lie as for Fig. 2.6(a) then flex neck and shoulders and hold as for Fig. 2.6(c).

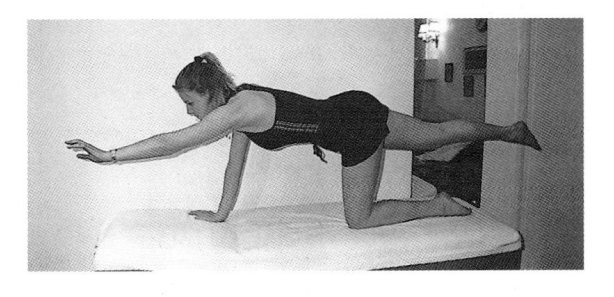

Figure 2.8 Super (wo)man. Hold neutral back, raise opposite leg and arm, but do not lose body tension. This exercises the pelvic and back muscle stabilizers.

(g) Running. Should be avoided until better as the impact compresses the disc and facet joints. When better, try to run 'tall', supporting the pelvis with the back and abdominal muscles. See Figs 2.9 and 2.10.

Home and workplace

The back and neck cause most problems whether sitting at a desk or bending over garden or household tasks. Many of these problems can be avoided if the patient observes the following:

(a) Do not wedge the telephone between the head and shoulder as this twists the neck sideways, producing facet and disc problems. The use of a shoulder holster or headset is recommended.

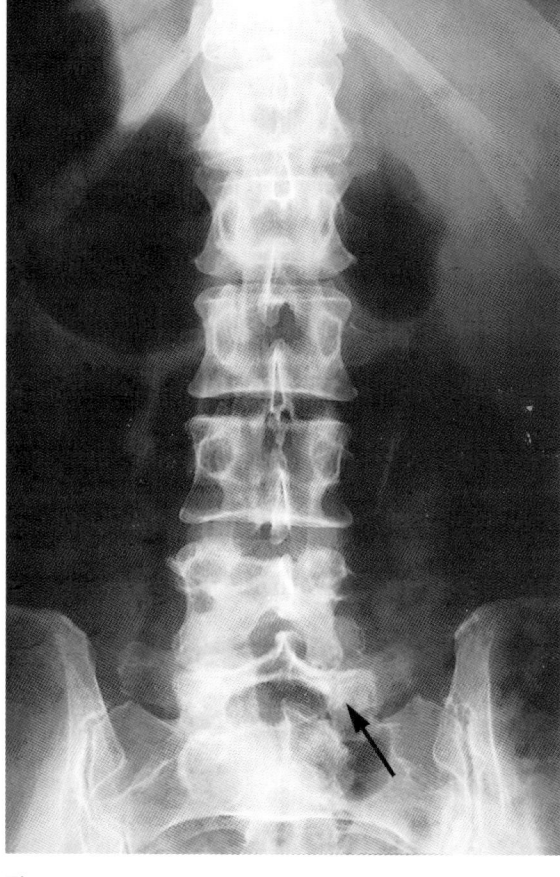

Figure 2.9 Hemilumbarization. The previous East German regime would not accept a congenitally abnormal spine for elite training because there were too many problems.

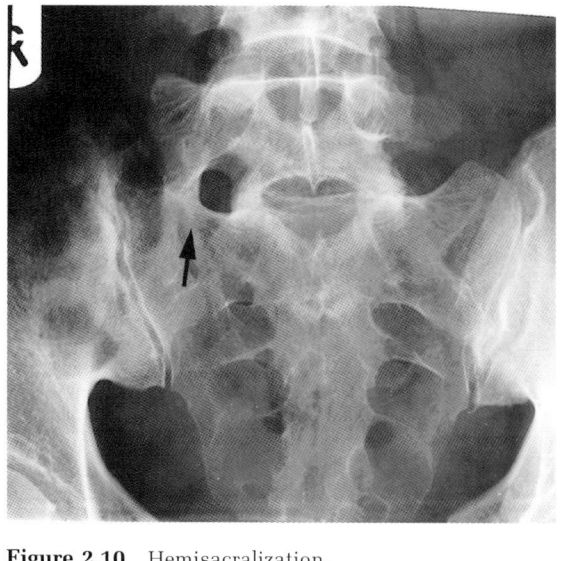

Figure 2.10 Hemisacralization.

(b) Adjust the computer and chair to the correct height. If the computer terminal is set too low on the desk and the chair is too high, or if the patient wears bifocals, they may sit slumped with a rounded back, hyperextending the neck for long periods during the day, to look at the computer screen.

(c) The computer screen should be about 15–30° below from the head position, and the keyboard and mouse operated with relaxed shoulders and bent elbows. If the screen and keyboard are offset from centre, then dorsal problems will also occur. Most people sit too slumped during a long day, and the lumbar

and dorsal spine need to be straightened so that the head is balanced – not looking up or down and not pushed forward.

(d) Office chairs should be fully adjustable – the tilt of the seat, and the back and height should all be adjustable to each individual use.

(e) A kneel-on chair or seat wedge (thinner at the front) and lumbar rolls help sitting pain with a rounded back, especially if it is eased by stretching backwards when the patient stands up after sitting. See *Correcting the posture*, p. 13

(f) Lumbar supports in cars are useless unless they adjust up and down to fit the lumbar lordosis of the patient in question. If no seat adjustments are available, adopt a sitting up tall position (whilst driving with bent elbows). Car seats, despite all the adjustments available, often leave arms too far from the steering wheel and the head against the roof. Those with back problems need to sit nearer the steering wheel with bent arms in order to take the tension out of the back and sit taller; however, if the seat is squabbed back to get the necessary head height then use a cushion to maintain lumbar lordosis.

(g) In the home, get the patient to sit to the front of the chair, or sideways on a sofa resting the back against the arm, and point one knee towards the ground, this will tilt the pelvis and comfortably straighten the back.

(h) No one goes out and runs 2–3 hours without any training, yet people will go into the garden and do 2 hours of weeding and digging, and wonder why they have back problems. They must learn to bend with a neutral lordotic back, buttocks out, hips and knees bent, and weight over the middle of the feet. See *Bending*, p. 14.

(i) Plan 5–10 minutes of bending jobs around the house and garden, followed by 5–10 minutes of standing and reaching jobs.

(j) Get patients to try vacuuming to the side and slightly behind their hips.

(k) Standing half bent over a sink, ironing board, etc., is a killer for the back. Standing with legs wide apart drops the height without bending the back or straining the knees – leaning the front of the thighs into the side of the sink enables a neutral back position to be held whilst reaching into the sink.

(l) Use the bottom out position for all half bent positions, from brushing the teeth to making the bed and emptying the car boot or oven.

Further reading

Cyriax, J. H and Cyriax, P. J. (eds) (1993) *Cyriax's Illustrated Manual of Orthopaedic Medicine*, 2nd edn. Butterworth-Heinemann, Oxford.

Palastanga, N., Field, D. and Soames, R. (1989) *Anatomy and Human Movement: Structure and Function*. Heinemann Medical, London.

Watkins, R. (ed.) (1996) *The Spine in Sports*. Mosby, St Louis, MO.

3

Neck

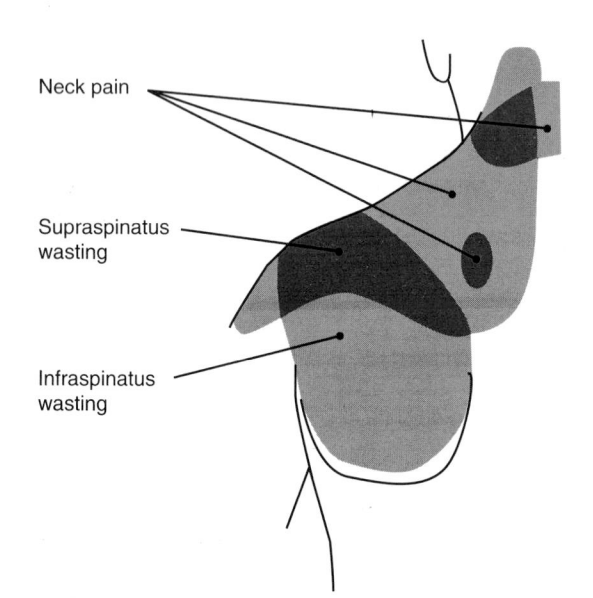

Neck pain

Supraspinatus
wasting

Infraspinatus
wasting

This book is not a First Aid or advanced life-saving
instruction book and should only be used as a
guideline – formal training is recommended for all
pitch-side support staff.

Injury on the pitch

Damage to the neck may be acute, traumatic and disastrous, and all pitch-side doctors must be aware of semi-rigid lock-on collars and log-roll techniques which should be applied to any player with a head and neck injury who has 'pins and needles', numbness or motor weakness. Five people must be involved with log-rolling and stretchering the patient, feet first, off the pitch, and the senior physician should control the head. Scoop stretchers are effective. The neck should be supported not only in a semi-rigid support to prevent flexion of the neck but also from side flexion. The airway must be guaranteed clear and supplemental oxygen administered. A neurological assessment should be recorded and the patient removed to hospital; preferably, in the case of a severe injury, to a neurosurgical unit. It is better to be safe than sorry [1, 2].

Whiplash injuries

Perhaps the whiplash effect can be appreciated by considering the effect on various tissues. Muscles around the neck that try and decelerate the movements will suffer a severe eccentric load which may tear a few fibres or produce DOMS (see Glossary). This comes on 24–48 hours after injury and can last up to 3 months. Anti-inflammatories and RICE (see Glossary) will help in the first place, followed by the usual electrotherapeutic modalities to control inflammation, e.g. ultrasound and interferential, and gentle stretching and exercises to regain muscle function.

If there is displacement of the vertebral column, then the pain may present at the time of the accident and represent facetal dysfunction. This is helped by corrective manipulation or mobilization. The displacement may also affect the cervical disc causing disc displacement, dural irritation and root compression. Wearing a collar, traction and root-blocks may be of benefit.

Finally the intravertebral and dural suspensory ligaments may be torn, often leaving an acutely sensitive neck where all movements hurt; however, MRI scans show little wrong, probably because scans are taken way after the acute inflammatory phase and only in the chronic adhesive phase.

This range of problems can all exist together and each element must be treated not only on its own merit, but in respect of its effect on the other elements. Protective muscle spasm is often provoked and if allowed to establish seems to produce myofascial pain.

The most common long-term effects are degenerative facetal changes which in themselves may produce pain but may also narrow the lateral canal and irritate the nerve root, but this also occurs with ageing.

Cervical disc

Findings
See MRI scan in Fig. 3.1.

(a) Mild. Asymmetrical pattern of neck pain with soft end feel to the neck range. Flexion may produce pain lower down the back and, if root compression is present, pain to the appropriate dermatome, flared by neck movement. Brachial nerve tensioning test may be positive. Adson's manoeuvre may be positive (see Glossary).

(b) With root signs. Root symptoms and signs may be present:

C2   Occipito-frontal headache (sympathetic signs of altered facial sweating may be present).

C3   Disc lesion is very, very rare.

C4   Trapezoid and anterior chest pain and hyperaesthesia.

C5   Altered sensation over lateral deltoid. Weak deltoid and biceps. Biceps power decreased.

C6   Altered sensation over shoulder to lateral forearm and thumb. Weak biceps and wrist extensors. Biceps and pronator power decreased.

C7   Altered sensation in fingers. Weak elbow extension and wrist flexion. Triceps power decreased.

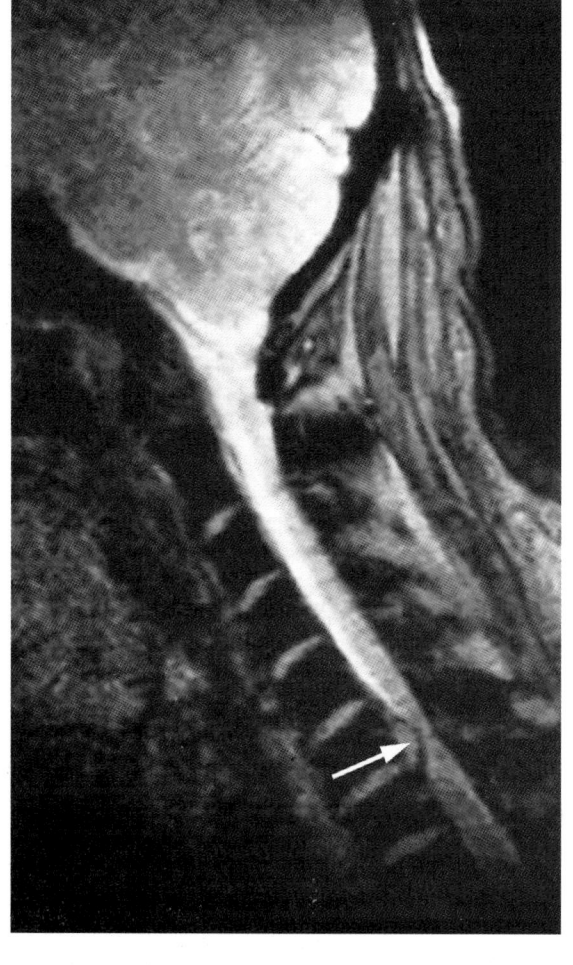

Figure 3.1 T1-weighted MRI shows a cervical disc causing dural compression and root palsy, but no cord compression. Conservative management was successful.

C8/T1 Altered sensation radiating to ulnar aspect of arm in fourth and fifth digits. Weak intrinsics of hand [3, 4].
(c) Cord compression shows symptoms and signs in the back and the leg that do not seem to fit with appropriate back examination. L'Hermitte's (Fig. 3.2) sign and Valsalva may be positive (see *Glossary*).

Cause
Prolapsed/herniated cervical disc.

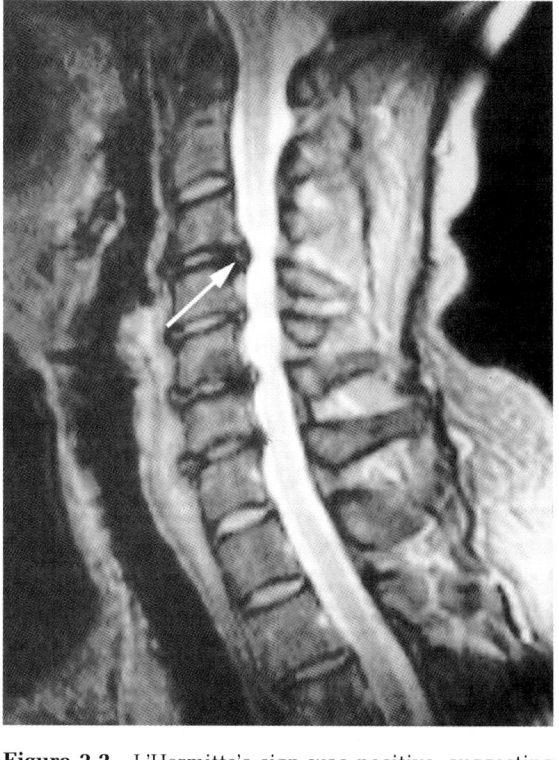

Figure 3.2 L'Hermitte's sign was positive, suggesting cord compression, and surgery was required.

Investigations
X-ray for bony problems. MRI and CT to display the disc lesion and exclude other intraspinal causes.

Treatment
(a) Mild. Mobilization techniques such as Maitlands, Mulligan's Nags and Snags, and traction to neck. Avoid 'head-hanging' posture over the desk or lying in bed reading with the head flexed forward on the chest. Specially designed neck pillows may help, but often switching between two ordinary pillows when lying on the side and one when lying prone or supine may be adequate, as may tying a cord around the pillow to form a butterfly wing shape.
(b) With root signs. Support the neck and limit the range of movement with a cervical collar, try traction. These disc lesions tend to settle over 6–12 weeks and the pain can be helped

by avoiding neural tensioning caused by stretching the arms up or outwards. A root-block and, sometimes, trigger-point injection or acupuncture will help, as, if needed, can a cervical epidural.

(c) Cord compression. Cord compression with signs and symptoms spreading towards the legs requires surgery.

Sports

Cervical discs should not be twisted or stressed. Even axial compression and impaction from running is painful so that, most times, the pain will not let the patient play. Once reduced and stable, start with running and build to extensions such as serve at tennis and badminton; however, rugby scrums and impact sport should be avoided for 6–9 months.

Comment

Thank goodness most cure themselves over time. Most treatments are directed to controlling the pain whilst the disc settles, usually over 6–12 weeks.

Cervical facet joint

Findings

Acute onset of neck pain, 'cricked neck' or more insidious onset through to persistent discomfort with an asymmetrical pattern of movement with a hard end feel to neck range. Only with root entrapment at the lateral canal will there be root symptoms flared by movement, when Adson's manoeuvre will be positive (see *Glossary*).

Cause

Either dysfunction between the vertebral segments or degenerative arthritis of the facet joints.

Investigations

X-ray with obliques to display lateral canal and encroaching osteophytes, but MRI and/or CT scan if a disc is also suspected; however, these investigations are probably not required clinically unless failing to make progress with treatment.

Treatment
Acute or root signs

(a) Electrotherapeutic modalities to ease inflammation and pain, root-block or facetal cortisone.

(b) Rest in a cervical collar if required then mobilization and manipulation when inflammation has settled.

Chronic

(a) The head must be held straighter on the neck because when the body is slumped forward, the neck is held in extension, especially whilst looking at computer screens through bifocal spectacles. Correct the posture by reforming the lumbar lordosis, reducing the dorsal kyphosis and resitting the head straighter on the neck, which decreases cervical facetal impingement. Holding a telephone between the ear and shoulder almost manipulates the normal neck and produces problems.

(b) Facetal injection.

(c) Rarely, surgery to the lateral canal if root involvement has occurred.

> **Caveat** – Congenital abnormalities (e.g. hemivertebrae, osteoid osteoma), which often present in the child or adolescent.

Sports

(a) In ball games the head is held still to focus on the ball whilst the body is moved. The neck provides this coordinating link which is so vital that neck pain invariably interferes with performance. During the acute phase, sport is best avoided.

(b) Chronic facetal osteoarthritis will provoke a change in technique, especially such as that required during the golf swing when a less full swing will have to be adopted.

(c) Tennis serving will have to be flatter and badminton may prove impossible.

(d) Most difficult are contact sports and the safe advice is to avoid the sport until better.
(e) Breathing during swimming freestyle into a flexed and then rotated neck, as when trying not to rise too high out of the water, can produce facetal problems.

Comment

Overall, one must be safe, and the best advice is to avoid contact sport until better. CT scans help to assess long-term problems of facet joints much better than X-ray or MRI. Manipulation of the correct cases is the treatment of choice. Facetal injection of cortisone can be effective.

Stingers and burners [3]

Findings

Type 1 Bilateral arm pain and temporary quadriparesis = cervical stenosis.

Type 2 Pain lasting up to or more than 15 minutes, dense paraesthesia (dead arm) = brachial plexus traction.

Type 3 Discrete transient root pain and traumatic motor weakness. Commonly, transient loss of function with searing, lancinating pain coursing down the arm. Temporary paralysis lasting 10–15 min. Often C6 numbness in the lateral three fingers can persist. Weakness of shoulder abduction and wrist extensors. Brachial nerve tensioning tests are positive.

Cause

Type 1 Axial loading of the neck.

Type 2 Lateral neck flexion away from and shoulder depression on the side of the pain.

Type 3 Hyperextension and rotation. Most commonly a combination of extension and lateral flexion, compressing the lateral canal on the ipselateral side, whilst causing traction of the roots on the contralateral side [5].

Investigations
CT, MRI and EMG.

Treatment
(a) Postural control and neck strengthening.
(b) Electrotherapeutic modalities for inflammation and pain.
(c) Facetal or root injections of cortisone.
(d) Surgery.

Sports
For American football, modify shoulder pads with a combined neck roll. Advise change of sport with cervical stenosis after analysis of spinal canal size [5].

Comment
Although rugby and wrestling occasionally have this injury, it seems much more prone to occur in American football, possibly because of the head-on tackle, even though 'spiking' is banned.

Ligamentous neck pain

Findings
A full range of movements or symmetrical limited range of movements which may be painful in full flexion and extension. There is tenderness to palpation over C7 T1.

The patient invariably has functional, or true dorsal kyphosis, and sits over a desk for long periods. There may be protraction of the head.

Cause
Overload of the neck ligaments – usually at C7 T1, occasionally at the nuchal crest, from constant neck flexion, the 'head-hangers' neck or as part of the whiplash complex (see Chapter 2).

Investigations
None clinically required apart from eliminating other causes.

Treatment

(a) Correct posture – especially first and foremost retraining a lumbar lordosis and reducing the dorsal kyphosis. This can be aided by raising the desk and lowering the chair, and sitting on a wedge seat or kneel-on style chair.
(b) Retraction exercises of the neck.
(c) Electrotherapeutic modalities to calm inflammation and ease pain.
(d) Muscle balance training.
(e) Sclerosant injections of the ligaments (see Glossary).

Sports

Activity helps these people.

Comment

Correction of posture should correct 95% of these patients.

Myofascial pain

Findings

Possibly accompanies an underlying cause (see *Cause*, below). The neck range may be full or symmetrically limited and/or painful with a soft painful end feel as muscle spasm is induced, preventing a full range of movement. There are tender trigger points, usually over the trapezius and rhomboids. These can produce radiating pain to the arms and localized muscle spasm may be palpated.

Cause

The muscle is held in constant tension, even when at rest. This may be post-traumatic or have become a habit to protect an underlying problem, such as a painful facet joint, disc or shoulder. It may, however, reflect psychological tension. The muscle spindle may be controlled by the gamma efferent tone.

Investigations

Only for the underlying causes, although previous root irritation may be relevant.

Treatment

(a) Explanation of muscle spasm, and how and why agonist and antagonist muscles work at rest, and in these cases are under constant tension even at rest, and therefore how the muscle may even appear to be fatigued doing nothing. Treat the underlying cause.
(b) Electrotherapeutic modalities to calm inflammation. NSAIDs.
(c) Spray and stretch.
(d) Dry needling or acupressure or ultrasound to the trigger spot. Injection of steroid or local to the trigger points.
(e) Hydrotherapy to encourage muscle exercises.

Sports

Most patients will not do any activity, but should be encouraged on a little and often basis, with the explanation that muscles will ache when first trained but that this is a good thing (see Chapter 20). NSAIDs may help at this time. Use hydrotherapy to encourage muscle work but reduce muscle load.

Comment

Probably this area is less well understood and the underlying mental fear or psychological problems must be handled at the same time. The principle of a primary injury, such as a shoulder, being followed by a secondary problem, such as hunching and contracting the trapezius, to protect from shoulder pain, but then becoming overloaded themselves, thus producing further pain, must be appreciated. Treat the primary cause and follow rapidly with treatment to the secondary cause which is the habituated muscle spasm.

Further reading

1. National Health and Medical Research Council (1995) *Head and Neck Injuries in Football*. Australian Government Publishing Service, Canberra.
2. Ryan, A. J. (1991) Protecting the sportsman's brain (concussion in sport). *Br. J. Sports Med.* **25**, 81–86.
3. Watkins, R. (ed.) (1996) *The Spine in Sports*. Mosby, St Louis, MO.

4. Cyriax, J. H and Cyriax, P. J. (eds) (1993) *Cyriax's Illustrated Manual of Orthopaedic Medicine*, 2nd edn. Butterworth-Heinemann, Oxford.

5. Castro, F. P., Ricciardi, J. R., *et al.* (1997) Stingers, the Torg ratio, and the cervical spine. *Am. J. Sports Med.* **25**, 603–608.

Bruckner P. and Khan K. (1993) *Clinical Sports Medicine*. McGraw-Hill, New York.

Reid, D. (1992) *Sports Injury Assessment and Rehabilitation*. Churchill Livingstone, Edinburgh.

4

Dorsal spine

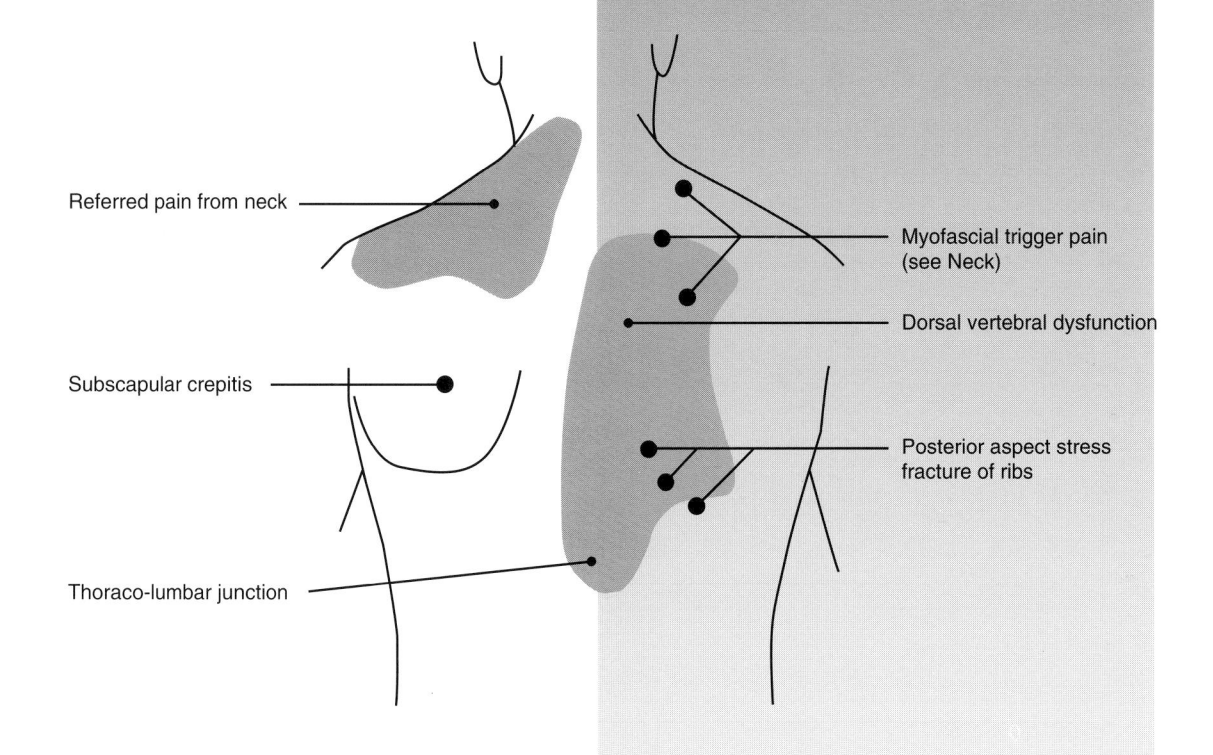

Referred pain from neck

Myofascial trigger pain
(see Neck)

Dorsal vertebral dysfunction

Subscapular crepitis

Posterior aspect stress
fracture of ribs

Thoraco-lumbar junction

Referred from neck

The thoracic spine provides lateral flexion and rotation with limited flexion and overload or trauma within these positions may cause dorsal spinal dysfunction. It is unusual for a disc displacement to occur in this area, though not impossible.

All examinations of the dorsal spine start with an examination of the movements of the cervical spine and the cervical spine should be considered as a cause if these tests produce discomfort or pain in the dorsal spine (see Chapter 2).

Dorsal vertebral dysfunction

Findings
The onset may be acute or chronic. Pain may be felt centrally, but often to one side of the spine or even radiating around the chest wall. Lateral or anterior chest pain, without spinal pain, may occur. The lower dorsal vertebrae refer towards the abdomen, D9 the umbiliacus and the thoraco-lumbar junction to the groin via the ilio-inguinal nerve, so pain may be referred to these areas. Often worse lying, better sitting or standing, so that the patient may sleep in a chair rather than in bed. Twisting to one side hurts. Breathing may hurt. The pain is worse with movement. The higher vertebrae may refer pain to the arm or shoulder. (During clinical practice one notices referred pain towards the arm from the dorsal spine even down at D8. This may appear during palpation of the facet joint or injection of the facet joint and one should not reject these histories, but realize that referred pain is still poorly understood.) Neck flexion may produce dorsal pain, but whether this represents classical referred pain or dorsal dural irritation, facet joint flexion or ligamentous stress is not clear. Rotation of the dorsal spine is worse to one side rather than the other and, whilst testing this, pelvic rotation may be prevented by sitting the patient with the legs hanging over the couch so that mainly dorsal rotation is tested. Stretching forward to touch the floor outside the opposite foot with the contralateral

hand may be painful and there may be local tenderness to palpation over the spine, facet joints or costo-vertebral joints.

Cause
The most common cause is usually from the facet joints and possibly from the costo-vertebral joints, but dorsal discs do occur. Ligamentous pain particularly from the interspinous ligaments is common. Many problems are postural in origin and are usually due to too much of a dorsal kyphosis.

Investigation
It may be important to exclude the differentials, especially intrathoracic, as these have such potentially serious consequences. Most common X-ray findings show a kyphotic spine, anterior osteophytes of no clinical significance, apart from reflecting dorsal discal degeneration. Schmorl's nodes reflect discal herniation into the body of the vertebrae and are probably of no clinical significance. Anterior wedge collapse reflects old Scheuermann's, or osteoporosis with a crush fracture, TB or secondaries. See Fig. 2.2.

CT or MRI may show intraspinal blood vessels which may be significant if enlarged.

Treatment
(a) Most commonly responds to manipulation. May have to be done frequently and then pain suddenly clears.

(b) Injection of cortisone to the facet joints.

(c) Mobilization and/or injection of the costo-vertebral joints.

(d) Sclerosant injections (see *Glossary*) of supraspinous ligaments and facet joints.

(e) Posture. Usually correction of excess lumbar lordosis by pelvic tilting and then extension of the thoraco-lumbar junction or in a rounded back by general increase in lordosis, especially over the dorsal spine (see Chapter 2, p. 12).

(f) Extension exercises to dorsal spine, and avoid flexion and rotation.

(g) Self-manipulation by lying on fist, handkerchief or tennis ball!

(h) A pillow in front of the chest may limit dorsal rotation when asleep and thus the stresses across the facet joints.

(i) Rarely surgery to a disc.

Sports

Dorsal facetal, or costo-vertebral, problems can occur outside sport and interfere with performance; however, sports with flexion and rotation, e.g. rowing, squash and golf in addition to contact sports, can produce facetal dysfunction.

Comment

Manipulation helps most dorsal problems which appear to be mainly facetal. The patient's relatives can be taught how to do a straight lift and extension of the dorsal spine. Facetal hydrocortisone and sclerosants will often settle the chronic cases. Do be aware that dorsal cord lesions may have few signs or symptoms in the dorsal spine but may cause apparent lumbar problems and that undiagnosed leg pain requires investigation of the higher levels of the spinal cord.

Scheuermann's epiphysitis [see Chapter 2, Part 1, Cartilage end plates]

Occurs in teenagers and presents with a painful dorsal spine which may have no mechanical signs (see *Posture and relative rest help*). Analgesics and NSAIDs may be given. This is often quite refractive to treatment until the spine has fully developed. See Fig. 2.2. May require spinal brace.

Comment

This is often quite refractive to treatment until the spine is fully developed.

Costo-vertebral joint

The upper ribs move in a bucket handle plane, whilst the lower ribs move in a pump handle plane and mobilization techniques employ this variance. Whether the examination techniques

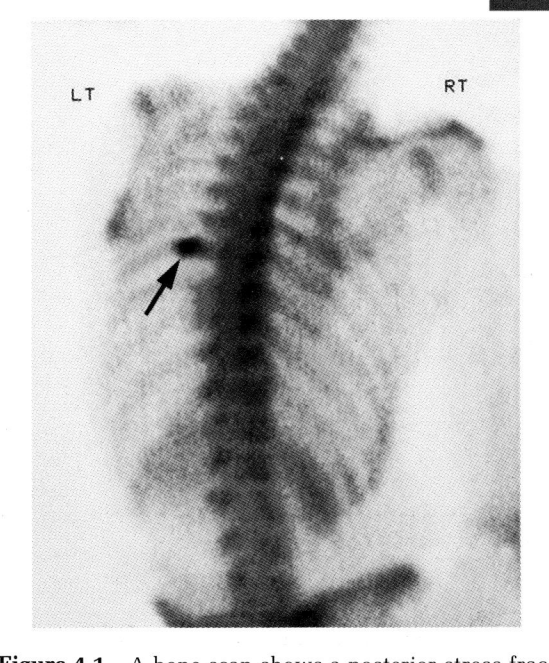

Figure 4.1 A bone scan shows a posterior stress fracture of the ribs in a golfer.

can accurately differentiate this diagnosis from facetal pain is of some doubt.

Myofascial pain

Myofascial pain has a local trigger point that may ease with continued acupressure from the fingers. See Chapter 3.

Fractured rib – traumatic or stress

A positive rib spring test raises the possibility of a rib fracture (Fig. 4.1). See Chapter 5.

Subscapular crepitus

Elicitation of this sign indicates rubbing between the scapular and thoracic wall. See Chapter 17.

Costo-sternal joint (Tietze disease)

Dorsal referred pain may radiate to the sternum but localized tenderness or swelling over the costo-sternal joints is suggestive this is the cause. It is not easy sometimes to differentiate as pressure on the sternum may irritate the spine and pressure on the dorsal spine may irritate the sternal joints. They are best tested with the patient sitting to prevent this effect. See Chapter 5.

Bony disease – primary or secondary

Constant pain not worse with movement and atypical findings, but fracture may be worse with minimal movement. If in doubt investigate further.

Intrathoracic problems

If pain on breathing, swallowing and exertion rather than movement occurs then consider intrathoracic problems such as pleural, myocardial, reflux oesophagitis or a mediastinal cause.

Further reading

Bruckner, P. and Khan, K. (1993) *Clinical Sports Medicine*. McGraw-Hill, New York.

Cyriax, J. H. and Cyriax, P. J. (1993) *Cyriax's Illustrated Manual of Orthopaedic Medicine*. Butterworth-Heinemann, London.

Hutson, M. A. (ed.) (1996) *Sports Injuries: Recognition and Management*, 2nd edn. Oxford Medical Publications, Oxford.

Reid, D. (1992) *Sports Injury Assessment and Rehabilitation*. Churchill Livingstone, Edinburgh.

Watkins, R. G. (ed.) (1996) *The Spine in Sports*. Mosby, St Louis, MO.

5

Lumbar spine

Part 1
Flexion-orientated lesions

Prolapsed or herniated disc

Findings

The typical history involves a period of slouching, straining, lifting or pushing, with the back in a flexed position, followed by the slow onset of pain, coming on over a few hours or sometimes overnight. Standing flexion and side flexion are painful, and there may be a catch or deviation of the spine when returning from flexion to neutral. Some may be deviated sideways. Straight leg raise, Lasegue's and slump test may be positive (see Glossary).

The following weak muscles indicate nerve root damage:

Psoas	L1/2
Quadriceps	L3/4
Knee jerk down	L3/4
Tibialis anterior	L4
Extensor hallucis	L5
Extensor digitorum longus	L5
Peroneals	L4 or 5
Hamstring/calf	S1
Ankle jerk absent	S1
Gluteals	S2 [8]

Cause

The nucleus pulposus is squeezed in a posterior direction by flexion of the spine (see Fig. 2.4). This happens gradually and is known as 'disc creep' [12]. Typically, flexion will cause the disc to move posteriorly towards the spinal canal where it will cause pain from the nerves in the

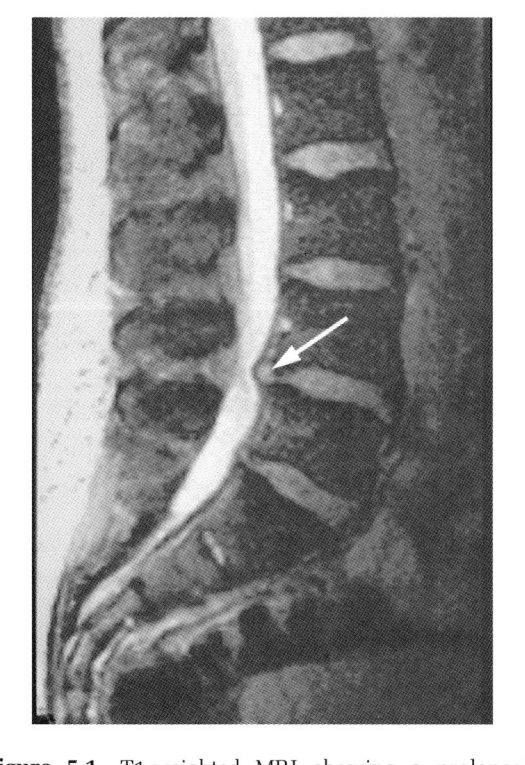

Figure 5.1 T1-weighted MRI showing a prolapsed lumbar disc impinging on the dura.

annulus and posterior longitudinal ligament, or it will impinge on the dura itself, causing intense pain. If the prolapse extends further then it will compress the nerve root causing radiation of pain to the appropriate dermatome, 'pins and needles', numbness, fasciculations, and muscle weakness (root palsy). See Fig. 5.1.

Caveat – Diminished or absent perineal sensation, or loss of control of anal sphincter or bladder, is a S3/4 lesion and requires emergency surgery.

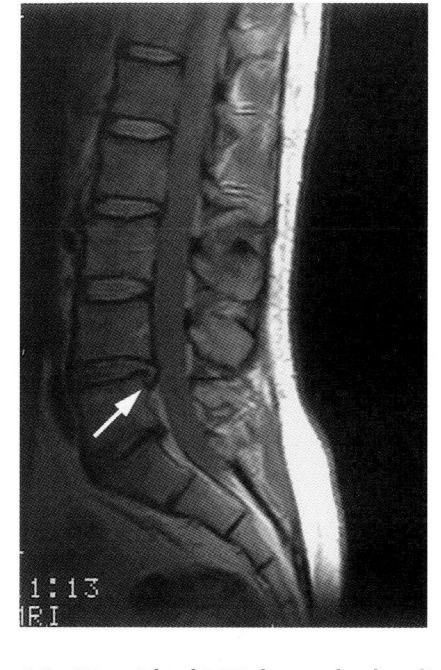

Figure 5.2   T1-weighted MRI shows a lumbar disc prolapse that has extended along the posterior aspect of the
vertebral body as a sequestrum, which is unlikely to
reduce with conservative measures.

(f)   Adverse neural tensioning techniques (at this
stage when the disc is still prolapsed will
increase the pain).

(g)   Surgery – discectomy.

> **Caveat** – Many so-called lumbar rolls built into
> seats are placed too low and push the pelvis
> forwards, thus increasing flexion of the spine.
> McKenzie's flexion exercises may make this type
> of disc worse (see *Glossary*).

Sports

Avoid all sports during a painful flare of a disc
herniation, but see *Annular disc or 'disc creep'* for
exercise when improvement has started.

Annular disc or 'disc creep'

Findings

The creeping disc, which some may call the
annular disc, will often exhibit itself after sitting
for a time when the patient gets up from a seat
with backache, is slightly stuck bent forwards,
but manages with extension exercises to
straighten up and reduce the pain, often entirely,
and then walks away with no problems. Examination may reveal nothing or minor backache on
flexion. Often the posture is a flat, straight spine
and the patient sits slumped into a lumbar
kyphosis. See Fig. 5.3.

Cause

See prolapsed or herniated disc (above). However,
note that the creeping disc usually does not
impinge on the dura or nerve root.

Investigations

None clinically required, but see *Prolapsed or herniated disc* if lesion progresses.

Investigations

Clinically not required if signs are sufficient to
make a diagnosis of a disc lesion. X-ray only to
rule out bony causes; however, if in doubt, or if no
progress with therapy, then MRI or CT scans to
establish the presence of a sequestrum (Fig. 5.2) or
the level of the disc involved and to exclude other
intraspinal pathology. If this fails use a surgical
disc probe to locate and establish whether and
which is the painful disc.

Treatment

(a)   Rest in its acute phase though activity should
be encouraged as soon as possible.

(b)   Posture to maintain extension.

(c)   McKenzie extension exercises (see Glossary).

(d)   Traction.

(e)   Epidural.

Treatment

Postural control to avoid flexions (see Chapter 2).

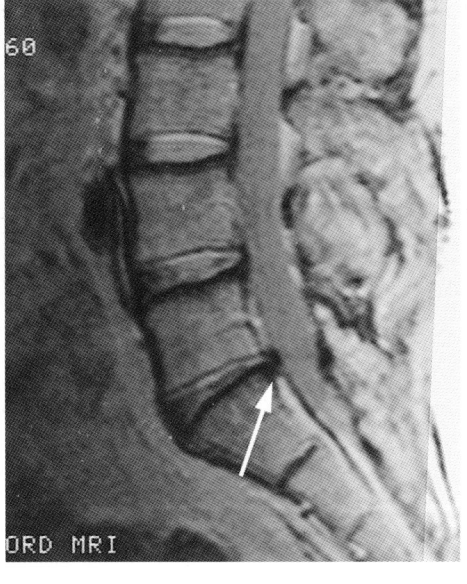

Figure 5.3 A small annular protrusion that may on T2-weighted MRI show an increased signal within the bulge.

Sports

(a) Instead of slumping in the changing room after a hard game, sit with the lumbar spine in extension.

(b) Cycling. Lengthen the frame, raise the handle bars, use tribars or a handle bar extension to lengthen the functional frame and maintain lumbar lordosis.

(c) Weightlifting. Emphasize the maintenance of lordosis or a neutral back during lifting or straining. As soon as the trunk and back are thrown in to help the lift then stop as this means that the muscle being trained is fatiguing and other muscles are being used to help out, frequently flexing the spine.

(d) Sailing. Maintain postural lordosis in a dinghy, and lumbar extension whilst lifting the anchor, winding the winch and pulling on the sheets.

(e) Wind surfing. The problems for beginners occur when the sailboard pulls the sailor into flexion and, dramatically so, whilst pulling up the sail out of the water. Experienced sailors, who use a harness and deep water start, usually can cope without too much flexion of the spine.

(f) Golf. Stand with the upper body more upright, bring arms closer to the body and sit as if on a shooting stick. Bend over one knee, resting the elbow on the knee for support with the other leg extended behind, to tee up or pick the ball out of hole. Pull the golf trolley with the hand palm up and close to the buttock.

(g) Hockey. Bend from the knees and emphasize lordosis or lumbar neutral.

(h) Rowing. Beware of over-reaching and try to maintain lumbar lordosis. Weight training with the 'upright row' risks overloading the flexed back – use an ergo instead.

Dural and nerve root adhesions

Findings

Adhesions will prevent the free movement of nerve or dural tissue and thus provoke pain on bending or sitting, especially with straight legs, such as lying in a bath and in bed, and will often wake the patient from sleep. Because the nerve is trapped, 'pins and needles', altered sensation and continual pain may be presenting symptoms. Some history of trauma, or disc pathology, preceding the current problems will therefore also exist and signs from this may co-exist at the consultation. see *Prolapsed or herniated disc.*

Cause

Formed following inflammation within the spine, most commonly following disc lesions. A vital principle to be understood is that the dura, spinal cord and nerves must be able to move freely to accommodate the changes in body and limb position. This is most easily understood by appreciating that the shortest distance between two points is a straight line. So stand with an absolutely straight back – thus the distance from the top of the brain to the tip of the filum terminale is shorter than when you bend forward to put your head on your knees. These tissues must be able to alter position to accommodate these changes. This same principle will apply to a bent leg or hip where the peripheral nerve must be free to move. The restriction of movement in the dura or the nerves forms the basic principle behind dural stress tests such as the straight leg raise, Lasegue's, slump and femoral stretch tests (see *Glossary*).

Investigations
MRI scan, followed by gadolinium MRI scan to differentiate fibrous tissue from disc (Figs 5.4 and 5.5).

Treatment
(a) Adverse neural tensioning (see *Glossary*).
(b) Epidural injections [7, 8, 10].

Sports
May have to gradually play and exercise clear of pain over several months, particularly avoiding positions of flexion or equivalent to straight leg raising. This is non-formal adverse neural tensioning! (see *Glossary*).

Comment
So often the patient who almost grabs you by the collar to enforce the fact they do have genuine pain, in spite of a paucity of findings, does have night pain and a slump test that is positive. Even if these findings are not present, an epidural will dramatically improve their pain. Those that do have dural tensioning signs will have the pain improved; however, the mechanical adhesions may not release and therefore adverse neural tensioning may be tried to free up and stretch out the nerve from the scar, but if over-stretched will again produce pain. I am not yet impressed by adverse neural tensioning as a treatment for this condition, although I can see the logic.

Lumbar ligaments

Findings – posterior lumbar ligaments
A ligamentous history is one of pain at rest improving with activities but returning if the activities are prolonged. Thus, pure ligamentous back pain is worse first thing in the morning,

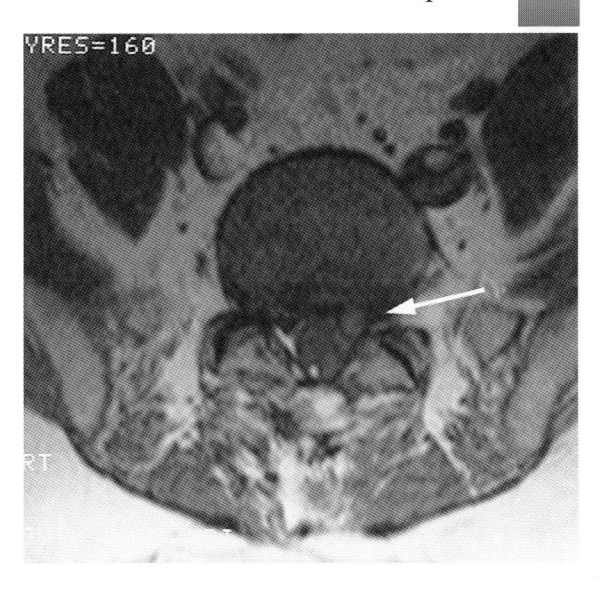

Figure 5.4 Pre-gadalinium MRI shows a lesion that fills the spinal canal (arrow).

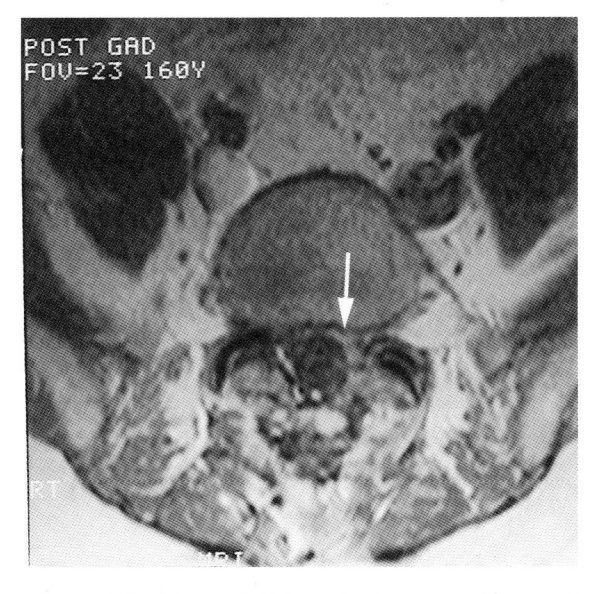

Figure 5.5 Post-gadalinium MRI shows increased signal within this lesion, suggesting fibrous scar tissue rather than a disc.

sitting for a long time, standing for a long time, but gives no trouble playing games or with activities. It has been christened the 'cocktail or theatre back', giving discomfort when the back is stationary but being relieved by movement. However, it does not always present in its pure form, but as an accompaniment to the mechanical problems of the facets and disc. Ligamentous pain can also refer down the leg, often to the back of the knee.

Findings – inter- and supraspinous ligaments

There is not a recognizable history that is diagnostic of inter- and supraspinus ligament injuries apart from flexion pain. It is not common and is usually a complication of more major problems.

Cause

Stress from flexion, rotation, sheering, and compression and distraction, to the pelvic ring on its posterior aspect, which may be more vulnerable around menstruation, or secondary to mechanical disc or facetal problems in the spine.

Investigations

None are clinically diagnostic for posterior lumbar ligaments, although interspinous tears have been displayed with contrast mediums.

Treatment

(a) Electrotherapeutic modalities to calm pain and settle inflammation, such as ultrasound, interferential and shortwave diathermy. NSAIDs.

(b) Sclerosant injections [1, 8, 10] (see *Glossary*).

Sports

(a) Compression of interspinous ligaments, or impingement of the spinous processes, occurs in gymnastics or acrobatics with severe local hyperextension as in 'hanging baskets', walkovers and gymnastic vaults.

(b) Females who get perimenstrual backache are more at risk around this period time. Avoid heavy training during this time.

Comment

Though acute flares are helped by NSAIDs and physiotherapy, sclerosant injections give long-term relief and indeed may be the only treatment to relieve some ligamentous backaches. I have cured pain behind the knees left after a back lesion and people who had full but negative investigations for renal causes of loin pain with lumbar ligamentous sclerosant injections.

Part 2
Extension-orientated lesions

This group is less homogeneous than the flexion-orientated lesions and the history must be listened to closely, as the minor elements give a clue to the lesion (Fig. 5.6).

Facet joint

See Fig. 2.3.

Findings

The lesions may be acute and tend to present as lumbar pain without referral. However, experimental irritant injections into facet joints have produced referred pain in similar dermatomal patterns as root lesions. The referred groin pain is often facetal in origin. As a disc degenerates, so the facet joints are brought into closer approximation and degenerative changes occur in the facets themselves, giving a pain that is more continuous, may have radiation, but invariably has a mechanical history of movement-induced pain. They may accompany or continue after disc pain has settled, but they themselves do not produce numbness or 'pins and needles', although their effect on the adjacent nerve root may. Extension and side flexion is painful, as may be full flexion. Dural stress tests are negative. Facet joint rocking and rolling hurts, as may local pressure over the relevant joint. Sacro-iliac stress tests which are non-specific may also hurt (see *Glossary* and Chapter 2).

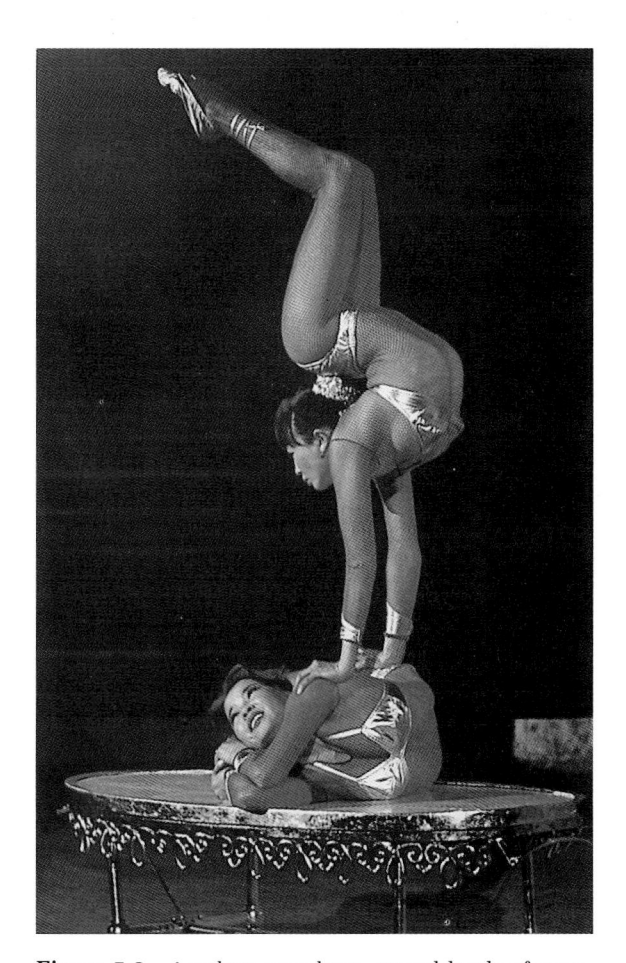

Figure 5.6 Acrobats may have several levels of spondylolisthesis.

Cause

(a) Impingement of one zygoapophysis on its adjacent pair from too much extension, which, posturally, is usually accompanied by lack of trunk and abdominal muscle tone and a slouched lordotic, standing posture.

(b) Often acute movements that disturb the alignment of the facet joints cause 'catching' pains.

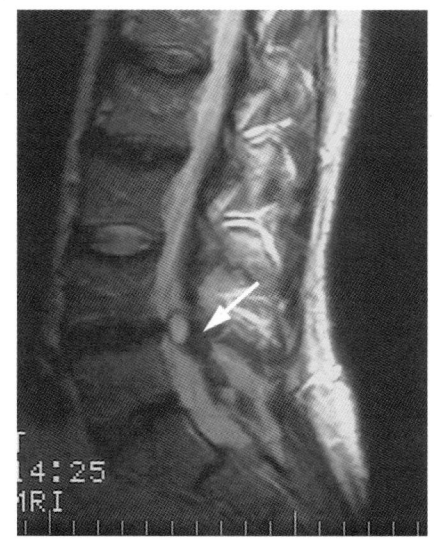

Figure 5.7 An intraspinal canal synovial cyst from the facet joint.

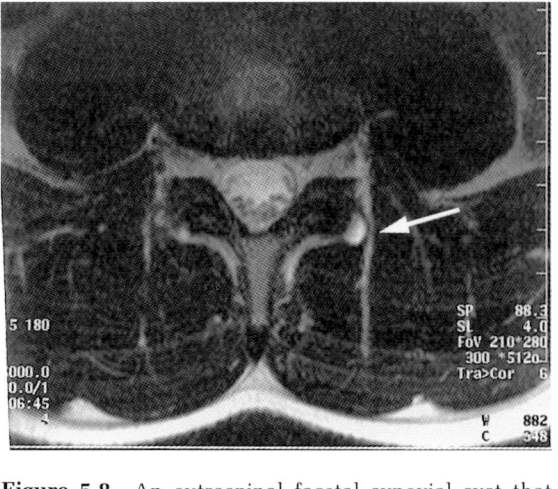

Figure 5.8 An extraspinal facetal synovial cyst that mimicked a spondylolysis in a teenaged tennis player.

(c) Pain may be secondary to an underlying disc lesion – the disc causing malalignment of the adjacent vertebrae, thus disturbing the facetal alignment or the vertebrae simply compressing the disc and, as it degenerates, allowing the facets to approximate.

(d) Osteoarthritis of the facet joints.

Investigations

X-ray will show established hypertrophic osteoarthritis, but CT scans are clearer than MRI for visualizing facet joints and early sclerosis. However, MRI can display the presence of intraspinal or extra-articular facetal synovial cysts. See Figs 5.7 and 5.8.

Treatment

(a) Manipulation. These respond well to flexion rotation manipulations. Self-manipulation and McKenzie flexion exercises will help. Massage helps as muscle spasm is often present.

(b) Electrotherapeutic modalities to calm inflammation, such as interferential and shortwave diathermy.

(c) Posture. Do not try and increase lordosis as for a disc but allow the patient to slump into flexion. Softer beds are more comfortable, as will be the patient standing with one foot raised on a box or the foot rail in a pub. Kneeling on chairs and extension exercises make extension problems worse. A shooting stick or a bar stool may make standing tolerable for facetal problems by allowing a half sitting position to be adopted.

(d) Perifacetal cortisone or intra-articular cortisone injections under screening give relief but perifacetal sclerosants may be required for long-term relief.

(e) Cryo or chemical rhyzotomy of the sinu vertebral nerve denervates the facets (see Chapter 2, p. 8).

> **Caveat** – In adolescents, in particular, exclude an early stress fracture of the pars interarticularis.

Sports

Can occur in all sports, but particularly extension-orientated sports (see *Spondylolysis*). Older sportspeople are more prone to facetal problems.

Comment

Facetal osteoarthritis occurs in many of the elderly, who should be allowed to slump or perch on a chair, have soft beds and who are improved by flexion mobilizations. Manipulation may produce dramatic improvement and may also help realign adjacent vertebrae, to allow the prolapsing nucleus pulposus to return centrally. Perifacetal sclerosants do seem to be successful and may even produce a chemical rhyzotomy.

Lateral canal entrapment

Findings

The history is of back pain and, almost invariably, root pain down the leg, that is made worse in extension or walking around. The patient relieves the situation by sitting down, half sitting parked on the edge of a desk or shooting stick, and leaning and squatting forward. The root may be irritated in the lateral canal by the facet joints especially when enlarged with arthritis, but also by a lateral disc, when the history will have elements of disc pathology and some flexion discomfort. Whilst testing extension, the position should be held, when this may bring on referred root pain. Flexion dural stress tests, straight leg raise, Lasegue's and slump may be positive if disc or adhesions are present, but they are usually negative (see *Glossary*).

Cause

Entrapment of the nerve root in the lateral canal, by a lateral disc, or more usually degenerate disc, and hypertrophic osteoarthritis of the facet joints narrowing the lateral canal. Rarely a facetal synovial cyst. See Fig. 5.7. Spondylolisthesis will also narrow the canal.

Investigations

Clinically not required unless failing to progress, then MRI or CT (see Fig. 5.12).

Treatment

(a) Flexion manipulations or mobilizations.
(b) Traction in Fowler's position and/or home traction such as a 'back swing', but a pillow under knees to maintain flexion may be required.

(c) Permit the patient to have a postural flexion slump (see *Facet joints*).
(d) Cortisone to the facets may settle inflammatory swelling around the nerve root.
(e) A paravertebral block placed in the lateral canal.
(f) Laminectomy.

Sports

Avoid extensions in sport and as this problem is most common in the older person, swimming and the tennis serve are most affected. The facetal problems prefer backstroke as diving into the pool and the other strokes produce extension of the spine. The tennis serve should have increased knee bend to reduce back extension. See *Spondylolysis*.

Comment

Most 'back books' advocate good posture which entails a lumbar lordosis, but this group is helped enormously when they are given permission to slump or slouch. Techniques of self-manipulation with the hips flexed can be really helpful in preventing recurrences.

Spondylolysis and stable spondylolisthesis

Also known as stress fracture of the spine, bowler's back and gymnast's back.

Findings

Both the acute and chronic when inflamed have persistent, usually unilateral, lumbar pain worse with movement, often presenting in an adolescent and can be sport related. Lumbar extension is painful and side flexion may be painful. Straight leg raise, Lasegue's and slump tests are all negative. There are no abnormal neurological signs. One-legged extension test and the Fitch catch are often painful. Facet joint rocking and rolling is often painful. There is local tenderness to palpation which may be unilateral or bilateral. See *Glossary*.

Cause

This may occur idiopathically in 5–6-year-olds without symptoms and only comes to the fore when the back is stressed with extension manoeuvres, when the facet above is thought to act like a chisel onto the pars interarticularis below. However, stress lesions of the pars interarticularis can be induced by sporting activities, especially repetitive rotation extension manoeuvres, and extension-orientated pain in an adolescent must always raise the possibility of this lesion. Possibly more common with a spina bifida occulta and a long isthmus of the pars interarticularis.

> **Caveat** – May heal at one level and fracture at the next level above (a climbing fracture).

Investigations

(a) Oblique X-ray. 'Scottie dog collar' which can appear sclerosed or lytic (Fig. 5.9).

(b) A planar bone scan may not display the lesion in the very early stages and a SPECT scan (Figs 5.10 and 5.11) will be more diagnostic and should be requested at the same time [2]. X-rays may show a lesion which is then shown to be non-active on the bone scan, which indicates that this particular lesion has probably healed with fibrous union. The bone scan may then display a further hot lesion on the other side, which is the new active lesion.

(c) CT scan with a reverse angle gantry is required to display the lesion.

(d) MRI scan will reveal the medullary oedema in the pars on the T2- and STIR-related sequences.

> **Caveat** – A positive lesion on X-ray may not be the cause of pain, and a bone scan will show whether this is active and may even show an active lesion that is not visible on X-ray. Generally, but not invariably, the bone scan-positive lesion is capable of healing and can be monitored on CT scanning. Medullary oedema can be seen on MRI but the cortical bone is not so easily visualized.

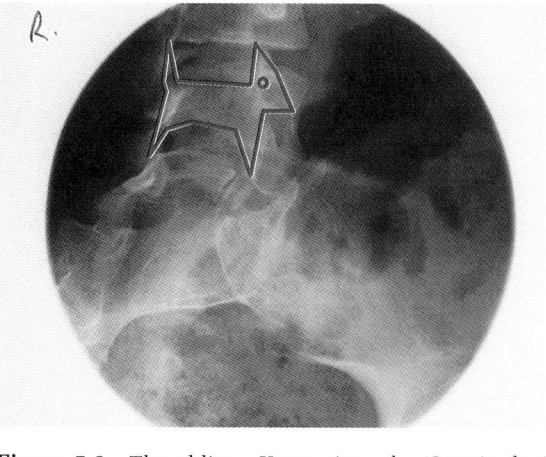

Figure 5.9 The oblique X-ray gives the 'Scottie dog' appearance. A collar is produced as a pars intra-articularis lesion.

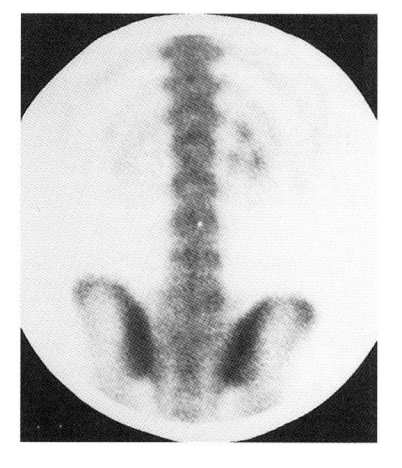

Figure 5.10 A planar bone scan in which the spondylolysis is easily missed (see Fig. 5.11).

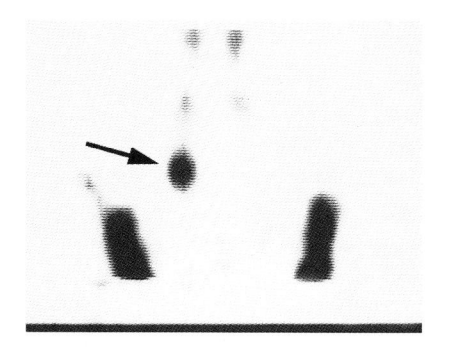

Figure 5.11 A SPECT scan of the patient shown in Fig. 5.10 where the spondylolysis is clearly displayed.

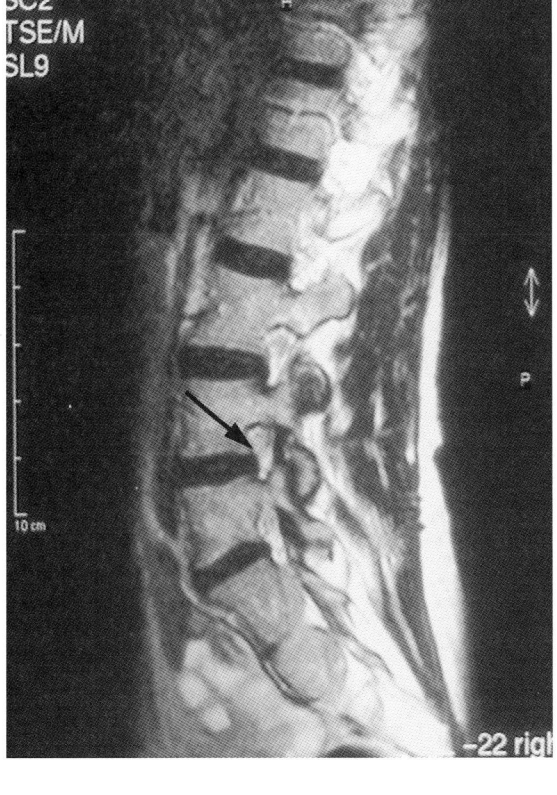

Figure 5.12 Sagittal T1-weighted MRI clearly shows the lateral canal with the nerve root and surrounding disc and facet joints (arrow).

Treatment

(a) Three months' rest from causative activity is usually sufficient. The lesion probably heals by bony union when the bone scan is hot and is considered to have healed by fibrous union if the bone scan is cold. CT scan is probably the best modality besides pain for monitoring healing.

(b) Cross-train for fitness using non-impact methods such as cycling and rowing, and avoid swimming except for backstroke. Avoid running, especially downhill, if it produces discomfort.

(c) A stable spondylolisthesis may respond to manipulation as there is often a facetal element to the pain.

(d) Alter any causative technique (see *Sports*).

Sports

(a) Gymnastics. Extensions must be avoided during healing. However, note that besides the generally accepted extension work, whipping giant circles on the rings to increase downward acceleration may force extension and be causative.

(b) Cricket. Fast bowlers at cricket, who have a mixed bowling style, are more prone to this injury. Bowlers should either be side on or front on, check with a coach. Youngsters should limit the number of fast balls they bowl, e.g. as recommended by the Australian Cricket Board [3]:

Under 12 Matchplay: A limit of two spells of four overs with approximately a 1 hour break.

Practice: 2 × 30 minutes of practice sessions per week: 5 minutes short run – reduced pace; 20 minutes match speed/coach controlled; 5 minutes specific technique development.

Under 16 Matchplay: A limit of two spells of six overs with approximately a 1 hour break.

Practice: 2 × 40 minutes practice sessions per week: 5 minutes short run, reduced pace; 25 minutes, match speed, coach controlled; 10 minutes, specific technique development.

Under 19 Matchplay: A limit of three spells of six overs with approximately a 1 hour break.

Practice: 3 × 40 minutes practice sessions per week: 5 minutes short run – reduced pace.

(c) Swimming. Avoid butterfly until healed. Other strokes are usually pain-free, but severe back extension with the pull phase in breaststroke may cause a flare. Diving into a pool may promote extension and therefore pain.

(d) Football. There is a fairly high incidence (10–12%) amongst the English Football Association selected youth at the National Training Centre. The cause is not yet understood but may be linked with jumping into extension to head a ball.

(e) Tennis. Serving with too much back extension. The player may have to develop more knee bend during the serve to compensate.

Comment

An awareness of the existence of this problem and recognition that certain sports can cause the problem is essential. Whether screening of children for spina bifida occulta, with which there is thought to be an increased incidence, is cost-effective remains to be seen. Rest from activities is essential, but it is difficult to know when the youngster should be returned to their sport. Rest for 3 months with a hot bone scan, which is thought to reflect healing is taking place, may be sufficient, but continuing pain, especially in sports like gymnastics, can be difficult to manage, as often during the period of rest the child grows faster, which may influence rotational speed, and parental and coach pressure to return the child to activities is extreme.

L5 S1 disc

A history of a disc, perhaps with dural tensioning signs, but worse in extension. See *Flexion-orientated problems* and *Mixed lesions* for L5 S1 disc.

L2/3 L3/4 disc and adhesions

Findings

The patient often presents stuck in flexion, bent over, and is happier sitting and lying with the knees bent. Probably the large prolapse necessary to cause problems is irritating the dura or nerve roots and straightening up produces the equivalent to a femoral stretch test. There is often referred pain in the L2/3/4 area on the front of the thigh. However, it is *flexion* that produces the prolapse and after the acute stage extension exercises will help. See Chapter 2, *Lumbar disc*.

Cause

These discs are not so common as L4/5 and L5 S1, but it is flexion manoeuvres that produce this problem and often in a person with a straight spine, which seems to divert the stresses to the higher segments. As there is more room in the spinal canal at this level, the smaller prolapses cause less problems.

Spinous process impingement

Findings

Has a mechanical history of repeated extension movements and is locally tender to palpation over the relevant spinous process. Worse on extensions; pain is located centrally.

Cause

Uncommon. Impingement of one spinous process on another during excess extension.

Investigations

Apart from trauma where the spinous process may be fractured, not relevant.

Treatment

Modalities to calm inflammation, such as ultrasound, laser and local cortisone.

Sports

In acrobatics, particularly the 'hanging basket', and in gymnastics walkovers, especially if the gymnast has a tendency to drop into extension at the low lumbar level L4/5, L5 S1 as opposed to extending upwards and then backwards, spreading the extension through all the lumbar vertebral segments. A whip into extension, as in circles on rings, or whip somersaults can produce this effect.

Comment

I have only seen this problem rarely and only in the sports above. Individuals respond to cortisone but must have the technique that produces the acute lordosis at one area corrected if possible. I have also seen congenitally absent spinous processes that permitted more facetal impingement.

Part 3
Mixed orientation

Some back histories will have a combination or a variance of problems between extension and flexion, often because the lesion is unstable or changes in pattern as it progresses.

L5 S1 disc

Findings

Normal pattern disc prolapse

(a) Flexion of the spine is painful; there may be an arc of pain, causing the flexing spine to deviate sideways through a small angle (swing round the lesion), or an arc of pain on returning from flexion which catches and causes the patient to place their hands on their knees or hips to push up through this arc of pain. This can occur with discs at other levels.

(b) Side flexion is more painful to one side than the other.

(c) Straight leg raise, Lasegue's and slump tests may be positive (see *Glossary*).

(d) Root signs will involve L5, extensor hallucis, extensor digitorum longus, extensor digitorum brevis, peroneals and/or S1, calf or hamstring. Absent or reduced ankle jerk (see Chapter 2).

(e) Extension manoeuvres ease the pain.

Collar stud disc

As for normal pattern disc, but extension is painful as well and may refer pain to the leg during this movement. See Fig. 2.5.

Cause

This disc, like the L4/5 disc, is commonly prolapsed but a percentage of these discs are accompanied by a retroposition of L5 on S1 and a collar stud deformity of the prolapsing disc. This disc therefore can also present symptoms mainly in extension; however, as the lesion regresses and the collar stud is less marked, the symptoms are more flexion orientated. This disc must be treated as a separate entity when considering management as it is common and its pain patterns vary throughout treatment.

Investigations

Lateral X-ray shows small retroposition of L5 on S1 and a hollow in the inferior surface of L5 caused by the disc, whilst MRI scan shows the disc often with a collar stud effect. See Fig. 2.5.

Treatment

This disc problem is often flared by extension or flexion exercises in the first place and rest or epidurals may be required. In the early stages flexion is easier, and traction in Fowler's position and manipulation may help, but the neutral position for movement and posture is required (not too far forward nor too far back). Later extension exercises may be tolerated.

Sports

See *Disc lesions*.

Comment

This is probably the most difficult disc to treat and there have certainly been cases where early extension exercises have seriously exacerbated the problem. Mixed lesions require the understanding that both flexion and extension can make them worse, but later one or the other McKenzie exercises (see *Glossary*) may be of help, whilst posture will have to be in the neutral position, not too far forward nor too far back.

Unstable spondylolisthesis

See *Spondylolysis*.

Findings

An unstable spondylolisthesis may usually have pain from the ligaments and facet joints; however, if the slip progresses to involve the dura or commonly the lateral canal, then nerve root signs and symptoms will follow, and dural stress tests and adverse neural tensioning will be positive even in flexion. If severe, dural or root signs of the appropriate root level may be elicited. There may be a palpable step in the lumbar spine. Sacro-iliac joint stress tests can be positive as this manoeuvre stresses the unstable vertebral segment (see *Glossary*).

Cause

Slip of one vertebra on another due to bilateral fracture of one level pars interarticularis. Defined as grade 1 up to 25% slip, grade 2 up to 50% slip and grade 3 beyond 50% slip. May present as an acute lesion or develop insidiously.

Investigations

(a) Lateral X-ray will display and grade the spondylolisthesis (Fig. 5.13).
(b) CT scans require a reverse angle gantry to display the pars, but this view is not good for showing any associated disc lesion.
(c) MRI scan if there are dural signs as it will display the extent of any disc involvement.

Treatment

Most athletes will present with a grade 1; very few reach grade 2 or grade 3 requiring surgical fusion.

(a) Gentle manipulation, if no dural signs, as this gaps the facetal encroachment.
(b) Traction moves proximal segment backwards [4] and try first in Fowler's position (see *Glossary*).

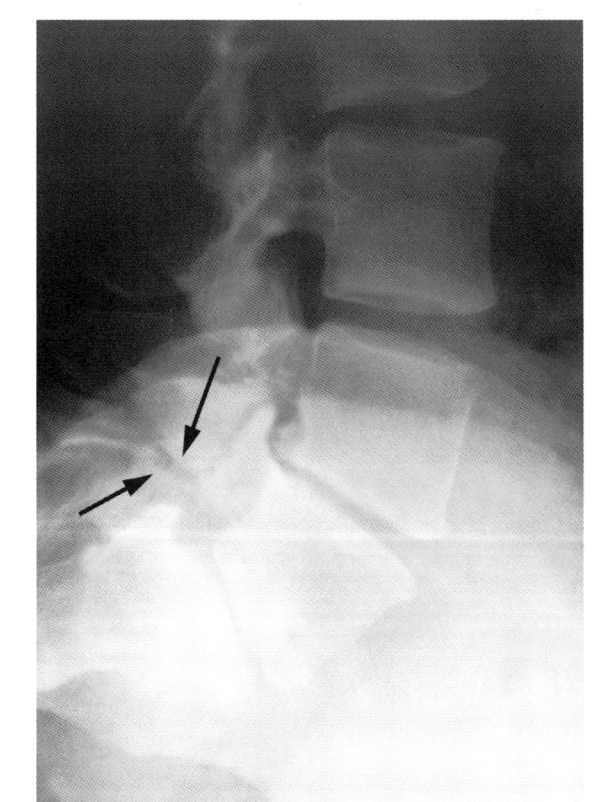

Figure 5.13 A lateral X-ray showing a grade one spondylolisthesis of L5 on S1.

(c) Sclerosant injections to stabilize the unstable segment.
(d) A lumbar corset does seem to give these people support and comfort.
(e) Home traction and sclerosants may produce long-term stability.
(f) Surgery for grade 3, and the unstable grade 1 and 2. Possibly a greater indication for professional sportspeople to have surgery if the sport increases loads on their back.

Sports

See *Spondylolysis*.

Comment

Spondylolisthesis may be pain-free and the problem is instability. Many sportspeople do not want surgical stabilization and can be controlled by home traction and sclerosants, plus avoidance of excessive extension exercises or axial weight bearing. However, certain sports or large training loads may require surgery to stabilize the back. Note that the pars interarticularis stress fractures may 'climb' as one level is healed or is fused so the stress is taken up to the level above and the stress injury appears in the segment higher.

Lateral canal with disc

The older sports person is more likely to have facetal osteoarthritis and narrowing of the lateral canal, so nerve root symptoms, worse with extension, suggest this possibility. See *Lateral canal*.

Sacro-iliac joint

Now accepted as having a nutational (nodding) movement in the L-shaped joint. CT and MRI scans show osteophytes and areas of sclerosis or lysis consistent with stress across the joint that is not associated with systemic problems or ankylosing spondylitis (Figs 5.14–5.16).

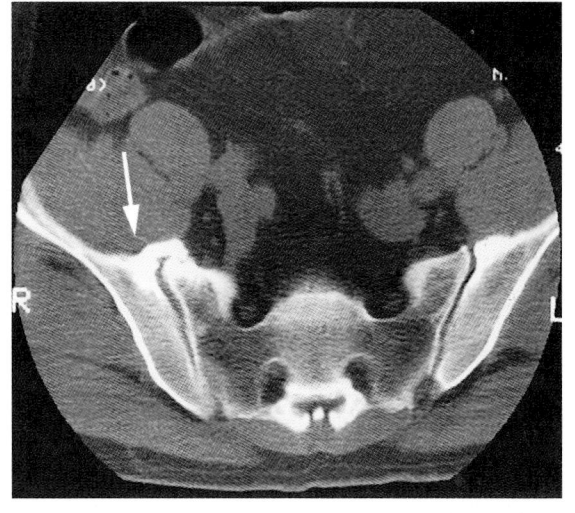

Figure 5.15 A CT scan with a large right and developing left anterior osteophyte.

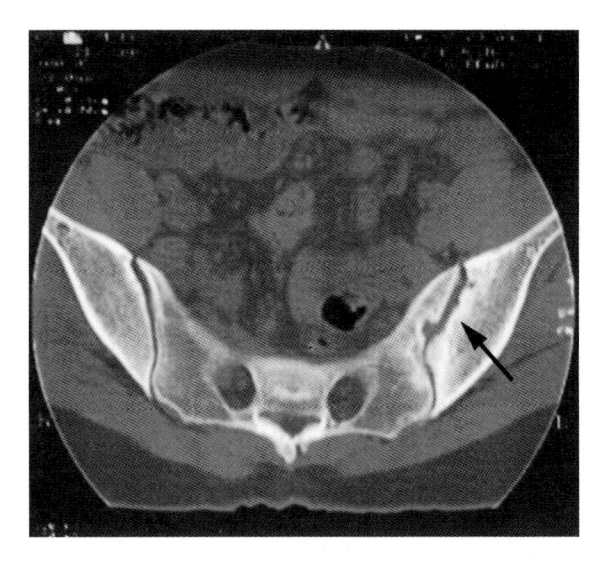

Figure 5.16 A CT scan showing ankylosing spondylitis. This 30-year-old HLA-B27-positive female had normal X-rays and MRI.

Findings

A history of trauma and pain associated with the following:

(a) Pain on running downhill.
(b) Riding a horse can force abduction of the hips to its limit which then will transfer this leverage onto the sacro-iliac joint.

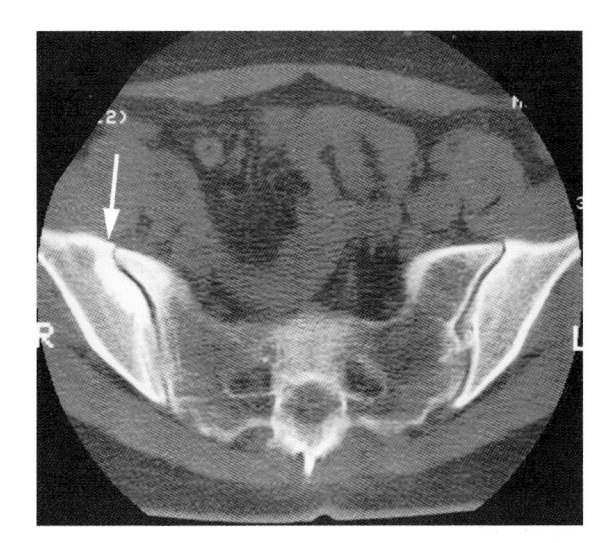

Figure 5.14 A CT scan with sclerosis on the right ilial side of the sacro-iliac joint.

(c) May be acute and debilitating after trauma and this severity of response suggests ankylosing spondylitis.

(d) May have an accompanying disc or facet joint or ligamentous history.

(e) Pelvic spring may be painful, but if the patient supports the L5 segment by lying on a hand and this relieves this sign, then it is probably negative for the sacro-iliac joint and rather suggests segmental dysfunction. Other pelvic stress tests may be positive (see *Glossary*).

(f) Hip flexion may be painful because full hip flexion tests will continue the flexion into the spine and pelvis after the hip has reached its limit of range.

(g) May be tender to local palpation and compression over the joint.

(h) Though pain may be referred down the leg from the sacro-iliac joint, there is no history of 'pins and needles' or numbness, and dural stress tests are negative (see *Glossary*).

(i) Extension and full flexion may be painful.

Cause

(a) Sacro-iliac stress from a vertical compression force transferring foot impaction up to the spine, but this may occur during a rear end shunt in a car when the driver's foot is on the brake and the force is transferred up to the sacro-iliac joint.

(b) A shear force in the vertical plane such as a foot caught in a stirrup wrenching the leg away from the pelvis.

(c) Distraction occurs when the leg is forced or accelerated into adduction, such as during martial arts kicking.

(d) Compression occurs when the hip is stretched into external rotation, such as stretches in aerobics or in the lithotomy position, martial arts and some aerobic routines (Fig. 5.17).

(e) Increased relaxation of ligaments around menstruation or the third trimester of pregnancy makes the sacro-iliac joint more vulnerable.

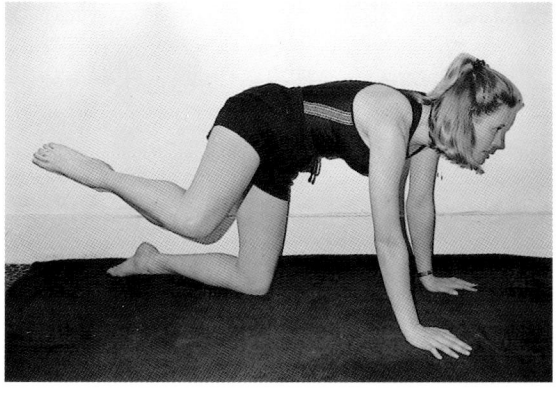

Figure 5.17 An aerobic routine involving hip abduction that can stress the sacro-iliac joint.

(f) Stress fractures have been reported in oligo/amenorrhoeic runners [5].

See Fig. 8.11.

Investigations

(a) X-ray for ankylosing spondylitis and bloods for HLA-B27 and ESR (Fig. 5.18).

(b) Bone scan if a stress fracture or bony pain is suspected. MRI or CT scan through sacro-iliac joints. See Figs 5.14–5.16.

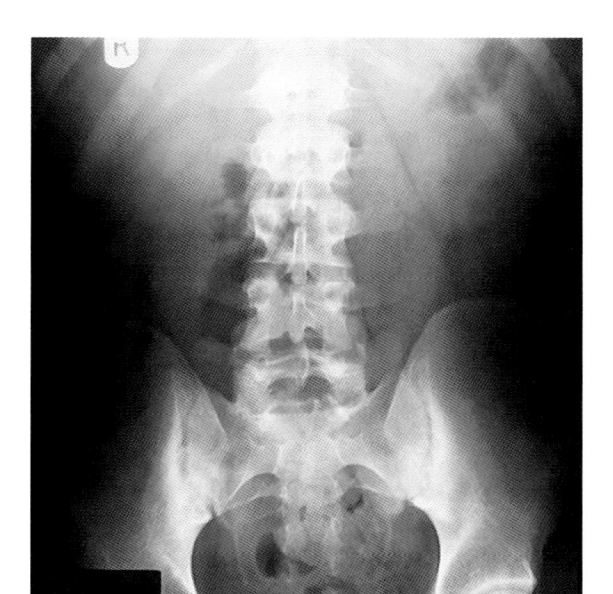

Figure 5.18 X-ray showing ileal sclerosis around the sacro-iliac joint typical of ankylosing spondylitis.

Treatment

(a) Manipulation.
(b) Sacro-iliac belt for distraction injuries.
(c) Sacro-iliac injections – cortisone, sclerosants [1, 6].
(d) Anti-inflammatory drugs.

Sports

(In particular, sacro-iliac joint pain is worse with:

(a) Martial arts, kicking.
(b) Running. Worse on running downhill and bend running. Running should be avoided until pelvic stress tests are negative.
(c) Pole vault. The take-off leg when the drive and extension compresses the sacro-iliac joint.
(d) Horse riding. External rotation – longer or shorter stirrups may be easier. Internal rotation which distracts the sacro-iliac joint may cause pain, in which case riding with very short stirrups may make this worse – ride longer until better. Shear forces can occur from the foot being caught in a stirrup during a fall.
(e) Aerobics. Hip abduction movements especially whilst kneeling must be avoided (see Fig. 5.17). Do low impact, not high impact training.
(f) Swimming. Breaststroke may flare the sacro-iliac joint, use a wedge kick or, if not a serious swimmer, just waft the legs.

Comment

Dysfunction of this joint is both over- and under-diagnosed. The pelvis is a ring and as a ring cannot be disturbed at only one point, so one injury may produce, or be associated with, another injury. Thus these sacro-iliac joint problems are often associated with facet, disc or ligamentous lesions. The standard views to investigate a back do not include the sacro-iliac joint and coronal obliques will be required for MRI or CT scanning. Sacro-iliac joint belts are of limited help. Manipulation may help the sacro-iliac joint (although often it is the accompanying facet that is probably being manipulated). Hydrocortisone has short-term relief but sclerosant injections provide longer term help and have proved of great value.

Further reading

1. Klein, R. G., Eek, B. C., DeLong, B. and Mooney, V. (1993) A randomised, double blind trial of dextrose–glycerine–phenol injections for chronic low back pain. *J. Spinal Disorders* **6**, 22–33.
2. Read, M. T. F. (1994) Single photon emission computed tomography (SPECT) scanning for adolescent back pain. A sine qua non? *Br. J. Sports Med.* **28**, 56–57.
3. Foster, D., John, D., *et al.* (1989) Back injuries to fast bowlers in cricket: a prospective study. *Br. J. Sports Med.* **23**, 150–154.
4. Freiberg, O. (1989) Lumbar instability in the young population; biomechanics, occurrence, new diagnostic and therapeutic methods. *Paarvo Nurmi Congress Book from Advanced European Course on Sports Medicine: 50th Anniversary of the Finnish Society of Sports Medicine*, pp. 208–210.
5. Bottomley, M. B. (1990) Sacral stress fracture in a runner *Br. J. Sports Med.* **24**, 243–244.
6. McGill, S. M. (1987) A biomechanical perspective of sacro-iliac pain. *Clin. Biomech.* **2**, 145–151.

Bruckner, P. and Khan, K. (1993) *Clinical Sports Medicine*. McGraw-Hill, New York.

Cyriax, J. H and Cyriax, P. J. (eds) (1993) *Cyriax's Illustrated Manual of Orthopaedic Medicine*, 2nd edn. Butterworth-Heinemann, Oxford.

Hutson M. A. (ed.) (1996) *Sports Injuries: Recognition and Management*, 2nd edn. Oxford Medical Publications, Oxford.

Palastanga, N., Field, D. and Soames, R. (1989) *Anatomy and Human Movement. Structure and Function*. Heinemann Medical Books, Oxford.

Reid, D. (1992) *Sports Injury Assessment and Rehabilitation*. Churchill Livingstone, Edinburgh.

Watkins R. G. (ed.) (1996) *The Spine in Sports*. Mosby, St Louis, MO.

6

Anterior chest pain

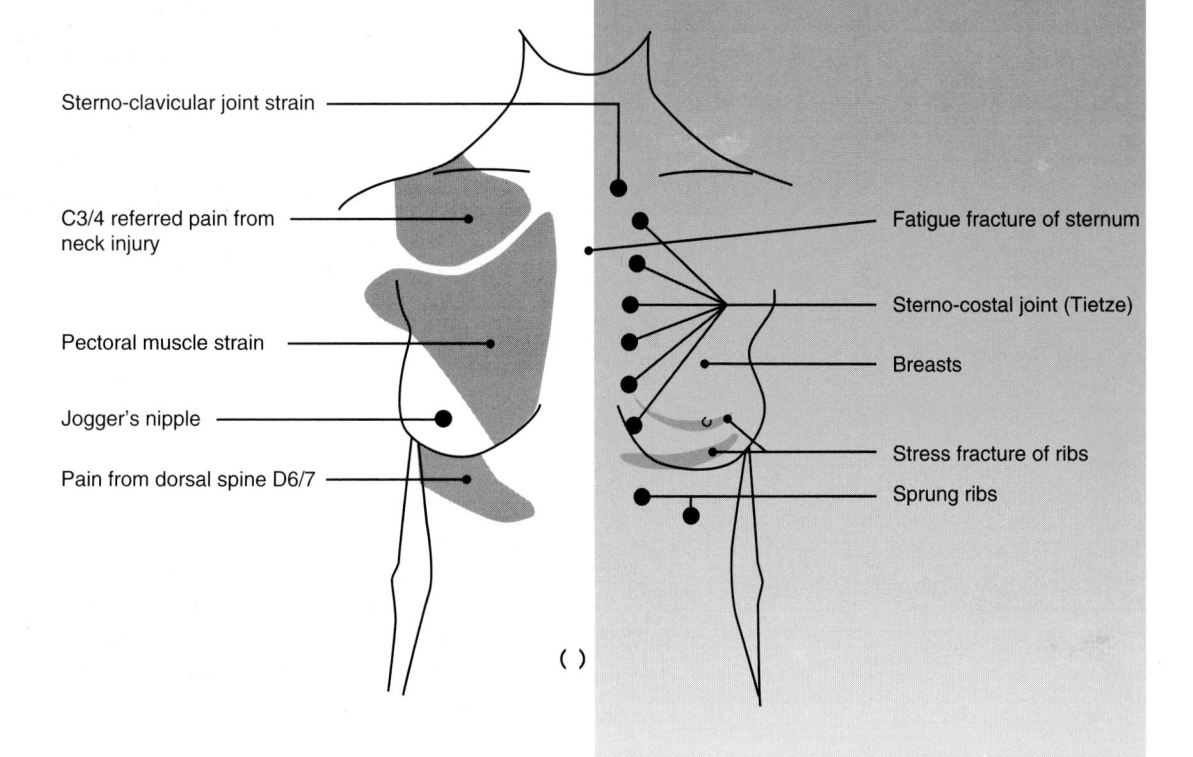

Sterno-clavicular joint strain

C3/4 referred pain from neck injury

Pectoral muscle strain

Jogger's nipple

Pain from dorsal spine D6/7

Fatigue fracture of sternum

Sterno-costal joint (Tietze)

Breasts

Stress fracture of ribs

Sprung ribs

( )

Systemic causes

Every history should be directed to eliminate any cardiovascular problem, particularly concentrating on exercise induced pain and shortness of breath. People do not faint during exercise unless there is a problem either with the heart, hypoglycaemia or hyperthermia.

Young people, under 30 years, are unlikely to have coronaries, but their cardiac problems are likely to be arrhythmias, valvular problems and hypertrophic cardiomyopathy, and these may present as problems during exercise. Long, tall streaks that play basketball and volleyball may have Marfan's and be prone to aortic medio-necrotic dissection. Chest infection, asthma and exercise induced asthma should always be considered, as should pulmonary embolus for those on the pill. Reflux oesophagitis in cyclists may be helped by antacids or even peppermint to reduce gastric distension, and fizzy drinks should be avoided.

Referred pain from the dorsal spine

Dorsal rotation with flexion and local palpation of the dorsal spine will indicate referred pain as a possibility (see Chapter 4).

Referred pain from the neck

Check neck rotation, flexion and extension, plus side flexion for referred pain over the front of the chest from C4 (see Chapter 3).

Fractured ribs – traumatic

Look for a history of trauma and in particular a sharp catching pain on inspiration or movement that is localizable over a rib. Check for haemoptysis, tension pneumothorax and surgical emphysema, and in particular flail ribs. Management of these severe complications is dealt with in advanced trauma life-saving and not in this book. The uncomplicated rib spring positive rib fracture will settle without treatment over 4–6 weeks, during which time non-contact sport may be played to pain tolerance.

Costo-chondral cartilage (Tietze)

Findings

Anterior chest pain that may be bilateral or located over one joint or several joints. It may produce confusion by hurting on inspiration and chest expansion but also on full expiration, coughing and slouching. It is locally tender to palpation over the costo-chondral joint. Tietze disease has also a swollen inflamed joint.

Cause

Tietze disease is a systemic inflammation of the costo-sternal joints, but in sport it is usually post-traumatic and occasionally idiopathic.

> **Caveat** – This rather unpatterned history of pain on expansion and compression of the chest, and therefore being flared with exercise, does confuse with angina. It may be very difficult to distinguish from referred dorsal pain as rotations can hurt the costo-chondral lesion as well. Local palpatory pressure must be applied with the patient sitting as pressure on the costo-chondral joint may also apply pressure on the dorsal spine when the patient is lying down and vice versa.

Investigations

None are clinically required to establish the diagnosis but investigations to exclude intrathoracic problems may be instituted as it is better to be safe than sorry. If the joint is swollen or not settling, look for systemic inflammatory disease.

Treatment

Avoid compression of the chest and shoulder exercises that require pectoral muscle work. Modalities to settle inflammation such as local ultrasound, laser and intra-articular cortisone. NSAIDs may help the Tietze.

Sports

No sport is obviously causative, but when present upper limb sports may have to be avoided until better.

Comment

It is probably confused with angina frequently but if the exercise ECG is normal then local tenderness will give the clue, as the history can be confusing with both opposites, i.e. chest compression and expansion, being painful. Ultrasound usually works over time but intra-articular cortisone can work rapidly.

Sterno-clavicular joint

Findings

Pain following trauma or with shoulder movements. Visible anterior subluxation of clavicle on sternum, or a joint that appears swollen. Shoulder girdle movements may all hurt and it is locally tender to palpation. The pain may be referred up the front of the neck to the angle of the jaw.

Cause

(a) Trauma.
(b) Shoulder girdle problems.
(c) Systemic inflammatory disease.

> **Caveat** – Posterior subluxation of the clavicle is rare but may involve the great vessels from the aorta and require surgical release.

Investigations

X-ray for fracture and disease changes. Full blood count, including CRP, ESR, anti-nuclear factor and rheumatoid factors.

Treatment

Modalities to settle inflammation, such as ultrasound, laser and cortisone injection into the sterno-clavicular joint. NSAIDs may be of value with inflammatory disease.

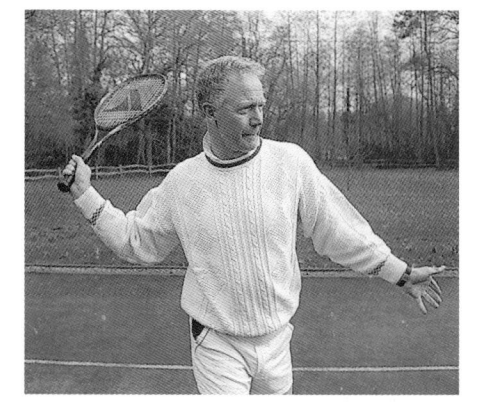

Figure 6.1 The player is too front-on, but has rotated the dorsal spine allowing full shoulder movement.

Sports

Often from trauma. However, when a racket player stands front-on to forehand or overhead shots and does not rotate the dorsal spine, but forces retraction of the shoulder girdle, then the whole pectoral girdle, including the acromio-clavicular and sterno-clavicular joints, may become painful. See Figs 6.1 and 6.2.

Comment

These really do very well with cortisone and, once calmed, often cause no more trouble, even on returning to racket sports. The above fault, (see Fig. 6.2) is often demonstrated by the aggressive player with poor technique who tries to hit hard from the front-on position, and must be corrected – this itself may be curative.

Stress fracture of ribs

Findings

Usually around the anterior to mid axillary line of rib 4–7 with associated pain during the relevant sport. Breathing and coughing may be sore and rib spring is positive. There is no referred tenderness from the dorsal spine though a posterior angle stress fracture of the ribs can occur. See Fig. 4.1.

Cause

Presumed irregular pull from serratus anterior and

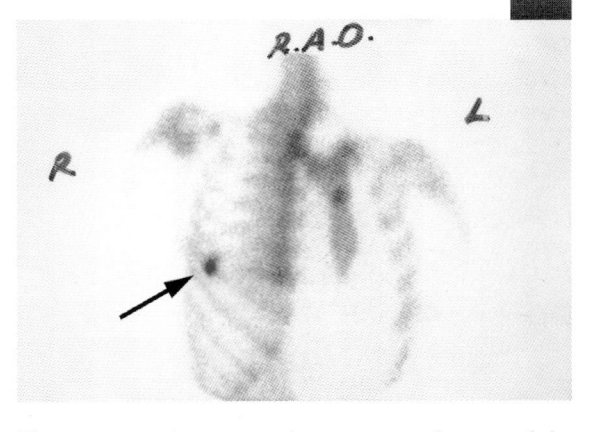

Figure 6.3 A bone scan shows a stress fracture of the ribs in a rower.

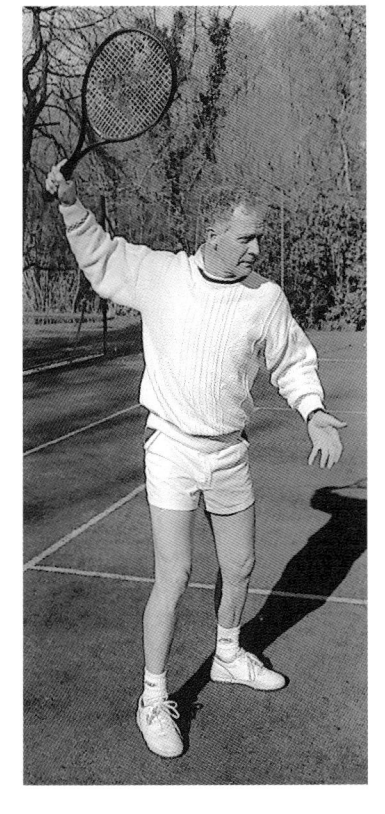

Figure 6.2 The player is front-on, but has retracted the shoulder and elbow. To achieve power, even more shoulder retraction is attempted and this severely stresses the whole pectoral girdle, particularly the anterior capsule, acromio-clavicular and sterno-clavicular joints. Either dorsal rotation or a side-on position must be used with the shot.

external oblique muscles plus rotational strains across the ribs cause the stress fracture of the ribs [1, 2].

Investigations
X-ray is often negative, even in the late stages. Bone scan – especially if a sport associated with this lesion is played by the patient (see *Sports*). See Fig. 6.3.

Treatment
Rest for 4–6 weeks from causative activity and alter the poor technique.

Sports
(a) Rowing. Possibly an oarsman that is used to rowing one side of the boat who then switches to the other side, pulls too soon with the 'inside hand' which does not coincide with the arc of rotation of the oar – blocking serratus anterior or the external oblique. A truncated arm pull through and a decreased lay back position plus a decreased lever arm may yield a decreased risk of stress fracture [1].
(b) Golf. Probably when the left side is blocked out to stop the left side breaking away and thus prevent hooking, either deliberately or accidentally, but the pull from the arms is still powerful [2].
(c) Paddlers/canoeists. Possibly pulling on the ipsilateral arm as opposed to pushing with the contralateral arm.
(d) It is reported in swimming [3].

Comment
Chest pain and rib spring positive in these above sports should warrant a bone scan if clinically unsure of the diagnosis.

Sprung rib

Findings
Surprisingly sharp localized pain over the ninth

costal cartilage, worse on full inspiration and expiration. Simply flexing at the waist and abdominal exercises hurt, and the pain may interfere with sport to a disproportional extent.

Cause

Usually the ninth costal cartilage becomes unstable and flicks over the eighth rib. Almost always traumatic.

Investigations

None clinically required; however, if worried, investigate to rule out other causes of abdominal or chest pain.

Treatment

Difficult to treat successfully. Modalities to settle inflammation, such as ultrasound, laser and local cortisone injection. Often requires rest from abdominal and pectoral girdle activities for longer than expected.

Sports

Usually occurs in contact sports and because breathing hurts – even aerobic training may prove troublesome.

Comment

Although physiotherapy and injections help, this injury can still require some time to settle and a return too soon to physical activity seems to flare the problem.

Pectoralis tear

Findings

Acute episode, followed by massive bruising and later a palpable gap in the pectoralis muscle around the anterior axillary line, may be present. Weakness and perhaps pain on resisted adduction of the arm.

Cause

Tear of usually pectoralis major with violent powerful adduction of the arm.

Investigations

Not clinically required, but ultrasound scan of muscle to assess size of tear may be appropriate.

Treatment

(a) Try strapping the arm or holding in a sling across the chest to shorten and approximate the pectoralis. The muscle does tend to re-attach to the thorax, but a gap may always be palpable and function weaker. After 3 weeks, start isometrics, and gradually increase isotonic and isokinetic abduction. Build to bench press and pectoralis decks (see Glossary).

(b) Surgery may be the appropriate treatment [4].

Sports

Judo and wrestling where the powerful adduction forces are resisted by the opponent.

Comment

I have only seen two – my surgical colleagues thought they could not approximate the muscle tear as the tissue was too friable. Later, local attachment had occurred with a palpable gap and separation, but a return to almost normal function. However, Wolfe et al. [4] feel surgery is the firstline treatment.

Fatigue fracture of the sternum

Findings

An acute injury with sit-ups. Acute chest pain, worse on coughing and movement. Locally tender to palpation [5].

Cause

An unusual stress fracture as a complication of sit-ups in a body builder possibly associated with pectoral muscle activity. Usually this fracture is traumatic.

Investigations

X-ray for the fracture and CT or MRI scan to exclude underlying neoplasia. Blood tests to exclude leukaemias.

Sports

Weight training.

Comment

I have not seen a case.

Further reading

1. Karlson, K. A. (1998) Rib stress fractures in elite rowers. A case series and proposed mechanism. *Am. J. Sports Med.* **26**, 516–519.

2. Read, M. T. F. (1994) Case report – stress fracture of the rib in a golfer. *Br. J. Sports Med.* **28**, 206–207.

3. Taimela, S., Kujala, U. M. and Orava, S. (1995) Two consecutive rib stress fractures in a female competitive swimmer. *Clin. J. Sports Med.* **5**, 254–257.

4. Wolfe, S. W., Wickievicz, T. L. and Cavanaugh, J. T. (1992) Ruptures of the pectoralis major muscle. An anatomic and clinical analysis. *Am. J. Sports Med.* **20**, 587–593.

5. Robertson, K., Kristensen, O. and Vejen, L. (1996) Manubrium sterni stress fracture: an unusual complication of non contact sport. *Br. J. Sports Med.* **30**, 176–177.

Bruckner, P. and Khan, K. (1993) *Clinical Sports Medicine.* McGraw-Hill, New York.

Reid, D. (1992) *Sports Injury Assessment and Rehabilitation.* Churchill Livingstone, Edinburgh.

7

Abdomen

Referred from the dorsal spine

Check for pain on rotation of the spine and on local dorsal spinal palpation (see Chapter 4).

Sprung rib

Localized tenderness over the ninth to 12th costal cartilage (see Chapter 6).

'Stitch'

Findings
Pain, often subcostal, that occurs early on during exercise, when this exercise is usually continuous and aerobic.

Cause
Not known, but possibly early splanchnic vascular contraction, diverting visceral blood to the muscular system and causing an ischaemic type of pain. A proper warm-up seems to prevent the onset.

Spighellian hernia

Findings
Quite severe abdominal pain on exercise and very localized tenderness with a small pit in the obliquus muscle about finger tip size that is tender to palpation.

Cause
Small anterior abdominal wall defect that reaches the spighellian fascia.

Investigations
None of clinical importance.

Treatment
Surgery.

Sports
None specifically relevant.

Comment
I have only seen three cases, but all had seen many doctors. The very local tender pit was pathognomonic and all were cured by surgery. Real-time ultrasound did not aid diagnosis.

Rectus abdominis

Findings
Localized tenderness in rectus abdominis, worse with sit-ups or resisted abdominals.

Cause
Strain of the rectus abdominis, usually at one of the aponeuroses or close to the lateral wall.

Investigations
Ultrasound scan may show unilateral hypertrophy or malfunction.

Treatment
(a) Electrotherapeutic modalities to settle inflammation.
(b) Stop sit-ups and correct any sporting technical faults.

Sports
(a) In general it is related to training too many sit-ups. Beware anabolic steroids may be being abused.
(b) Tennis. The serve may produce a unilateral, enlarged rectus abdominis, possibly because the left hip is pushed forward at the throw up, when the weight is transferred to the left side. The left hip cannot clear out of the way during the hitting phase and the rectus abdominis must 'pull the body through' the serve. Purely pulling harder with the abdominal muscles to get top spin may increase the loading and cause the strain.

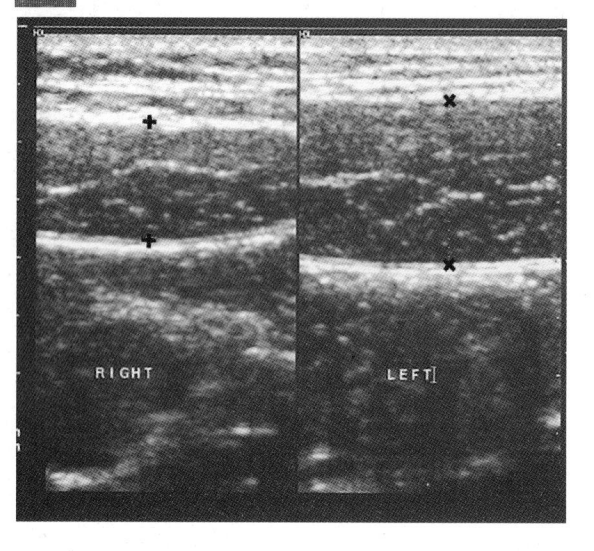

Figure 7.1 Ultrasound scan of a tennis player showing unilateral enlargement of the rectus abdominis (between the two crosses).

Comment

Not common. I wonder if too many people work too hard on their abdominals and to what end? Probably it is more common in tennis in its unilateral form (Fig. 7.1).

Epigastric discomfort

Rule out dorsal vertebral referral, a coronary and, in the elderly, an aortic aneurysm. It often reflects tension, but in sports like cycling can indicate some reflux or subdiaphragmatic compression from the stomach. An antacid, peppermint or charcoal biscuit will get rid of the wind and reduce this discomfort. Check at tournaments whether the athlete is drinking fizzy drinks which may contribute to the condition.

Conjoined tendon

Disruption of the conjoined tendons of the abdominal muscles causes groin pain that is also felt in the low abdomen. Tenderness to palpation through the inguinal canal at the external ring, which is dilated (see Chapter 8).

Pubic tubercle

Tenderness over the tubercle rather than the symphysis suggests conjoined tendon disruption (see Chapter 8).

Pubic symphysis

Low abdominal ache with exercise, especially associated with groin or perineal pain and tenderness over the pubic bones (see Chapter 8).

Abdominal pains

Apart from the usual medical problems check for melaena which can be associated with long-distance running.

Renal pain

Check for haematuria and myoglobinuria which are associated with long periods of exercise or high-intensity exercise (see *Glossary*).

Further reading

Bruckner, P. and Khan, K. (1993) *Clinical Sports Medicine*. McGraw-Hill, New York.

Reid, D. (1992) *Sports Injury Assessment and Rehabilitation*. Churchill Livingstone, Edinburgh.

8
Groin

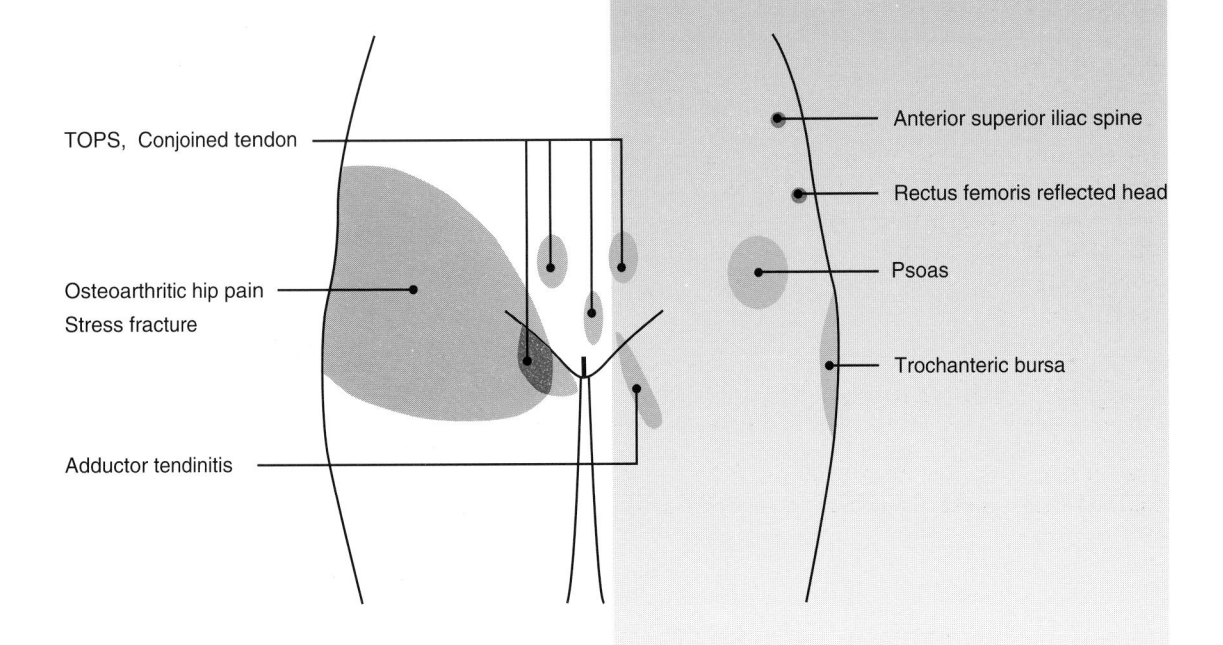

TOPS, Conjoined tendon

Osteoarthritic hip pain
Stress fracture

Adductor tendinitis

Anterior superior iliac spine

Rectus femoris reflected head

Psoas

Trochanteric bursa

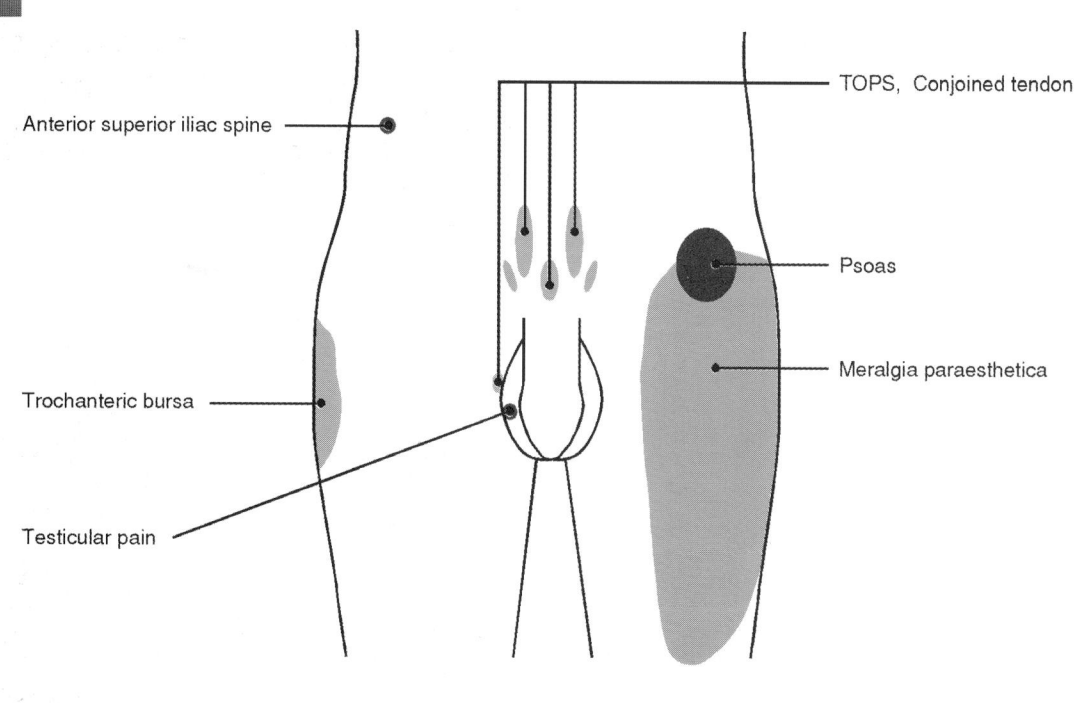

Anterior superior iliac spine

TOPS, Conjoined tendon

Psoas

Meralgia paraesthetica

Trochanteric bursa

Testicular pain

Referred pain

Always check for referred pain from the spine, particularly thoraco-lumbar junction with the ilio-inguinal nerve supplying the groin (see Chapter 4). Also check the fourth and fifth lumbar segment for facetal problems which refer to the groin (see Chapter 5). These segmental problems can be associated with sacro-iliac and ligamentous problems. They may be the cause of the pain or be in association with the pain. This is because the pelvis is a ring and a ring cannot be disturbed in only one spot, so there is always some minor or major associated problem within the ring, besides the main injury (see Chapter 5).

Osteoarthritis of the hips

Findings
Generally presents with pain in the hip or groin, but may present with generalized knee pain and no hip pain. A low buttock ache may also be present and therefore it can be difficult to distinguish between a back or a hip. If initial back

movements, tested whilst standing, bring on the pain, then sit the patient on the couch and repeat the tests for back movements, which should be pain-free. Equally the extreme range of normal hip movements can load the pelvis and the back, and cause pain referred to the hip. Arthritic joint movements should hurt at the end of the range, which may be restricted either mechanically or by pain. The Trendelenburg gait and tests may be positive (see *Glossary*). When the hip is tested sitting, passive external and internal rotation of the hip are painful; when tested lying, passive abduction is reduced from the normal 45–50° and painful, adduction is limited and painful as are flexion and extension, to add to the limited external and internal rotation. Lying prone with the knees bent allows rotation of one hip to be compared with the other.

Cause
Degeneration of articular cartilage with cysts and sclerosis in the femoral head and/or acetabulum (see Glossary). It is possible that sportsmen are more prone to this problem than the general population, but it seems worse with impact sports, such

as running and jumping. However, total rest in plaster of Paris produces articular chondral degeneration of the adjacent surfaces as no synovial fluid can flow up the nutrient cannaliculi to nourish the cartilage so non-impact exercise is beneficial.

Investigations

X-ray of the hips looking for osteophytes, narrow joint space, cysts, sclerosis and the flattened femoral head of an old Perthes (see Glossary; Fig. 22.18). MRI can show osteochondral damage before it is visible on an X-ray, but as the treatment is not altered by this investigation, it is probably not warranted.

> **Caveat**
> (a) An os acetabulare may limit hip range, which may affect martial arts, reducing the kicking range, but the pain is usually unidirectional (Fig. 8.1).
> (b) Stress fracture of the femoral neck in the young active, especially the oligo/amenorrhoeic runners.
> (c) A patient with a fractured hip lies with the foot externally rotated.

Treatment

(a) Electrotherapeutic modalities to calm the soft tissue inflammation, such as shortwave diathermy and interferential.
(b) Maintenance of muscle strength and fitness by non-impact training (see *Sports*).
(c) Inject the hip joint with cortisone to calm any capsulitis.
(d) Surgical replacement.

Sports

(a) An arthritic joint must be moved within the pain-free range, but avoid extremes of range. Stop stretching, martial arts and movements into this painful range.
(b) Non-impact training with a bike, which may need the saddle raising if flexion of the hip is limited, or a rowing machine or rowing within the pain-free range. When swimming, avoid the breaststroke. If this is the only stroke

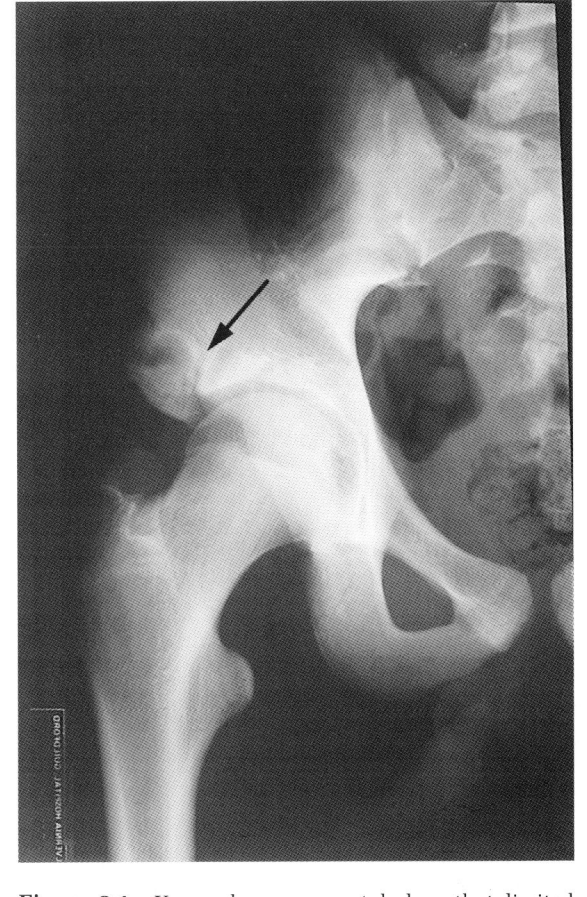

Figure 8.1 X-ray shows os acetabulare that limited the range of kicking and thus caused pain in a karate player (arrow).

available then wedge kick rather than full frog kick to avoid pain.
(c) Maintain quadriceps strength with closed plus open chain exercises; however, the osteoarthritic find open chain exercises less painful (see Chapter 20).
(d) Golf, left arthritic hip. Advise the patient to open the stance, use more arm swing and play a fade shot. Right hip osteoarthritis restricts the swing, so that a hand and arm shot is required.
(e) Tennis. Restrict oneself to doubles.

Comment

Physiotherapy and a switch to non-impact sports will help most people. Reserve injection of the hip, which is particularly useful in those with a lot of pain but little to see on X-ray, for special occasions, travel, holidays, etc. The story of being in a field surrounded by barbed wire (run around inside the field with no trouble but try to run outside that range and run into pain) helps a lot of patients understand how to manage hip movement with smaller paces, and swing both legs together in and out of the car, thus limiting the range of hip abduction required.

Adductor muscle strain

Findings
Acute or chronic groin pain. Locally tender over the adductor longus origin or the musculo-tendinous junction about 6 cm off the origin. The tenderness may extend along the inferior pubic ramus to the ischeal tuberosity if the adductor magnus is involved. This lesion does not tend to have lower abdominal pain (see *Groin pain*, *Traumatic osteitis pubis symphysis* and *Conjoined tendon*). Resisted inner and outer range of adductor muscles is painful. Resisted adductors are painful with the hip flexed.

Cause
Overuse of the adductor longus or magnus. Side steps or blocked adductor contraction such as a side foot tackle, kicking, twisting, turning movements or a slide into abduction. An entheseal spur may form – the horse rider's spur.

> **Caveat**
> (a) Exclude hip joint pathology.
> (b) An adductor tendinitis may still be part of a TOPS or conjoined tendon complex, when resisted adductors are painful on testing, but resisted adductor pain without palpable tenderness is not likely to be caused by the adductor itself.

Investigations
Usually not required, but an enthesopathy may have a positive bone scan and specific MRI views can display localized inflammation and possible bony oedema. Occasionally myositis ossificans can occur.

Treatment
(a) Electrotherapeutic modalities to settle inflammation.
(b) Local hydrocortisone.
(c) Massage techniques to reduce and realign scar tissue such as deep or cross-friction.
(d) Adductor stretches to limit scar tissue contraction.
(e) Isometrics to the adductors to help organize fibrocytes and maintain strength.
(f) Cross-train for fitness and start swinging movements, in and out of abduction.
(g) When fit to run, add the Achilles ladder through to sprints.
(h) Karioke and figure of '8' movement. Start the kicking ladder.
(i) Rarely surgical debridement.

See Chapter 20.

Sports
(a) Acute injuries occur when side stepping, stretching for a tackle or a blocked kick. Chronic injury often ensues but can come from recurrent twisting and stretching.
(b) In track and field, block starts and acceleration require hard work from the adductors and if the psoas is weak, limiting the drive from hip flexion, then the adductors are required to work harder. Strengthening the psoas will thus help.

Comment
This is a lesion that is often seen in its chronic phase. A steroid at the adductor longus origin accompanied by immediate rehabilitation often settles this lesion in 2 weeks, when it is ready for running and side steps rehabilitation. This procedure can also help to distinguish the adductor lesion from the conjoined tendon and TOPS – the adductor improving with the injection, the others remaining the same.

Conjoined tendon injury

See in conjunction with *Traumatic osteitis pubis symphysis* (TOPS).

Findings

Usually, a history of groin pain and suprapubic abdominal pain. May be severe enough to be bent double and may have accompanying adductor lesion, but the conjoined tendon lesion is not tender to palpation at the adductor origin, although resisted adduction does produce the pain. Swimming backstroke or front crawl hurts, as well as breaststroke, and turning over in bed may hurt in the low abdomen.

Resisted abdominals hurt, as does palpation of the external ring through the invaginated scrotum. If the external ring is not tender but no diagnosis is made, then one may have to run the patient over 2 weeks through the Achilles ladder (high knees and sprints) to provoke the injury. Sometimes after 2 weeks the patient breaks through the pain and is cured, whilst with others the external ring becomes increasingly painful to palpation and the diagnosis is confirmed. Often the contralateral side may produce symptoms after treatment of the primary side.

Cause

Disruption, degeneration of the conjoined tendon of the abdominal muscles at the attachment of the pubic tubercle. A crypt hernia may be present. The pelvis may be considered as a ring so there may be two injury sites in conjunction, such as the sacroiliac joint and the pubic symphysis. The cause may be from performing excessive sit-ups and twisting or backing off movements, such as in basketball, or a midfield soccer player in defence who has the ball played across him and back again. Possibly a limited hip range will predispose to this condition as the rotation is limited at the hip forcing the load onto the pelvis. TOPS may be the end stage of a continuum of damage.

Investigations

(a) Bone scan in the squat position with a pubic humeral ratio of less than 5:1 (see *Glossary*).

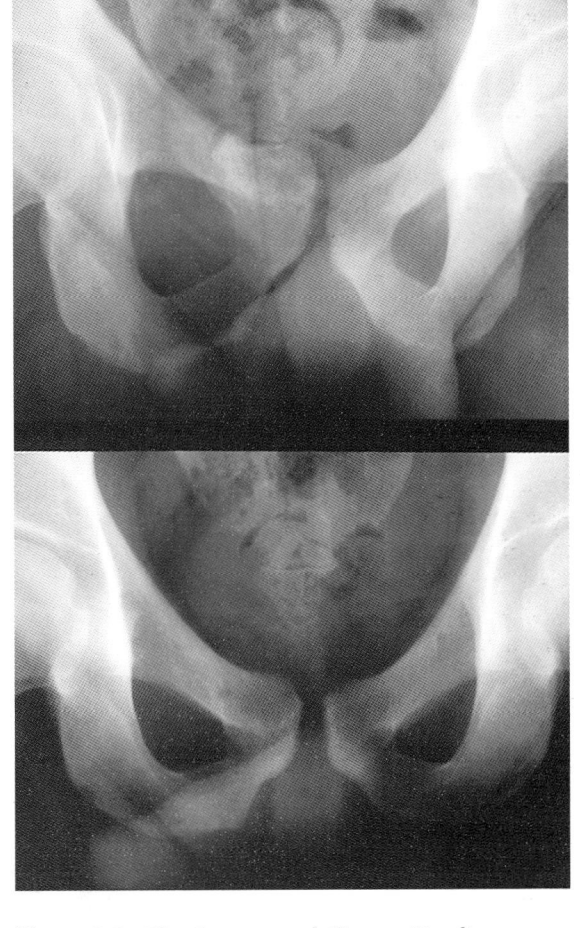

Figure 8.2 Flamingo or stork X-rays. Standing on one leg and then the other shows movement in the pubic symphysis greater than 2 mm.

This investigation excludes all stress fractures.

(b) X-ray. Flamingo/stork/one-legged standing views are normal and will exclude osteoarthritis of the hip (see *Glossary*) (Fig. 8.2).

(c) Abdominal herniograms may be positive but are of debatable value.

(d) Specific MRI views can show disruption and increased signal over the conjoined tendon (see *Traumatic osteitis pubis symphysis*).

Treatment

(a) Inject the pubic tubercle with local and hydrocortisone for temporary relief.

(b) Surgical plication of conjoined tendon.

(c) Rest, which may take 12–18 months to heal, but with controlled exercise may be the treatment of choice when surgery is not available.

(d) Controlled exercise. Cross-training on a bike (rowing or swimming may cause problems). Achilles ladder then add karioke runs plus figure of '8' and kicking ladder. Reduce sit-ups and certainly avoid rotational sit-ups.

> **Caveat** – There may be pubic tubercle or inguinal nerve sensitivity post operation, when a local injection with local anaesthetic and hydrocortisone will help.

Sports

This lesion has been reported as TOPS in many sports; however, they may be a continuum – the conjoined tendon being the precursor of TOPS, but the overall impression is that twisting and turning movements with one foot fixed, such as stretching out for a ball, is the major problem, for with good footwork the conjoined tendon sufferer can often play squash (see *Traumatic osteitis pubis symphysis*).

Comment

This is still a difficult diagnosis to make and sometimes comes down to no other diagnosis being available, plus a failure to rehabilitate. There seems to be an increased diagnosis of this problem. Are there in fact more of these injuries or are they being recognized more frequently? I do believe too many sit-ups are trained, especially with twists, for no improvement in performance. Some professionals are returned too soon after surgery to their sports when they either break down again or get a contralateral injury.

Traumatic osteitis pubis symphysis (TOPS)

Findings

See *Conjoined tendon*. The TOPS sufferer may use

phrases referring the pain up into the perineum or rectum as well.

Cause

Degenerative changes in pubic symphysis, which may be part of a disturbance of the pelvic ring. The pubic symphysis becomes unstable.

Investigation

(a) X-ray. Stork/flamingo/one-legged standing views show an unstable pubic symphysis with greater than 2 mm shift (see Fig. 8.2). X-ray shows areas of lysis and sclerosis in the pubic symphysis.

(b) Bone scan. Squat views may be hot and have a pubic humeral ratio greater than 5:1.

(c) Blood tests for HLA-B27, anti-nuclear factor and rheumatoid factor should be performed if the gracilis margin is fluffy or eroded (Fig. 8.3).

(d) Specific views on MRI will show bony oedema, disruption of the symphysis capsule both inferior and superior, and confirm antero-posterior translation of the pubic symphysis.

> **Caveat** – Fluffy erosion of the gracilis margin may be from either ankylosing spondylitis or rheumatoid arthritis (see Fig. 8.3), but ankylosis of the pubic symphysis is caused by ankylosing spondylitis (Fig. 8.4).

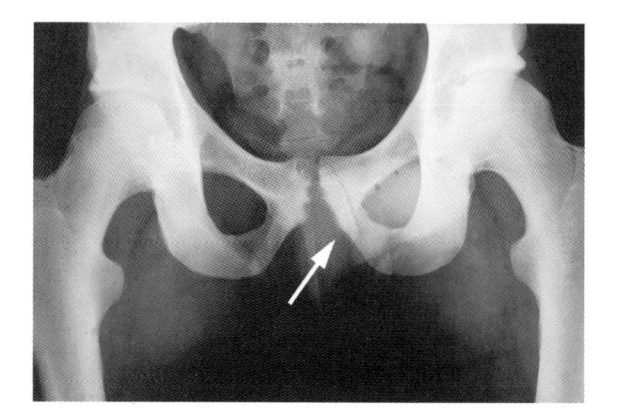

Figure 8.3 X-ray shows cysts and sclerosis with erosion of the gracilis margin in the pubic symphysis of a young footballer with ankylosing spondylitis (arrow).

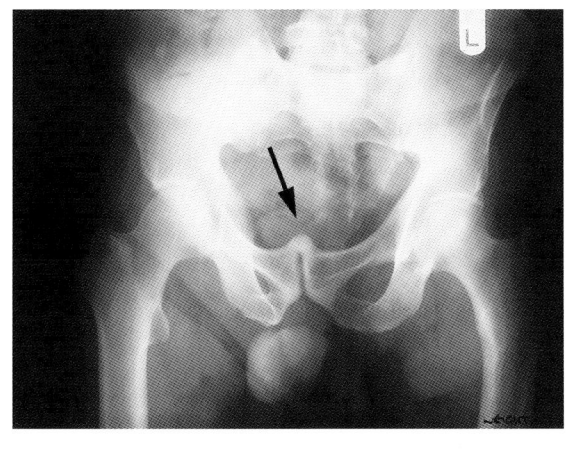

Figure 8.4 Ankylosis of the pubic symphysis.

Treatment

(a) Local anaesthetic and hydrocortisone into the pubic symphysis for temporary relief [1].
(b) Rest and cross-train for 12–18 months.
(c) Try conjoined tendon repair if less than 3 mm shift on stork views.
(d) Sclerosants to the sacro-iliac joints, to strengthen the other part of the pelvic ring, and possibly also to the pubic symphysis.
(e) Surgery to fuse the pubic symphysis if it remains unstable after the appropriate rest (rare).
(f) Treat any systemic cause.

Sports

(a) Change of direction sports may cause the problem if the side to side movement is not accompanied by good footwork. When the movement goes from side to side across the player, as in a midfield footballer, but the player has to stretch for the ball or make a tackle, then forced external rotation of the hip may stress the pubic symphysis. Players may have to channel the opposition in one direction to avoid the ball being played across them.
(b) When TOPS has occurred then swimming is painful, and not just breaststroke, but backstroke and front crawl produce abdominal pain.

(c) Cross-training should be on a rowing ergo to maintain equal pressure on both sides of the pelvic ring and then introduce asymmetry of load by cycling and, later, running.
(d) Sit-ups should be avoided.
(e) Running probably should not start for 12–18 months, and sprinting and high knee raises may be difficult until truly stable.

Comment

This may be the end-point of an unstable pelvic ring where the conjoined tendon strain is the early phase. Do we do too many sit-ups and are they relevant, or is it twisting across the pubis that causes the problem? The erosion of the gracilis margin certainly must lead to investigation for ankylosing spondylitis in the young and this sign is often not picked up on X-ray. This lesion can be considered as being equivalent to a fractured pelvis and it will take 18–24 months to heal. In several cases of mine, sclerosants to the sacro-iliac joints have helped stabilize the pubic symphysis. This may be utilizing the ring theory where a ring cannot be disturbed in only one place and at least two sites will be disturbed, therefore if two sites are stabilized (the sacro-iliac joints), the third (the pubic symphysis) will be helped.

Rectus femoris origin and hip pointer

Findings

Although the history may be of weakness when running or kicking, a careful history shows injury or an acute incident or low-grade pain with these activities and in an adolescent they particularly occur with kicking or sprinting. There is local tenderness over the anterior acetabulum or anterior superior iliac spine. Resisted straight leg raise is weak and painful, as may be resisted flexion of the hip. Quadriceps stretch is reduced and painful, and the modified Thomas test is positive (see Glossary). There may be variable passive hip signs that are not diagnostic. In an adult, a slip, stumble or kicking may cause the injury, as well as gradual overload.

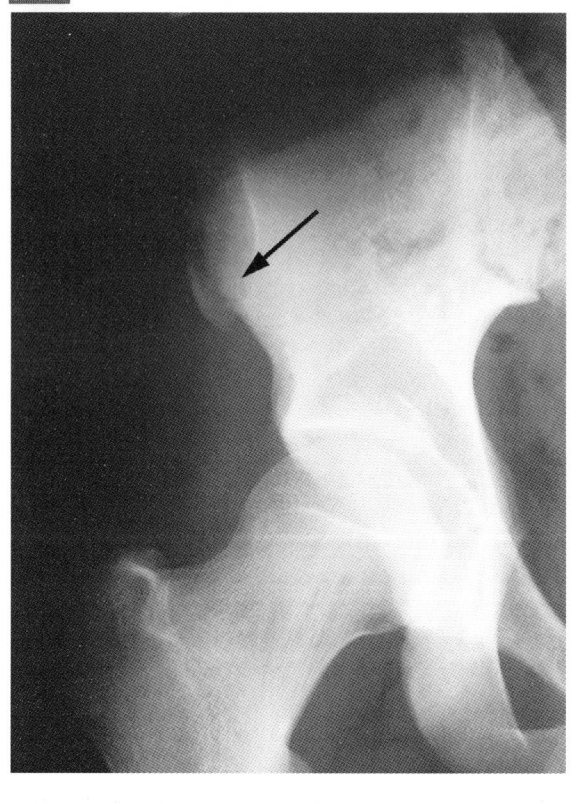

Figure 8.5 Anterior inferior iliac spine avulsion in an adolescent following a sprint race (arrows).

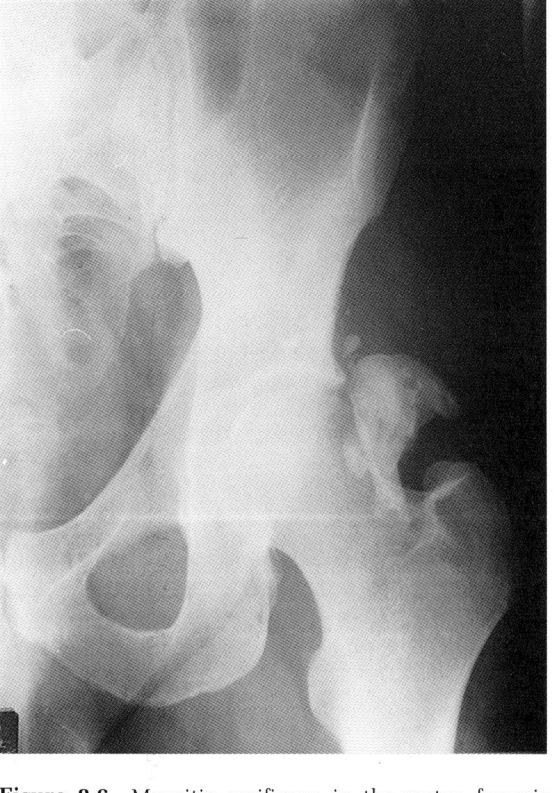

Figure 8.6 Myositis ossificans in the rectus femoris origin.

Cause

Enthesopathy or avulsion apophysitis, especially in the growth phase (Fig. 8.5). Usually at the acetabular reflexion or anterior inferior iliac spine.

> **Caveat**
> (a) This injury is prone to myositis ossificans. X-ray the patient who has a history of getting worse with treatment about 5 days post-injury (Fig. 8.6).
> (b) Weakness – check L3/4 nerve root of the lumbar spine.
> (c) The hip pointer occurs in baseball, particularly when sliding into base over this area which causes trauma or even a haematoma which may need aspiration but the injury is located more over the outer iliac crest.

Investigations

X-ray to display avulsion or myositis ossificans (see Fig. 8.6). Diagnostic ultrasound if 'hip pointer' haematoma is suspected.

Treatment

(a) RICE. May need crutches initially.
(b) TENS or interferential to provide minimal contractions of the rectus femoris in the early treatment of adolescents limited by pain.
(c) Stretch the quadriceps, especially with hip extension.
(d) Lying supine to extend the hip and then raise a straight leg with no added weights until the patient can manage 20–25 repetitions without pain, then add weights when free of pain.
(e) Quadriceps ladders.

(f) Kicking ladder (see Chapter 20).

(g) If myositis ossificans is developing, then rest and stretch only plus prescribe an anti-inflammatory such as indomethacin.

(h) This injury often takes a while to heal and is assessed clinically as weakness of straight leg raise rather than pain in the later stages.

Sports

(a) This appears with kicking, but may also be seen in the first few 100 m sprint races of the summer, especially in the adolescent.

(b) Baseball sliding on the iliac crest can produce trauma to this area.

Comment

This is more common than expected and often the persistent hip pain is rectus femoris weakness. The adolescent often has an avulsion or enthesitis and takes several weeks to settle. Myositis is quite common in the adult. Mini rugby used to have this injury a lot until tackling over the try line was abolished. The try scorer would often kneel down to score, and the tackler would pull the back and hip into extension.

Psoas strain/bursitis

Findings

Groin pain with, or following hill running, high knee drills or running on muddy ground, when the foot has to be pulled out of the ground. Sometimes running bent over as in field hockey. Passive hip flexion beyond 90° produces groin pain and resisted hip flexion at 90° is painful. There is tenderness to palpation about two fingers breadths lateral to femoral artery at the groin. Psoas stretch is tight and painful (see Glossary). Straight leg sit-up, or leg raise, may cause pain. Note, a weak psoas may cause anterior knee pain or adductor tendinitis as this weakness reduces active hip flexion thus encouraging a low knee, valgus movement, pattern (see Chapter 11).

Cause

Uncommon inflammation of the psoas bursa, occasionally avulsion or enthesopathy of the lesser trochanter.

Investigations

Clinically not required, but X-ray and bone scan of the lesser trochanter if not progressing to exclude avulsion of the lesser trochanter.

Treatment

(a) Electrotherapeutic modalities to settle inflammation of the bursa, such as ultrasound and interferential.

(b) Local injection of the bursa with cortisone.

(c) Massage and stretching of the hip and isometric hip flexion at 90° to control scar tissue.

(d) Cross-training and rest from hip flexion, especially if there is an enthesitis or avulsion of the lesser trochanter.

(e) Isometric hip flexion at 90° for strength.

(f) High knee drills stationary.

(g) Achilles ladder. Concentrate on high knee section (see Chapter 20).

Sports

(a) Usually running, especially with runners who carry their knees low and often into valgus, who start speed drills or hill running requiring a higher knee lift.

(b) Field hockey and cross-country skiing can produce the problem in the unfit – one by a crouched running style, the other by an overload when the leg is swung forwards.

Comment

The psoas weakness which reduces hip flexion, and therefore speed and acceleration, may go unnoticed, but it should be looked for in many knee, leg and ankle problems. Rehabilitation of this muscle may be the key to settling the other problems. The lesser trochanteric enthesitis takes patience and time to settle.

Stress fracture of the femoral neck

Findings

Often has a period of just an ache in the groin when running, but may have an acute exacerbation. The pain may radiate to the knee or even be referred to as sciatica. Sitting lumbar spine movements are pain-free but there are capsular signs in the hip or bizarre protection of hip movements.

Cause

Overload of the femoral neck through impact training or running where two types are recognized, the superior surface (tensioning type) in Babcock's triangle and the inferior surface (the compression type) in Ward's triangle (see Glossary). The superior is prone to complete fracture and avascular necrosis even after surgical pinning. Beware mid- to long-distance female runners with oligo/amenorrhoea as they may be more prone to osteoporosis and atypical stress fractures.

Investigations

Atypical hip pain in runners and army recruits [2] should be bone scanned, but X-ray as a first line. This may be negative or difficult to visualize. Bone scan if there are any doubts over diagnosis. Consider a CT scan for further assessment of the extent of the lesion.

Treatment
Tensioning type (superior surface); see Figs 8.7 and 8.8

(a) Increment non-weight bearing until the patient can stand without pain then walking with crutches then stick and finally unsupported. Later add non-impact cross-training such as rowing, swimming or cycling.

(b) When pain-free walking is obtained, gradually introduce running, on soft ground, with shock-absorbing shoes.

(c) Achilles ladder.

(d) Observe frequently, this is the problem stress lesion, if CT has shown an extension of the lesion beyond the cortex into the medulla, or

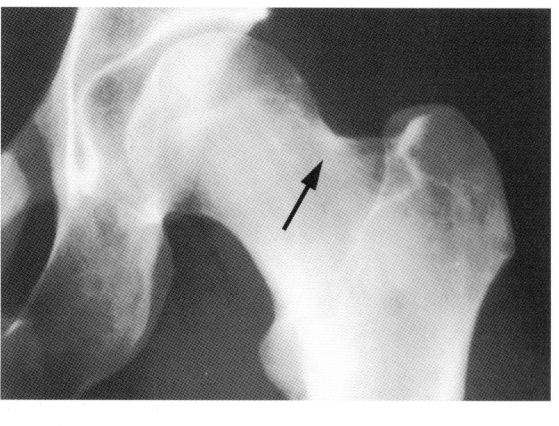

Figure 8.7 Fortunately the area of sclerosis in the superior surface of the femoral neck suggests healing of this stress fracture. CT scan would be required to exclude non-union (arrow).

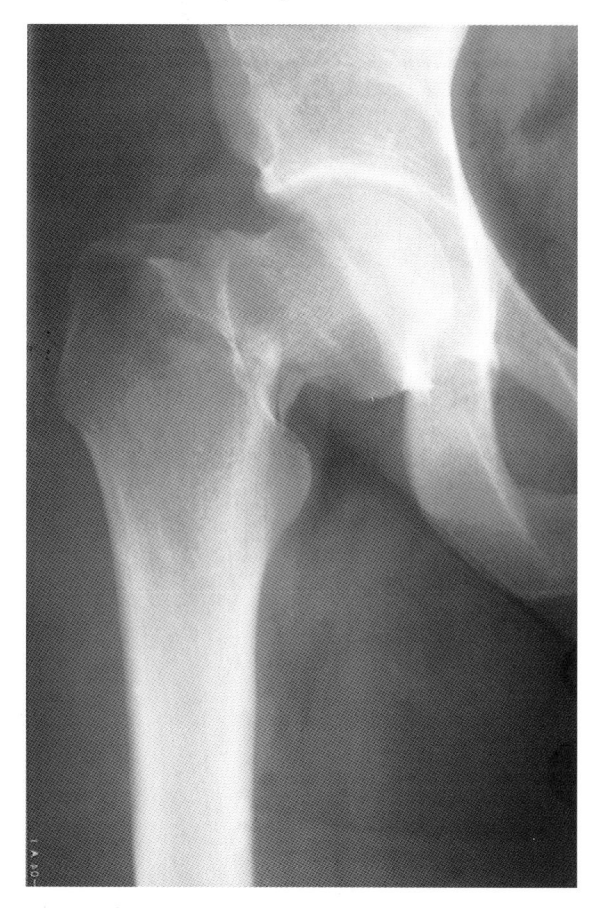

Figure 8.8 A disaster in a young athlete. This tension stress fracture has completed and will need surgical pinning. Avascular necrosis may still occur.

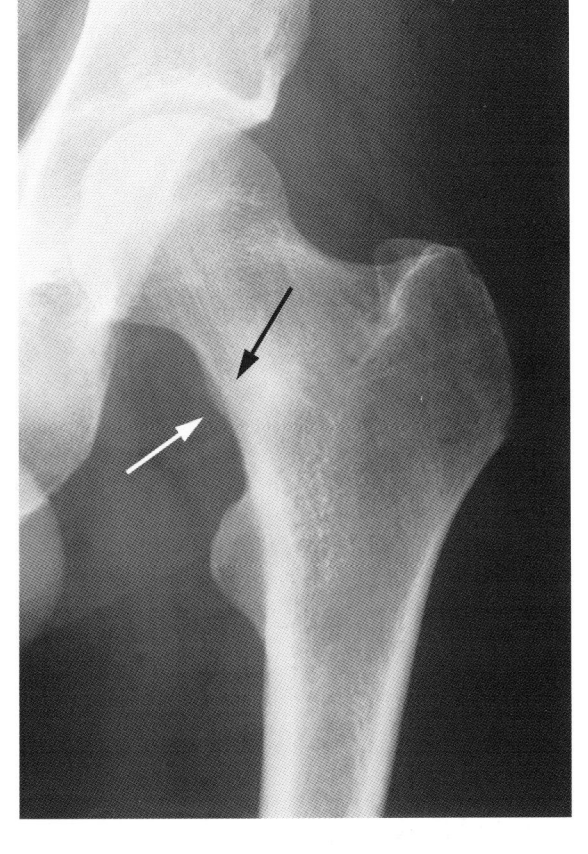

Figure 8.9 X-ray shows a healing compression stress fracture (arrows).

failure to progress, then surgical pinning is required.

Compression type
Treat similarly to the tensioning type but this usually heals without surgery (see Fig. 8.9).

Both types
Both types require:

(a) Training advice on how to increase distance and speed (see Chapter 20).
(b) Advise runners to cross-train for endurance training, only using running for speed work.
(c) Check on diet and weight, particularly oligo/amenorrhoeic runners, and consider an hormonal assay.

Comment
Because of the disaster of avascular necrosis it is better to bone scan and put the patient on crutches if you have the slightest doubt of the presence of a stress fracture. Subtrochanteric stress fractures are reported [3].

Stress fractures of the pelvis: sacrum

See Chapter 5.

Findings
Sacro-iliac pain, worse on impact. The back movements are pain-free but sacro-iliac and pelvic compression tests are positive.

Cause
Rare. Overuse fracture, possibly from unaccustomed repetition sprints on a Tartan surface in oligo/amenorrhoeic track and field athletes (see Chapter 5) [3].

Investigations
Bone scan (Fig. 8.10). Note that the sacro-iliac joint can appear hot, so CT if in doubt.

Treatment
Non-impact cross-training for 8–12 weeks. Check diet and hormonal status of oligo/amenorrhoea and include bone densitometry.

Sports
Long-distance female road runners, but has been seen in men, extending into the ileum [4].

Comment
A rare lesion. One athlete who, 1 month before a major championship, realizing these high level races were won by sprinting at the end of a 5000 or 10 000 m race, suddenly added large numbers of repetition sprints around the bend to her training with disastrous results.

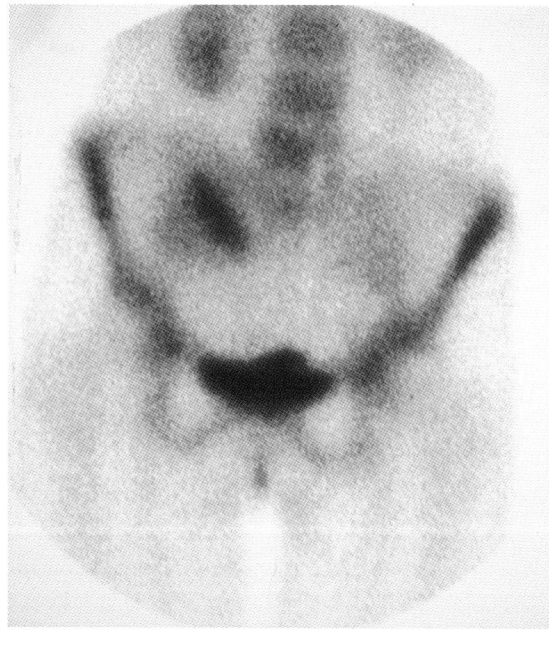

Figure 8.10 A bone scan shows a stress lesion across the right sacro-iliac joint (Dr Malcolm Bottomley).

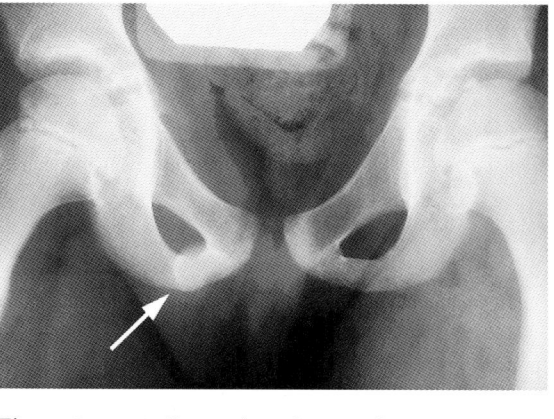

Figure 8.11 Callus in the inferior pubic ramus from a stress fracture (arrow).

Check the hormonal state and diet of the oligo/amenorrhoeic athlete.

Stress fractures of the pelvis: pubic ramus

Findings
Atypical pelvic pain, which may refer to the pubis and perineum or down the leg. It is worse with activity. Examination must exclude lumbar referral, hip, adductors and hamstrings.

Cause
A rare overuse fracture, usually of the inferior pubic ramus but occasionally in the superior pubic ramus. Invariably in long-distance oligo/amenorrhoeic female runners.

Investigations
X-ray may show callus because of the generally chronic onset (Fig. 8.11); however, the bone scan is positive.

Treatment
Cross-training without impact for 6–8 weeks, then go on to the hamstring ladder (see Chapter 20).

Sports
Long-distance female road runners.

Comment
I have only seen this lesion in oligo/amenorrhoeic long-distance female runners.

Neuroma

Many sportspeople have suffered trauma around the pelvis and some superficial nerve may be caught in scar tissue. Check for local point tenderness, especially over the iliac crests and in any inguinal hernial or conjoined tendon repair.

Meralgia paraesthetica

Pain over the anterior aspect of the thigh with local point tenderness sighted somewhere from the iliac crest to the upper mid thigh (see Chapter 10).

Os acetabulare

Probably seen on X-ray incidentally (see Chapter 22) (see Fig. 8.1), but can limit the range of movement.

Inguinal glands

Apart from the usual systemic, perianal and genital causes, athletes should be checked for tinea pedis and tinea cruris, plus infected or chronic lacerations from opponents' studs.

Inguinal hernia

A bulge and cough impulse over the internal ring. See medical textbooks.

Femoral hernia

Tenderness and perhaps a swelling in the femoral triangle, usually in a female. See medical textbooks.

Torsion of the testis

A painful testis lying in the horizontal plane. Seek urgent medical/surgical help if the pain is persisting.

Further reading

1. Holt, M. A., Keene, J. S., *et al.* (1995) Treatment of osteitis pubis in athletes. Results of cortico steroid injections. *Am. J. Sports Med.* **23**, 601–606.
2. Stoneham, M. D. and Morgan, N. V. (1991) Stress fractures of the hip in Royal Marine recruits under training: a retrospective analysis. *Br. J. Sports Med.* **25**, 145–148.
3. Leinberry, C. F., McShane, R. B., Stewart, W. G. and Hume, E. L. (1992) A displaced subtrochanteric stress fracture in a young amenorrheic athlete. *Am. J. Sports Med.* **20**, 485–487.
4. Bell, P. Joint consultation.

Bruckner, P. and Khan, K. (1993) *Clinical Sports Medicine.* McGraw-Hill, New York.

Reid, D. (1992) *Sports Injury Assessment and Rehabilitation.* Churchill Livingstone, Edinburgh.

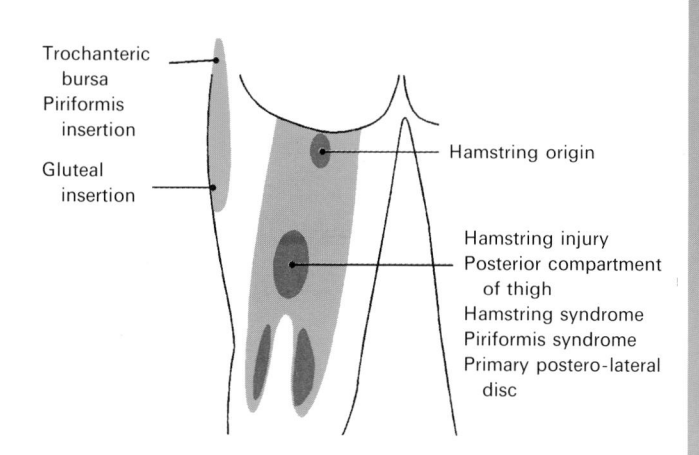

Trochanteric bursa
Piriformis insertion

Gluteal insertion

Hamstring origin

Hamstring injury
Posterior compartment of thigh
Hamstring syndrome
Piriformis syndrome
Primary postero-lateral disc

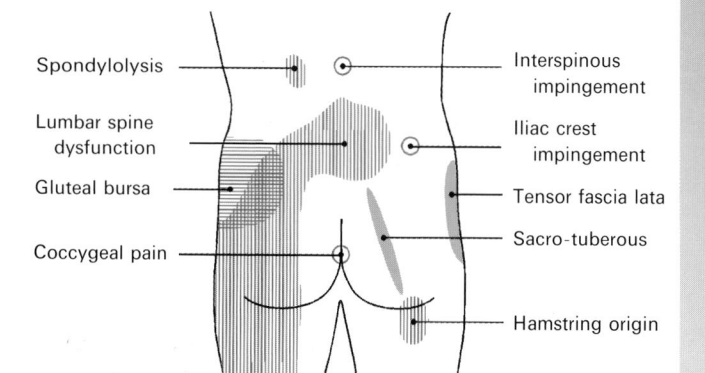

Spondylolysis

Lumbar spine dysfunction

Gluteal bursa

Coccygeal pain

Interspinous impingement

Iliac crest impingement

Tensor fascia lata

Sacro-tuberous

Hamstring origin

9

Buttock and back of thigh

Referred pain

Pain from the primary postero-lateral disc may exist in the back of the thigh without accompanying back pain and examination of the spine must be the first part of the clinical examination. Both facet joints and the sacro-iliac joint can also refer pain to the thigh and must be excluded before examining for more local causes (see Chapters 2 and 5).

Hamstring syndrome

Findings
A history of sciatica – night pain, leg pain, 'pins and needles' and numbness, worse with exercise. This is differentiated from spinal sciatica by testing the patient whilst sitting, when back movements do not hurt. Peripheral nerve stress tests, straight leg raise and Lasegue's test are positive, but the slump test makes no difference to the pain as the dura is not involved (see Glossary). Straight leg raise may be worse with internal rotation of the hip as this bows the biceps femoris and thus the sciatic nerve. Local tenderness over the lateral ischeal tuberosity may be palpated.

Cause
The sciatic nerve is bowed and irritated by the biceps femoris hamstring attachment to the ischeal tuberosity.

Investigations
X-ray to exclude avulsion of the ischeal tuberosity but, if in doubt, bone scan for a tuberosity lesion, or MRI scan of the lumbar spine to exclude a disc lesion. The MRI probably does not display the problem at the origin. EMG is probably not much help.

Treatment
Adverse neural tensioning with the leg internally rotated together with perineural cortisone injection around the lateral ischeal tuberosity to reduce inflammation. Surgical release of the biceps femoris origin [1].

Sports
None of clinical relevance. Rehabilitate via the hamstring ladder (see Chapter 20).

Comment
Rare. I have only seen two cases, and both did well with adverse neural tensioning and cortisone around the tuberosity, although in several cases in Finland surgery was successfully used [1].

Piriformis syndrome

Findings
Similar to the hamstring syndrome but no ischeal tenderness is palpated. It may be worse with resisted external rotation of the flexed hip or passive internal rotation of the flexed hip.

Cause
The sciatic nerve is compressed between the gemelli or as a variant, passes through, as opposed to beneath the piriformis.

Investigations
(a) X-ray to exclude bony cause such as the hip and ischeal tuberosity.
(b) Bone scan to exclude stress fracture and ischeal enthesitis.
(c) MRI to rule out other causes, especially disc lesions.

Treatment
Adverse neural tensioning and possibly a cortisone injection of the piriformis origin at the sacrum may help. Surgery to free the nerve.

Comment
Very rare and difficult to diagnose. I do not think this is the same problem that occurs after an established disc and sciatica where an injection over the inferior border of the sacrum may help.

Hamstring muscle injury

Findings

A history of a non-traumatic acute injury, during activities, with bruising tracking down to the back of the knee or appearing 3–4 days later. There is pain on stretching or resisted testing of the hamstring. Test the hamstring with the patient lying prone. A chronic injury with no bruising is more difficult to assess as straight leg raising will be painful and Lasegue's test is often ambiguous, but the slump test should not be relieved by raising the head whilst in the slump position. Resisted knee flexion or hip extension prone are painful. Local tenderness over the ischeal tuberosity suggests possible avulsion [2, 3] or enthesitis, whereas local tenderness to the muscle is usually 6 cm off the origin or over the muscle lesion itself.

Cause

A tear or sprain of the hamstring. The hamstring crosses two joints. Contraction of the hamstrings should extend the hip and flex the knees. Occasionally the hip is flexed whilst the knee is flexed and this paradoxical movement is known as Lombard's paradox. This paradoxical movement is stressed on change of cadence from the acceleration to cruise phase of sprinting (about 30–40 m into the race), bending whilst running (reaching for a ball, dipping for the line) or checking hard for a side step. Although the quadriceps/hamstring ratio is often quoted at 70% on isokinetic testing at 90° per second, the balance in fact alters at faster speeds depending on the sport, becoming less quadriceps dominant, and indeed runners may become hamstring dominant. Tests in the prone position (extended hip) may display a weakness not displayed whilst tested sitting (flexed hip). Tests also suggest that the weak or strong leg may be damaged, the strong leg over working to make up for the weak leg, so rehabilitation may have to be designed as well for the weak, non-damaged muscle to strengthen it. EMG studies show that the hamstring decelerates the extending knee ready for impact (co-activation of the hamstring and quadriceps) so that downhill running or a sudden dip in the ground can upset this

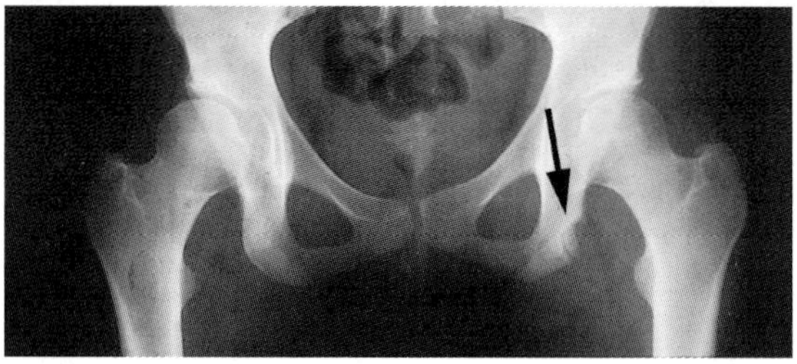

Figure 9.1 X-ray shows a discrete avulsion of the ischeal tuberosity caused by stretching into front and back splits.

coordination, producing a tear [4]. Thus a forced hurdles style stretch can often provoke contraction of the hamstring, the very muscle one is stretching, and produces an avulsion of the hamstring origin at the ischeum (Fig. 9.1). A violent fall into hip extension can avulse the hamstring origin [3].

Caveat – Primary postero-lateral disc (may have no back pain, only leg pain) – straight leg raising, Lasegue's and slump test may be positive, and resisted hamstrings should not hurt. A history of gradual onset and no acute hamstring episode suggests a disc lesion. Any history of 'pins and needles' or numbness suggests a nerve lesion.

Treat with long, strong traction, McKenzie's extension, extension posture (see Chapter 5).

Very occasionally, a tear may keep bleeding within the fascial compartment and produce an acute compartment syndrome. Increasing pain must be taken seriously (see *Posterior compartment of thigh*).

Investigations

(a) X-ray and/or bone scan if avulsion of the ischeum is suspected [3] (Figs 9.1–9.3).
(b) Real-time ultrasound and MRI scan will display a haematoma, and the MRI can show intratendinous lesions and an ischeal bursitis (Fig. 9.4). Ultrasound may show scarring.
(c) Isokinetic dynamometry at varying speeds both sitting and prone can display a weakness.

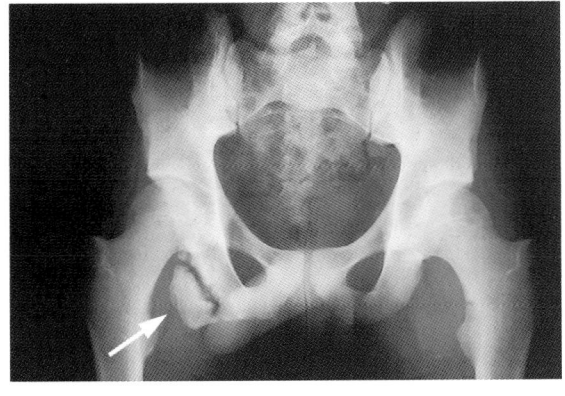

Figure 9.2 This avulsion of the ischeal tuberosity is chronic having remained detached and continued to grow.

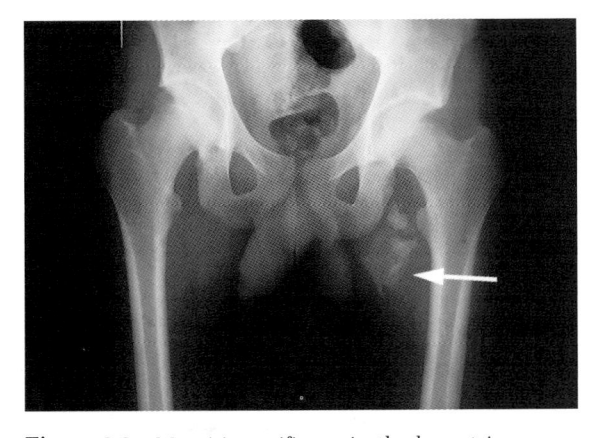

Figure 9.3 Myositis ossificans in the hamstring.

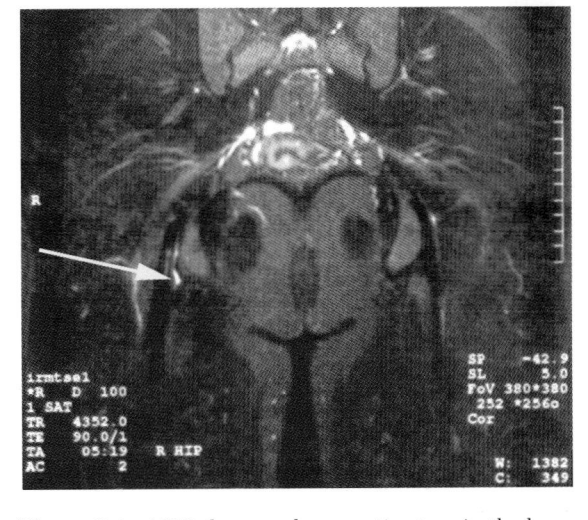

Figure 9.4 MRI shows a degenerative tear in the hamstring tendon and an ischeal bursa.

is adhesive, but the latter must be accompanied by stretching and the ladders.

(g) Surgical debridement of the tuberosity or resuture of avulsion [4].

(h) Occasionally, sacro-iliac joint manipulation is thought to alter the relative position of the pelvis and thus the relation of the ischeal tuberosity, but this therapy may only be treating referred pain.

(i) Aspiration of any haematoma under ultrasound screening control will hasten recovery.

(j) Early resuturing of avulsed hamstring origin ruptures [3].

Treatment
(a) RICE.

(b) Electrotherapeutic modalities to calm inflammation.

(c) Massage techniques to remove fluid and haematoma, and encourage fibrocyte orientation, such as effluage and frictions.

(d) Stretching to prevent scar contraction.

(e) Hamstring ladders – bottom and top. Note that sometimes the injured leg may be the strong leg, and the weak undamaged leg must be strengthened and trained (see Chapter 20).

(f) Cortisone to the ischeal tuberosity if the ischeal bursa is inflamed or the scar tissue

Sports
This injury can occur in most sports and rehabilitation should be completed before attempting match competition.

Comment
This is a common injury. The primary posterolateral disc is often misdiagnosed as a hamstring lesion and I have seen ischeal avulsion several times from just stretching exercises. The hurdle style stretch should not be forced but relaxed into using expiration to help. It is important to see if the weak or strong leg is damaged for full rehabilitation to be planned. I feel ballistic

stretching should also be used to train up hamstring co-activation (see Chapter 20).

Piriformis muscle

Findings
Pain in the buttock and towards the greater trochanter at its posterior aspect, where it is tender to palpation. Weakness of external rotation of the hip and resisted external rotation of the hip may be painful.

Cause
Tear or strain of the external rotators and hip stabilizers, usually at the insertion on the greater trochanter, but the whole muscle may be involved and may be part of the hip external rotator group causing the problem.

Investigations
None clinically relevant unless progress or diagnosis is in doubt, when an MRI may show inflammation of the external rotators of the hip including the quadratus femoris [5].

Treatment
(a) Treatment to calm inflammation, such as ultrasound or laser, and cortisone injections to the insertion. Occasionally injecting the origin may help.
(b) Massage techniques to organize scar tissue, such as frictions, to the insertion.
(c) Stretching of piriformis into internal rotation to prevent scar contraction.
(d) Isometrics to resist external rotation of the hip for scar organization and strength.
(e) Balance on one leg, but do not let the trochanter stick out with the femur in varus. Hold a half squat on one leg, but do not let the pelvis swing forwards on the ipsilateral side, which happens if the piriformis and external rotators are weak, and therefore cannot maintain the external rotation of this hip (Fig. 20.11, 10.12).
(f) Orthotics will help limit internal rotation of the hip during function and thus the work required by the piriformis.

Sports
Learn to run 'tall' by not letting the pelvis and hip collapse into internal rotation during heel strike and lift off.

Golf
Hitting into a closed left hip may cause a problem – open out the left foot.

Comment
This muscle group may be as important for the hip stability as the rotator cuff is for the shoulder and must be rehabilitated as emphatically.

Gluteal bursa

Findings
Diffuse pain over the upper and outer quadrant of the gluteals which is worse with active hip extensions and therefore running. Pain on resisted prone straight leg extension and perhaps passive hip flexion. Local tenderness in the upper and outer quadrant of the gluteals to deep palpation.

Cause
Overuse of the gluteals with unaccustomed exercise. Usually from running, climbing and walking, but may be from aerobics and martial arts.

Investigations
None clinically required.

Treatment
(a) Electrotherapeutic modalities to settle the inflamed bursa, such as ultrasound and interferential.
(b) Local cortisone over the tender area adjacent to the bone where the bursa lies.

Sports
Probably occurs more in aerobic and fitness classes and some martial arts when training for back kicks. Occasionally in stiff-legged style of running.

Comment

Not common. Usually from exercise that has concentrated on the gluteals. Any injection must be placed in the upper outer quadrant to avoid the sciatic nerve.

Trochanteric bursa

Findings

Gradual onset of pain over the greater trochanter which hurts to lie on or with crossed legs. The lumbar spine is pain-free and most hip movements are pain-free, but passive adduction and internal rotation may hurt. Resisted abduction may be painful and is locally tender to palpation over the greater trochanter. Ober's sign may be positive and the ileo-tibial tract tight. Check for pronation at the feet (see *Glossary*).

Cause

Inflammation of the bursa between the ileo-tibial band and greater trochanter caused by increased functional femoral anteversion producing a functionally tight ileo-tibial band. Sitting crossed legged, standing on one leg, running on a camber when the lower leg becomes inflamed, twisting dances and direct trauma.

> **Caveat** – Trauma over the greater trochanter may produce a haembursitis that requires aspiration.

Investigations

None are clinically relevant unless failure to progress, when a diagnostic ultrasound scan may show the bursa, especially a haembursitis, and, in the chronic case, MRI may have T2-weighted or STIR-related sequences positive (Fig. 9.5).

Treatment

(a) RICE.
(b) Electrotherapeutic modalities to settle inflammation, such as ultrasound, laser and interferential.
(c) Cortisone injection of the bursa.
(d) Massage techniques to relieve adhesions such as frictions.

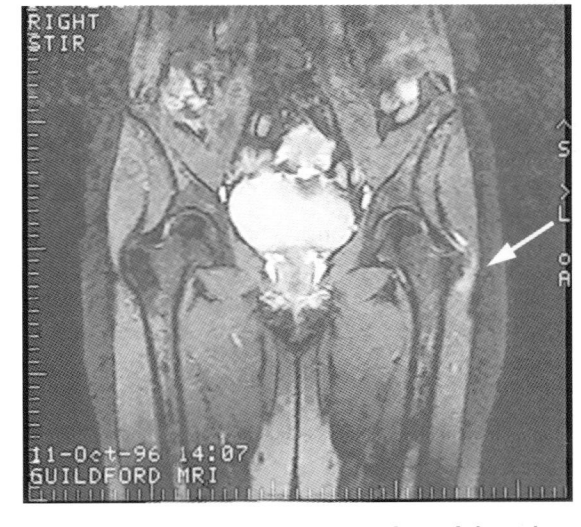

Figure 9.5 STIR sequence MRI displays a left trochanteric bursitis (arrow).

(e) Stretch ileo-tibial tract to reduce friction.
(f) Avoid sitting with crossed legs and standing on one leg with the hip out. Avoid carrying a child on the hip.
(g) Orthotics to reduce femoral anteversion.
(h) Strengthen external rotators of the hip including piriformis and gluteals.
(i) Surgical Z plasty to the ileo-tibial tract.

Sports

Race walkers rarely get this problem although the 'rolled through' running style that mimics the race walkers may be causative. The causes above may give a clue to the problem during exercise but camber running should be avoided (see *Glossary*).

Comment

Not common. Responds well to cortisone, but not desperately well to physiotherapy. Avoidance of the cause is important to prevent recurrence.

Sacro-tuberous ligament strain

Findings

Deep buttock pain exacerbated by the movement described in *Cause*. Tender on palpation over the superior surface of ischeal tuberosity and along the ligament to the sacrum.

Cause

Strain of the sacro-tuberous ligament that runs from the ischeal tuberosity to the sacrum. Occurs when the body weight is on one leg which is flexed at the knee and hip, at which stage the body is externally rotated and extended towards that leg, such as whilst digging a hole and throwing a spadeful sideways and backwards.

Investigations

None clinically required but bone scan or MRI to exclude other problems.

Treatment

(a) Electrotherapeutic modalities to settle deep inflammation, such as interferential.
(b) Injection of the superior surface of the ischeal tuberosity with cortisone.
(c) Passive hip flexions.
(d) Avoid causative factors as specified above or in sport.

Sports

Squash – not usually during the game, but occurs in a coach playing repeated backhand high clearance from close to the front wall – coach remains watching the shot. It is safe to play with this problem.

Golf – see also piriformis.

Comment

Not common but produces long-lasting deep buttock pain. Steroid to the superior surface of the ischeal tuberosity definitely helps.

Tensor fascia lata strain

Findings

Mainly long-distance runners but also in some martial arts. Resisted abduction of the thigh is painful and it is locally tender to palpation under the iliac crest at its origin. Check for over-supination, camber running, downhill running and various round head kicks. Piriformis and hip stabilizers may be weak.

Cause

A rare strain of the muscle origin under the iliac crest from overuse.

Investigations

None clinically required.

Treatment

Electrotherapeutic modalities to settle inflammation, such as ultrasound and laser. Local cortisone and local anaesthetic. Reduce loads and correct faults as in *Findings*.

Sports

(a) Mainly in untrained long-distance runners, when the other hip stabilizers are weak and supination is strong.
(b) Round the head and abduction kicks may cause problems in martial arts.

Comment

A rare problem that does well with cortisone but correction of hip stabilizer weakness is essential.

Posterior compartment of the thigh

Findings

Uncommon injury with a history which is indicative of long-distance running, being worse when the speed is increased and when running on roads. It settles with rest and slowing down, although if severe may last for 24 hours. Clinical examination reveals little. The differential, of hamstring pain, is sore with repetition sprinting or with resisted testing. Continued bleeding after a hamstring tear, accompanied by increasing pain, tenderness and swelling will need urgent surgical release.

Cause

(a) Chronic. Possibly increased vascularity of the hamstrings with exercise and therefore swelling of the muscle which is confined by the fascia. This compression reduces the blood flow causing a relative ischaemia.

(b) Acute. Continual bleeding from a hamstring tear (see *Hamstring muscle injury*).

Investigations

Required to rule out differentials as no tests are positive:

(a) X-ray.
(b) Diagnostic ultrasound – especially if continued bleeding is the cause.
(c) MRI of the back and leg.
(d) EMG to exclude neuromuscular causes.
(e) Bone scan to exclude bony causes.

Treatment

(a) Urgent surgery for ongoing bleeding.
(b) Stop running long distance and/or a surgical fascial split for chronic cases [6].

Sports

Long-distance running.

Comment

Very uncommon. I have only seen two and both went to surgery with variable results. I have only had one case of ongoing bleeding – a medical student, son of a doctor!

Coccygeal ligament

Tenderness with palpation of the coccyx externally and per rectum, and local tenderness alongside the coccyx over the sacro-coccygeal ligaments. Responds well to local ligamentous cortisone. See Chapter 2.

Iliac crest impingement

An extension problem in gymnasts and acrobats associated with walkovers when local tenderness to palpation develops over the iliac crest. Improved by rest, cortisone injections and electrotherapeutic modalities to settle inflammation. The walkover is often performed with acute extension at the lower lumbar segments as opposed to spreading the extension over the whole lumbar spine.

Further reading

1. Puranen, J. and Orava, S. (1988) The hamstring syndrome. A new diagnosis of gluteal sciatic pain. *Am. J. Sports Med.* **16**, 517–521.
2. Kurosawa, H., Nakasita, K., Saski, S. and Takeda, S. (1996) Complete avulsion of the hamstring tendons from the ischeal tuberosity. A report of two cases sustained in judo. *Br. J. Sports Med.* **30**, 72–74.
3. Oravo, S. and Kujala, U. M. (1995) Rupture of the ischeal origin of the hamstring muscles. *Am. J. Sports Med.* **23**, 702–705.
4. Osternig, L. J., Hamill, J., Lander, J. E. and Robertson, R. (1986) Co-activation of sprinter and distance runner muscles in isokinetic exercise. *Med. Sci. Sport Exercise* **18**, 431–435.
5. Klinkert, P., Porte, R., de Rooje, T. P. and de Vries, A. G. (1997) Quadratus tendinitis as a cause of groin pain. *Br. J. Sports Med.* **31**, 348–350.
6. Peltokatho, P. and Harjula, A. (1983) Posterior compartment syndrome of thigh in runners. *Sports Medicine in Track and Field Athletics: Proc. 1st IAAF Medical Congr.*, Finland, pp. 57–59.

Bruckner, P. and Khan, K. (1993) *Clinical Sports Medicine*. McGraw-Hill, New York.
Hutson M. A. (ed.) (1990) *Sports Injuries: Recognition and Management*. Oxford Medical Publications, Oxford.
Reid, D. (1992) *Sports Injury Assessment and Rehabilitation*. Churchill Livingstone, Edinburgh.

10
Anterior thigh

FRONT

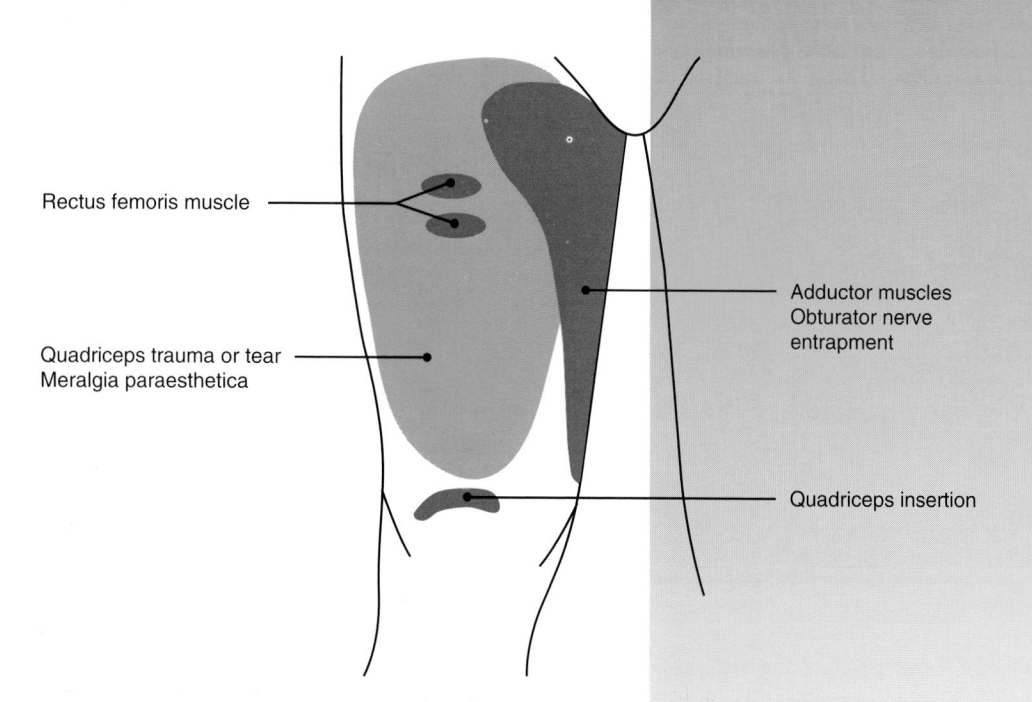

Rectus femoris muscle

Quadriceps trauma or tear
Meralgia paraesthetica

Adductor muscles
Obturator nerve
entrapment

Quadriceps insertion

Referred pain: lumbar nerve root L3/4

Findings

May or may not have lumbar pain, but pain may refer onto the anterior shin and top of the foot, which may have 'pins and needles' and numbness or hyperaesthesia. There may be painful fixed lumbar flexion and back movements which provoke pain. Femoral stretch is positive as is prone lying knee flexion (see Glossary). The knee jerk may be absent and the quadriceps weak, but this is not a pain-induced weakness. Hip rotation tested in the sitting position so as not to involve the back is pain-free. There is no history of trauma, swelling or bruising (see Chapter 5).

Cause

L3/4 disc or lateral canal entrapment of the L3/4 root; L2/3 is more groin.

Referred pain: hip

Findings

Sitting on the couch, lumbar movements are pain-free, but hip rotations, flexion, abduction and adduction are painful, and refer through to the knee (see Chapter 8).

> **Caveat** – Thigh and knee pain is a common presentation of the slipped capital femoral epiphysis in adolescents.

Trauma to the quadriceps

Findings

History of an acute episode of direct trauma or blocked quadriceps muscle action. Swelling of the thigh may occur and if the bleeding is extra-fascicular (peripheral muscle bundle tear) then the bruising will track down under gravity towards the knee. This early bruising is indicative that the injury will heal fairly rapidly, whereas swel-ling with no bruising, indicative of a central tear or haematoma, heals much more slowly. Painful resisted quadriceps, and pain that is worse on stairs, squats, straightening the knee and kicking. There is a limited quadriceps stretch and the Thomas test is reduced (see Glossary).

Cause

Direct trauma to quadriceps, especially whilst contracting the muscle. Blocking of fast quadriceps movement such as a kick blocked by a tackle, which then tears the muscle (see Glossary).

> **Caveat** – If sitting passive knee flexion remains less than 90° after a few days it is more likely to develop myositis ossificans, especially if the injury is near the femur. Increasing pain after 5 days suggests myositis ossificans, whereas increasing swelling and pain over 12–24 hours means bleeding is continuing into the muscle. See Fig. 10.1.

Investigations

Diagnostic ultrasound scan for any haematoma and myositis ossificans or X-ray for myositis ossificans.

Treatment

(a) Pressure and RICE.
(b) Aspirate any haematoma under ultrasound control in the early stages.
(c) Electrotherapeutic modalities to encourage healing and removal of tissue debris, such as ultrasound.
(d) Massage to remove tissue debris and realign healing fibroblasts.
(e) Electrotherapeutic modalities to encourage early muscle contraction within the pain-free range such as interferential.
(f) Stretch the quadriceps to prevent scar contraction.
(g) Isometric exercises followed by isotonic exercises (see Chapter 20).
(h) Quadriceps ladders (see Chapter 20).

A Practical Guide to Sports Injuries

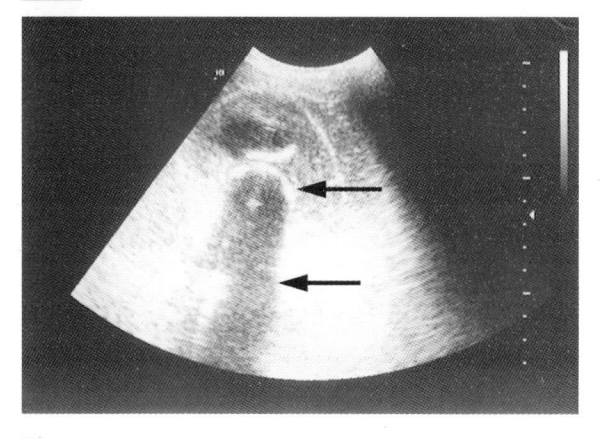

Figure 10.1 Real-time ultrasound displays a dark haematoma with bright reflection from the myositis ossificans near the bone. The bone shows as a white line with shadow beneath (arrows).

Sports

Occurs in sports where a quadriceps movement may be interrupted or blocked extrinsically.

Comment

Early management of this lesion has to be observed for the onset of myositis ossificans when rest must be instituted and NSAIDs (such as indomethacin) can be very beneficial.

Torn rectus femoris muscle

Findings

Acute or chronic history with pain in the upper mid quadriceps which is worse on running, kicking, squats and stairs. Sometimes the history is not of pain but weakness or incoordination during the above movements. The lesion is locally tender with two gaps, invariably palpable, about 6 cm apart in the upper mid thigh. Resisted knee extension with the hip flexed may be pain-free but supine lying and resisting a straight leg raise is weak or painful and the Thomas test is tight (see *Glossary*).

Cause

As for quadriceps trauma but also can develop insidiously, presumably from microtears. Kicking and sprinting are often causative as this muscle exhibits Lombard's paradoxical movement (see *Glossary*).

Investigations

None clinically required. Real-time ultrasound scan to monitor progress of the lesion.

Treatment

(a) The chronic phase is difficult to manage, usually maintaining quadriceps stretching, the quadriceps ladder for training and playing within tolerance or rest from sport whilst maintaining stretch and quadriceps rehabilitation.

(b) The acute tear is treated with pressure, RICE and then as for a quadriceps tear (see *Trauma to quadriceps*).

Sports

No specific sporting injury, but it may be concomitant with weakness of the psoas.

Comment

The chronic phase seems to niggle on without getting totally better, but then if the tear gets worse and completes, it seems to get better.

Ruptured quadriceps

Findings

Total separation of a muscle produces a painless muscle contraction on resisted muscle testing but this is unusual in the quadriceps where a partial tear occurs and resisted quadriceps is painful. There is bruising and swelling in the acute phase with a deformed quadriceps on contraction (Fig. 10.2; see *Trauma to quadriceps*).

Cause

An uncommon rupture of the quadriceps often from the patella insertion.

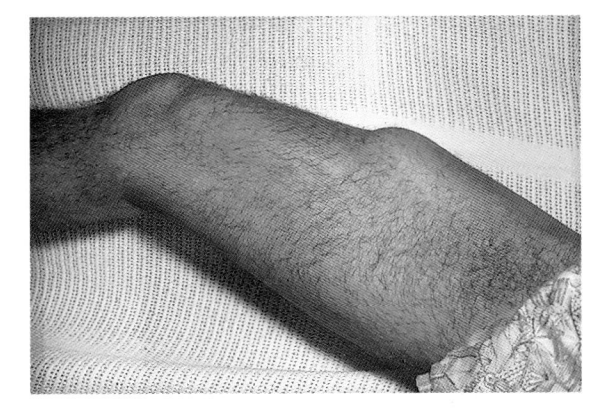

Figure 10.2 A previous ruptured quadriceps now functioning perfectly normally in spite of the deformity.

Investigations

(a) None clinically required. Minor quadriceps expansion lesions may require diagnostic ultrasound or MRI to display them.
(b) Ultrasound scan if you believe there is a drainable haematoma or wish to monitor the lesion (see Chapter 11).

Treatment

(a) Pressure RICE.
(b) Electrotherapeutic modalities to settle inflammation and remove tissue debris.
(c) Isometric exercises to organize scar tissue and build muscle strength.
(d) Stretching to prevent scar contraction.
(e) Closed chain exercises to maintain proprioceptive control and to strengthen muscle.
(f) Quadriceps ladders plus kicking ladder if required.
(g) Possible surgical repair.

See Chapter 20.

Sports

None particularly relevant.

Comment

Not common and certainly function appears normal without surgery; however, if the rupture is close to the insertion into the patella, then it may benefit from surgery.

Meralgia paraesthetica

Findings

Pain and numbness over the front to the lateral side of the thigh but the focal point of tenderness may range from the anterior superior iliac spine to the upper one-third of the thigh.

Cause

Compression of the lateral cutaneous nerve of the thigh, usually as it passes from deep to superficial, through the subcutaneous fascia.

Investigations

None clinically required. EMG is rarely of value.

Treatment

Relieve the cause of pressure and if required inject cortisone around the tender focal compression area of the nerve. Surgery to release the fascia.

Comment

Time and time again in sports players the compression is caused by the tight elastic around the top of the leg from shorts and the tender spot may be palpated under the compression band left in the skin by the elastic. Alteration of the elastic compression cures most!

Stress fracture of the femur

Findings

A history of pain in the hip, thigh or knee that is worse with activity, which is invariably running or marching. Onset of acute pain must be treated as a potential fracture, not a stress lesion, as the signs may be difficult to interpret and in fact no clinical abnormalities may be found, although transaxial stress across the femur may be painful.

Cause

A rare stress lesion across the femur.

Investigations

(a) X-ray is the first-line investigation, but is often negative.

(b) The bone scan in sports people is often a watershed investigation to differentiate bony causes from soft tissue and is required if any doubt about the lesion exists.

Treatment

Non-weight bearing with gradual introduction of weight bearing but beware this lesion can fracture [1].

Sports

A possibility in all impact sports but none particularly noted for this injury apart from the amenorrhoeic athlete.

Comment

A rare stress fracture, but why it should occur in the subtrochanteric region as opposed to the femoral neck is not understood. Beware of pathological fractures.

Further reading

1. Leinberry, C. F., Mcshane, R. B., Stewart, W. G. and Hume, E. L. (1992) A displaced subtrochanteric stress fracture in a young amenorrheic athlete. *Am. J. Sports Med.* **20**, 485–487.

Bruckner, P. and Khan, K. (1993) *Clinical Sports Medicine.* McGraw-Hill, New York.

Reid, D. (1992) *Sports Injury Assessment and Rehabilitation.* Churchill Livingstone, Edinburgh.

11

Knee

LEFT LEG (FRONT)

Pre-patella bursa

Hoffa's syndrome

Pes anserine bursa

Intra-articular swelling

Meniscal cyst

Pre-tibial bursa

Part 1
The swollen knee

A. Hot swollen knee

Infection, gout and inflammatory arthritis

Findings
All may present with the bulge test, ballottement or patella tap positive but gout may only have soft tissue thickening (see Glossary). The knee is warm and usually painful to the touch, and painful on all movements either active or passive.

Investigations
Aspirate and send the aspirate for microscopy culture and sensitivity. Polarized light for crystal arthropathy, gout or pseudogout and autoimmune antibodies.

Blood test for rheumatoid factor, HLA-B27 if *Salmonella*, *Shigella* diarrhoea as this could be an acute reactive arthritis, autoimmune profile and Lyme disease.

Treatment
Not covered in detail in this book. Refer to medical or rheumatological textbook for details (see *Slow swelling after 4–6 hours*).

B. Acute swelling within 4–6 hours of trauma

General

The bulge test, ballottement or patella tap are positive for intra-articular swelling (see Glossary). Assume a haemarthrosis until proved otherwise but can aspirate to confirm; however, the aspirate should be left standing for 5–10 minutes to allow fat globules, if present, to form. If seen, then a fracture has occurred.

Anterior cruciate ligament tear

Findings
The acute episode has a history of acute swelling within 4–6 hours after a twist, fall or impact on the knee which is painful on active and passive movement. The subacute or chronic has a history with a causative injury in the past and rapid knee swelling. The knee 'jumps', 'gives way' or is 'unstable'. The patient is 'unhappy' or cannot 'trust' the knee. Ballottement or patella tap is usually positive in the acute or subacute, whereas the bulge test may be positive in the chronic case as this sign is present with less fluid. Anterior draw and Lachmann test are positive, and the arthrometry

to measure translation is indicative. The pivot shift may be positive. The quadriceps and hamstrings are often weak (see *Glossary* for the various tests).

Cause

Direct trauma and/or a twisting fall ruptures or partially ruptures the anterior cruciate ligament. It may be part of O'Donaghue's triad [1] (see Glossary). Incorrect sporting technique such as sitting on the back of skis then standing upright whilst moving can be causative.

> **Caveat** – O'Donaghue's triad may have had dislocation of the knee, so check for popliteal artery damage.

Investigations

(a) Diagnostic aspiration of the haemarthrosis which has no fat globules unless there is an accompanying fracture.
(b) MRI scan with sagittal obliques at about 15°.
(c) Examination under anaesthetic and arthroscopy.

Treatment

For the professional sports person at the end of the season – early surgical repair. Otherwise, trial of conservative management for at least 6–12 weeks [2]. This consists of:

(a) Settle the fluid by aspiration, electrical modalities and NSAIDs.
(b) Stabilize the joint with a brace or elastic support.
(c) Quadriceps and hamstring strength, particularly hamstring [3] – should be trained by isometrics and electrical modalities progressing to closed chain exercises.
(d) Balance and proprioceptive exercises.
(e) Zig-zag hopping.
(f) Hamstring ladders (see Chapter 20).
(g) Cross-train for aerobic fitness.

If the knee is still unstable in general life or sport then consider surgical repair [4].

Sports

(a) Knee braces cannot be worn during competition whilst playing rugby or football and other contact sports, but may be of help in other sports.
(b) Ski bindings must be able to release upwards as well as sideways at the toes as well as the heel so that the backwards fall may be released [5]. Falling techniques may be taught to prevent cruciate ligament damage in skiers [6], and techniques such as sitting on the back of the skis and then standing up whilst on the move have been blamed.

Comment

Many elite games players, even in rugby, play with absent anterior cruciate ligaments [7] and one often finds clinically lax cruciate ligaments when examining the knee for something unrelated and only then discover a history of damage years ago that has left no functional knee problems. Whilst the muscles around the knee are working the knee is held under control. It is at rest when the knee is relaxed, or when checking a ball in soccer, or releasing the skis from the slope before turning to stop, that trouble may occur. The functionally stable knee seems to be able to prevent the pivot shift from occurring (except under anaesthetic) and the clinical persistence of the pivot shift during rehabilitation may be a warning that this knee will not do well with conservative management.

Tibial spine avulsion

Findings

Acute swollen knee following a history of trauma and the fluid is displayed by the bulge, ballottement or patella tap being positive. The anterior draw and Lachmann tests are positive, but the patient may protect the knee from these tests because of pain (see *Glossary*).

Cause

As for anterior cruciate ligament, but in children and adolescents the tibial attachment of the anterior cruciate is weaker than the ligament and avulses before the ligament tears.

Investigations

(a) Diagnostic aspiration of haemarthrosis which should display fat globules present.
(b) X-ray with tunnel views to display tibial spine.
(c) CT or MRI scan.

Treatment

Early surgical reattachment and the rehabilitation as for the anterior cruciate ligament tear (see Chapter 11).

Sports

See *Anterior cruciate ligament tear.*

Comment

This emphasizes the advantage of diagnostic knee aspiration because the fat globules are diagnostic of a fracture and X-ray or CT will display the underlying cause, so always leave the aspirate of any haemarthrosis in a container where it can be visualized after 5–10 minutes. The fat globules rise to the surface. The reattached tibial spine should heal entirely and leave no long-term problems.

Tibial plateau fracture

Findings

A history of acute swelling following trauma with the bulge test; ballottement and/or patella tap positive (see *Glossary*). There is pain on active or passive movement of the joint.

Investigations

Diagnostic aspiration of the haemarthrosis which should display fat globules as being present. Then X-ray of the knee with tunnel views and CT or MRI scan if required.

Treatment

Refer for orthopaedic surgical opinion.

Peripheral meniscal tear

Findings

An acute swollen knee after a twisting, falling injury which may then have a history of locking and/or clicking or giving way. McMurray's or Apley's sign may be positive and there is tenderness on palpation of the joint line (see *Glossary*).

Cause

Tear of the peripheral attachment of the meniscus.

Investigations

(a) Diagnostic aspiration of a haemarthrosis that shows blood and no fat globules.
(b) MRI – may show the meniscal tear or because the lesion is peripheral it may be difficult to interpret.
(c) Arthroscopy should be diagnostic.

Treatment

Surgical repair is the treatment of choice and then follow the knee ladders for rehabilitation (see Chapter 20).

Sports

May use non-impact cross-training until recovered and ready for knee ladders.

Comment

Probably the best outcome is following early repair, within a few weeks, so take an early surgical opinion as arthroscopy provides a reliable diagnosis and the best mode of treatment.

Dislocated patella

Findings

(a) The patella dislocates to the lateral side of the knee but may reduce spontaneously or with pressure on the patella or require sedation to achieve reduction.
(b) The patient may present after the incident because of pain, but with a history of immediate swelling. However, this may in fact be a description of the displaced patella or a

haemarthrosis and because the capsule ruptures, the swelling may be general around the knee and not confined to the joint. Bruising may occur later.

(c) Pain on quadriceps loading.

(d) When the patella is reduced, Clarke's sign remains positive for some time after.

(e) May have positive ballottement or bulge test some time after.

(f) Apprehension test is positive for some time after.

(g) Tender patella facets – usually medial, to palpation for some time after.

(h) Tender lateral femoral condylar articular surface to palpation for some time after.

See *Glossary* for the various tests.

Cause

(a) Traumatic – a blow dislocates the patella.

(b) Recurrent (see below).

> **Caveat** – Many normal knees that suffer patellar dislocation will develop chondral or osteochondral damage on the deep surface of the patella or lateral femoral condyle [8], whereas the abnormal lax patella may suffer recurrent dislocation because of hypermobility but cause no underlying bony damage because the tissues are lax (Fig. 11.1).

Investigations

None clinically required unless the patient fails to progress, then X-ray and MRI to display osteochondral damage. Consider arthroscopy for osteochondral damage and a possible loose body.

Treatment

(a) Reduction of dislocation and aspiration of haemarthrosis if present.

(b) Possible open repair of ruptured lateral capsule [9, 10].

(c) Electrical and physiotherapeutic modalities to relieve pain, settle soft tissue swelling and maintain muscle strength.

(d) Low load, high repetition exercises and increase the loads as improvement in pain tolerance permits.

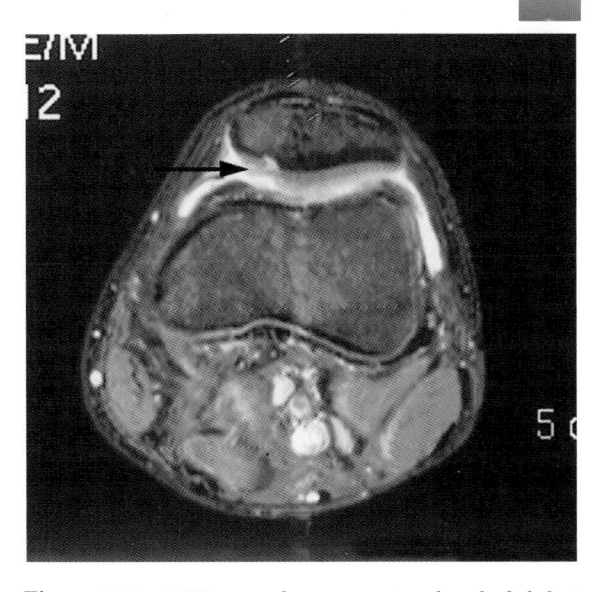

Figure 11.1 MRI scan shows an osteochondral defect in the medial facet confirmed at arthroscopy following traumatic patella dislocation in the normal knee.

(e) Correct any pronation or functional valgus at the knee, as this will hinder healing, by promoting lateral tracking of the patella.

(f) Control patella tracking with a patella brace, McConnell strapping techniques, as lateral capsule is usually ruptured.

(g) Cross-train. Rowing, cycling, backstroke or freestyle swimming (not breaststroke).

(h) Closed chain leg exercises.

(i) Progress to knee ladders.

See Chapter 20 and *Glossary* for details.

Sports

Osteochondral damage will take much longer to heal, and may prevent deep knee bends and a lot of power being applied to the knee until healed. Cross-training and low load, high repetition weights may have to be maintained for a considerable time.

Comment

Acute dislocation is a severe injury and only 60% may return to their previous sporting activity with no or minor limitations [8].

Posterior cruciate ligament tear

Findings

(a) Acute. Acute swelling following a history of trauma.

(b) Subacute and chronic. A history of trauma and an unstable knee (see *Anterior cruciate ligament tear*). The posterior tibia subluxes with the knee flexed at 90°, the sag sign is apparent and the posterior draw which increases the sag sign is positive (Fig. 11.2).

> **Caveat** – Anterior draw test may appear positive as the knee moves forward from the posterior subluxed position to the normal position. Check the popliteal artery is intact.

Cause

Trauma to the knee and rupture of the posterior cruciate ligament which may be part of a major ligamentous disruption.

Investigations

(a) Diagnostic aspiration of any haemarthrosis where there are no fat globules present unless accompanied by fracture.

(b) MRI scan to visualize the posterior cruciate ligaments.

(c) Diagnostic arthroscopy.

Treatment

(a) Usually conservative when a similar pro-gramme as the anterior cruciate ligament tears may be followed with a greater emphasis on quadriceps strength in proportion to the hamstring strength which is required for the anterior cruciate ligament.

(b) Surgical repair.

Sports

See *Anterior cruciate ligament tears*.

Comment

Far less common than anterior cruciate ligament tears and requirements for surgery are much more debatable [11].

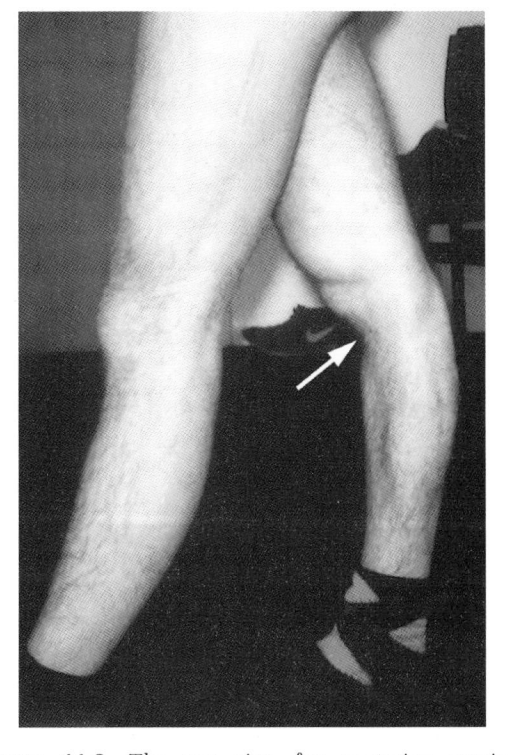

Figure 11.2 The sag sign for posterior cruciate damage is positive in this knee even when standing.

C. Slow onset swelling after 4–6 hours (cold)

Consider the cause of a hot swollen knee, as some of the causes can appear cold to the touch when seen in the early stages (see *Hot swollen knee*).

(a) Intra-articular swelling

Osteoarthritis of the knee

Findings
A history of previous damage or trauma or gradual onset of pain. The knee appears larger, although it may or may not have synovial swelling. The bulge test, ballottement or patella tap may be positive if synovial fluid is present. There is pain and limited extension and flexion at end of the range with a hard end feel. There can be a secondary valgus or varus effect at the knee. There may be ligamentous pain from colateral ligament strains. See Fig. 11.3.

Cause
Degeneration of the articular cartilage, more frequent after meniscectomy, cruciate ligament damage or intra-articular trauma.

Investigations
(a) X-ray – note uni-, bi- or tri-compartmental degeneration may occur.
(b) MRI or CT scan for early osteoarthritis or chondral flap, which may show on these scans when the X-ray is virtually normal.

Treatment
(a) Electrical modalities to ease pain and swelling.
(b) Activity rather than rest [12].
(c) Isometrics to quadriceps to maintain strength but not work the joint surfaces.
(d) Low load repetition weights as isotonic or isokinetic exercises, particularly to the quadriceps.
(e) Non-impact loading of the joint (rowing, cycling or swimming, not breaststroke) with low load, high repetitions.
(f) Possibly orthotics for the feet and posterior tibialis rehabilitation to prevent valgus stress at the knee.
(g) Injection of cortisone to settle the swelling and pain from the synovium.
(h) Intra-articular injections of hyaluronan.
(i) Knee brace if the valgus or varus stress is causing ligamentous pain.
(j) Arthroscopic washout.

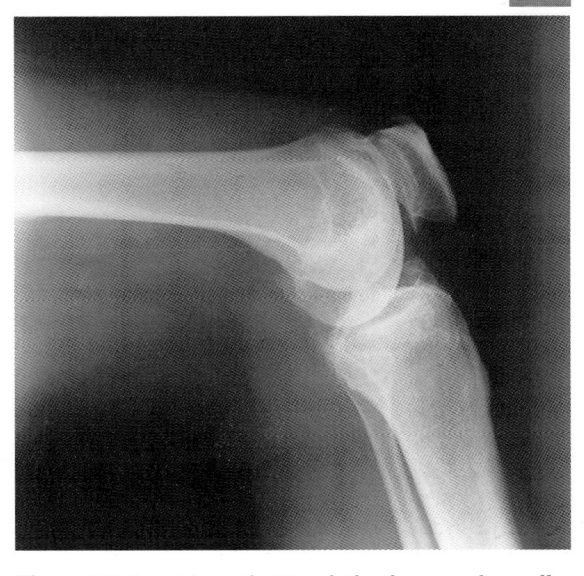

Figure 11.3 Osteoarthritis of the knee and patello-femoral joint.

(k) Arthroscopic debridement and drilling, and surgical correction of varus and valgus at the knees.
(l) Replacement prosthesis.

Sports
(a) Impact loading is not desirable – rowing, cycling and swimming are the most suitable activities.
(b) Play doubles at tennis rather than squash or badminton.
(c) Avoid running.
(d) Weight training should use low loads and high repetitions.
(e) Aquaerobics reduces the stresses across the joints but maintains mobility.

Comment
Orthotics may help to rebalance the knee but a vicious cycle of pain, inactivity and weak quadriceps must be broken by relief of pain and static quadriceps exercises. The rowing machine, swimming and cycling are very useful. Chairs should be higher than the knees to reduce the quadriceps loads required for standing up. Intra-articular injection of cortisone may dramatically relieve discomfort and just an arthroscopic washout can

prove very effective. A 'wet' knee seems to survive better than a dry knee where eburnation seems to occur faster (see *Glossary*).

Meniscal tear

Findings

(a) The history may be of slow onset pain but usually follows a more acute episode involving twisting in a flexed, loaded knee position.

(b) The knee may stick, lock, click, and have pain on twisting and turning. Episodic catching, with long periods clear suggests a parrot beak tear.

(c) Fluid may or may not be present.

(d) McMurray's test is usually positive but a negative test does not exclude a tear. Apley's grinding test is positive but a negative test does not exclude a tear.

(e) The joint line is tender to palpation.

(f) A unilateral block to extension in a non-osteoarthritic knee is a meniscal tear until proved otherwise.

(g) The duck waddle test is positive.

See *Glossary* for details of the tests.

Cause

Degeneration and then fimbrillation of the meniscus which often follows a traumatic twist of the knee, usually from a stumble or a blocked twisting movement or extraneous force, and these can tear the meniscus as can rapid squatting as in bunny hops or an awkward squat with rotation. There are various types recognized: bucket handle, parrot beak and radial tear (associated with meniscal cysts), and a horizontal cleavage tear (Fig. 11.4).

Investigations

Undiagnosed swelling and pain on twisting movements requires an MRI (Fig. 11.5); however, a complete full history of swelling and locking, findings of an extension block, and normal cruciate ligaments should go straight to arthroscopy.

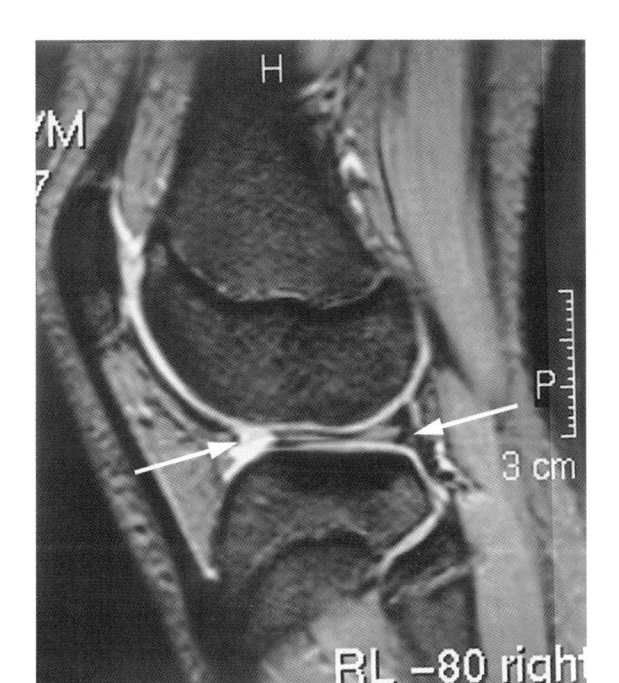

Figure 11.4   T2-weighted MRI shows a horizontal cleavage tear in a discoid meniscus between the arrows.

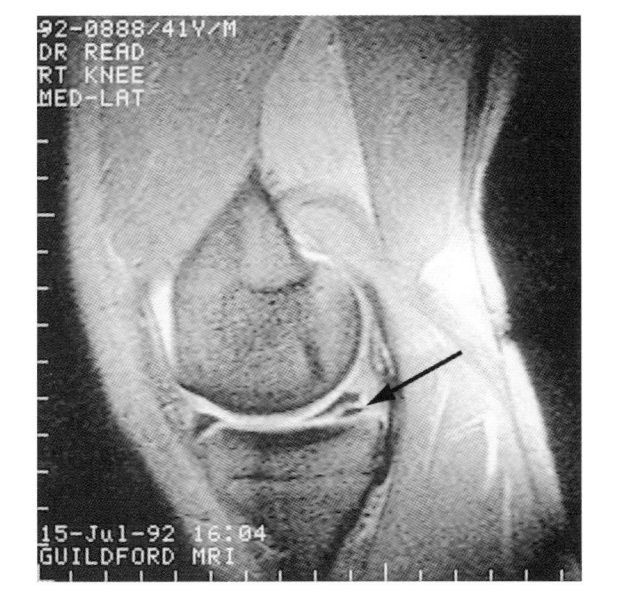

Figure 11.5   T2-weighted MRI with a posterior horn tear.

Treatment

A parrot beak or radial tear may settle with time, but arthroscopic resuturing or partial meniscectomy is usually required.

Comment

The history often gives the diagnosis, but a block to extension is a most important sign. An unstable knee (posterior/anterior cruciate ligament disruption) may lead to meniscal damage. MRI grades of meniscal damage exist where degeneration may be intrasubstance and mistaken for a tear. A tear should be visible on T2 or STIR sequences as well as T1; if not, it is more likely to be degeneration of the meniscus. Clot implantation may be the way to preserve the meniscus [13].

Loose body

Findings

Diagnostic history of episodic locking or catching of knee movements. Synovial swelling may be present. However, see *Osteoarthritis of the knee*, *Meniscal tear*, *Osteochondritis dissecans* and *Cruciate ligament tear*, which can all produce loose fragments.

Cause

A fragment (or fragments) of meniscus, chondral cartilage or bone is detached and interferes with joint articulation. If the loose body remains in the intercondylar notch it may cause no trouble.

Investigations

X-ray with tunnel views, CT and MRI. All may still be negative in the presence of a loose body.

Treatment

Arthroscopic removal and management of the causative lesion.

Sports

See *Osteochondral lesions*.

Comment

The history is more diagnostic as all investigations may be negative even in the presence of a loose body.

Osteochondral defect and osteochondritis dissecans

Findings

This is mainly found in teenagers and it is often the final diagnosis in undiagnosed knee pain. There may be synovial swelling and a history of a loose body (see *Loose body*). An osteochondral defect may have a history of degeneration following wear and tear and/or trauma.

Cause

Localized separation of small area of articular cartilage and underlying bone. Osteochondritis dissecans is almost always found on the convex surface of a joint, the femoral condyles in the knee, and this may represent a compression stress fracture. However, an osteochondral defect may occur on all surfaces, as it may follow trauma or precede osteoarthritis.

Investigations

X-ray, but progress to MRI. CT if not seen on X-ray but suspected clinically. MRI displays early osteochondral damage particularly well.

Treatment

If the fragment is unseparated, avoid impaction exercises until healed, otherwise arthroscopic debridement and removal of the loose body.

Sports

Osteochondritis dissecans is an adolescent injury that may be more frequent on artificial playing surfaces, such as with field hockey, where the surfaces are harder, there is less slide of the foot and the knee is used in a deeper squat to make a tackle. Osteochondral lesions may be treated by non-impact, low load exercises, but surgery may allow the patient to return to impact sports sooner.

Comment

It is often a missed diagnosis – remember active sporty adolescents do not have psychological painful knees and athletes whose pain prevents them playing a sport have a physical problem somewhere – osteochondritis is often the hidden agenda. A joint's only protection from osteoarthritis is by maintaining articular cartilage and it must be preferable to maintain articular cartilage as long as possible by giving time for this to heal by incremental loading of the joint rather than surgical debridement of the articular cartilage. If cartilage fragments are locking or catching the knee, then arthroscopic lavage and articular cartilage trimming may help, but we must ask ourselves what debridement and cartilage drilling does long term that is more advantageous than giving time for articular cartilage to repair, especially in the young.

Recurrent dislocation or subluxation of the patella

See *Anterior knee pain* syndromes.

Unstable knee

The patient complains of feeling that the knee gives way or they cannot trust the knee (see *Anterior and posterior cruciate ligament tears*, *Meniscal tear*, *Subluxing patella* and *Loose body*).

Baker's cyst

The patient has a feeling of tightness behind the knee, especially on squatting (see *Posterior knee pain*).

(b) Rheumatology

Synovial chondromatosis

Diagnosed on X-ray and requires surgical clearance of loose bodies if symptomatic (Fig. 11.6). See rheumatology books for further details.

Pseudogout

Calcium pyrophosphate deposition (Fig. 11.7). Cortisone may produce dramatic relief with

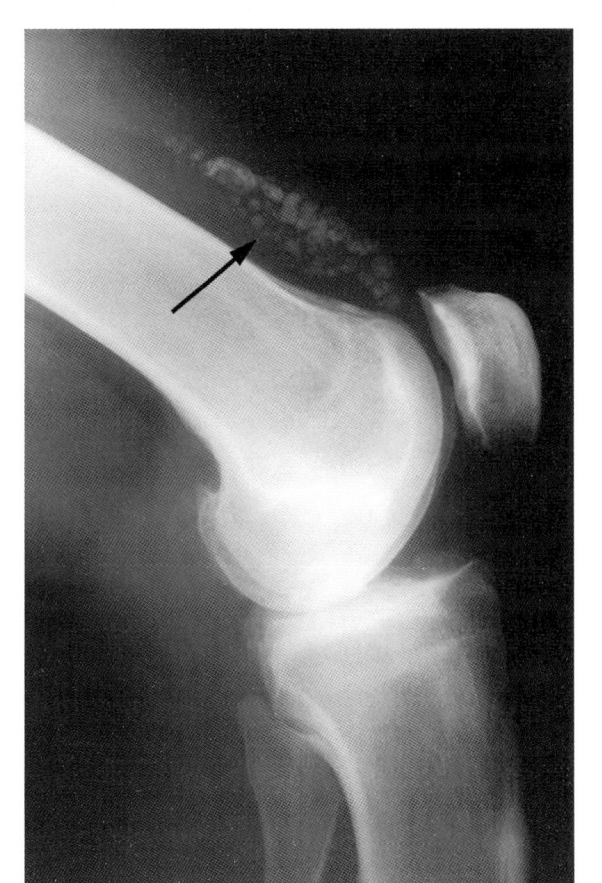

Figure 11.6 Synovial chondromatosis requiring surgical washout.

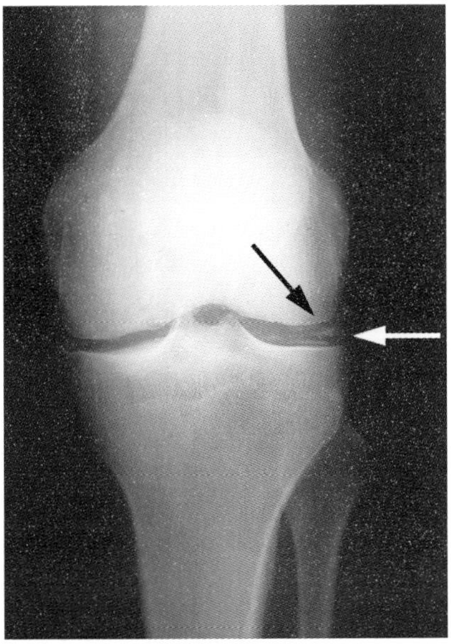

stiffness and pain, insidious onset and no history of trauma. Take a rheumatological opinion. See rheumatology books for further details.

Figure 11.7 Calcium pyrophosphate, pseudogout, within the meniscal substance.

intra-articular deposition. Take rheumatological opinion. See rheumatology books for further details.

Reactive arthritis

Often in HLA-B27-positive individuals following *Salmonella*, *Shigella*-type infection. Take a rheumatological opinion. See rheumatology books for further details.

Rheumatoid arthritis

Seropositive arthritis. Take rheumatological opinion. See rheumatology books for further details.

Other seropositive or seronegative arthritides

Monarthritis or multiple joint pains, with morning

(c) Extra-articular swelling

Pes anserine bursa/ semimembranosus bursa

Pain and swelling over the proximal medial tibia (see *Medial knee pain*).

Hoffa's fat pad

Swelling limited to either side of the patella tendon which is larger with the knee in extension and may be tender to touch (see *Anterior knee pain*).

Meniscal cyst

Firm localized palpable swelling over the lateral joint line of the knee, but it may be antero-medial or antero-lateral on the joint line (see *Lateral knee pain*).

Deep infrapatellar bursa

Painful swelling around the sides of the tibial tubercle (see *Anterior knee pain*).

Pre-patellar bursa (housemaid's knee)

Swelling localized superficially over the patella (see *Anterior knee pain*).

Effort-induced thrombosis (Paget–von Schroetter syndrome)

Pain and swelling at the back of the knee and the calf, worse with exercise (see Chapter 12).

Part 2
Anterior knee pain

B. Anterior knee pain syndromes

A. Referred pain

General

Always check all knee pain for referred pain from the third and fourth lumbar segment and from the hip (see Chapters 5 and 8).

Maltracking of the patella

General findings for faults at the hip, knee and foot
(a) Diffuse, poorly localized anterior knee pain.
(b) All have functional valgus at the knees on half squat test (Figs 11.8 and 11.9).
(c) Patella apprehension is usually positive.
(d) Medial patella facets are tender to palpation.
(e) Clarke's test is painful.
(f) The running style tends to be a low knee carry with windmilling effect of the lower leg so that when the patient is seen soon after exer-

LEFT LEG (FRONT)

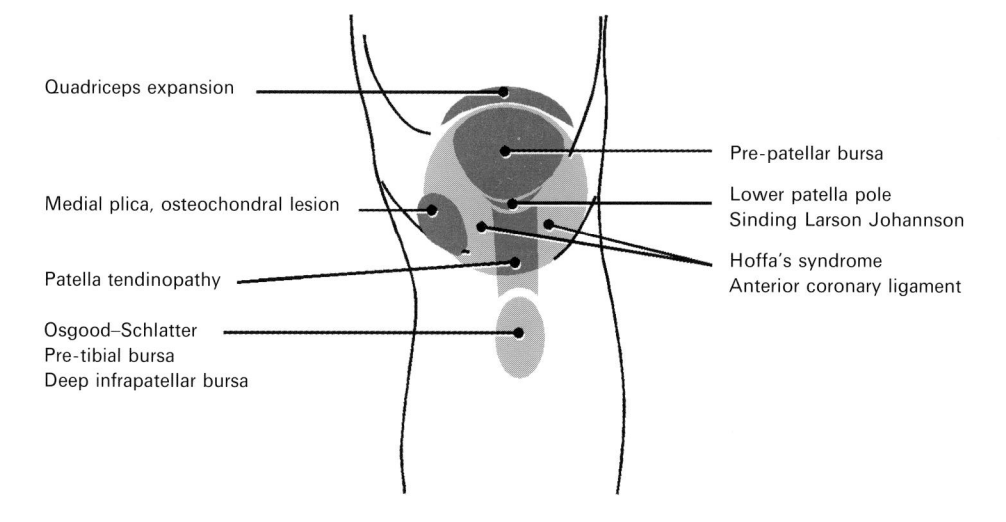

Quadriceps expansion

Medial plica, osteochondral lesion

Patella tendinopathy

Osgood–Schlatter
Pre-tibial bursa
Deep infrapatellar bursa

Pre-patellar bursa

Lower patella pole
Sinding Larson Johannson

Hoffa's syndrome
Anterior coronary ligament

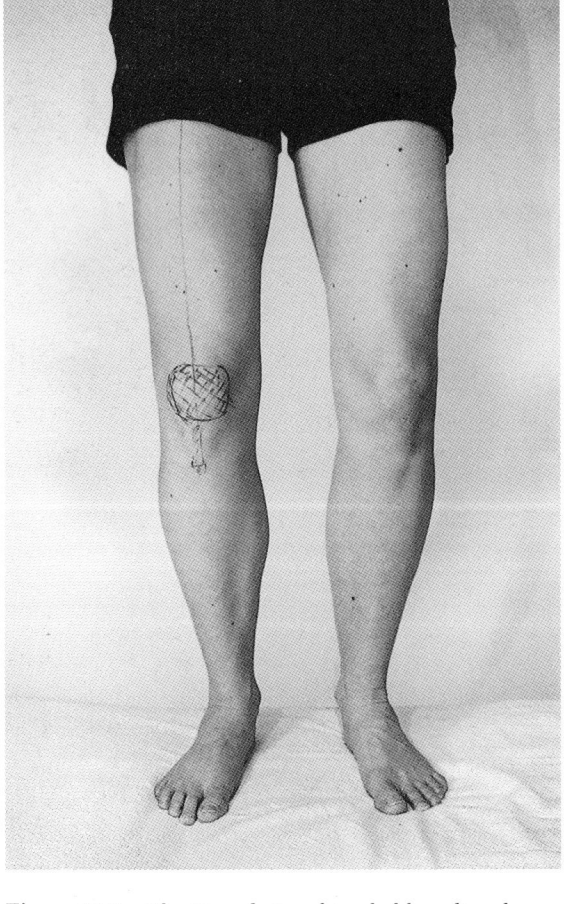

Figure 11.8   The Q angle is subtended by a line drawn from the femoral head to the middle of the patella and from this point to the insertion in the tibial tubercle. The Q angle is normally less than 15°. During this half squat test the knees have remained over the feet maintaining normal patella tracking.

cise, they may have tender capsular ligaments of the knee as well.

(g) Pain whilst sitting with knees bent. These patients often sit with their legs drawn up under themselves in valgus and kneel, sitting in between their feet.

See *Glossary* for various tests.

Fault at the hip

Problems are as described in general findings plus the patient stands with feet together and straight legs, but has patellar squinting, because of

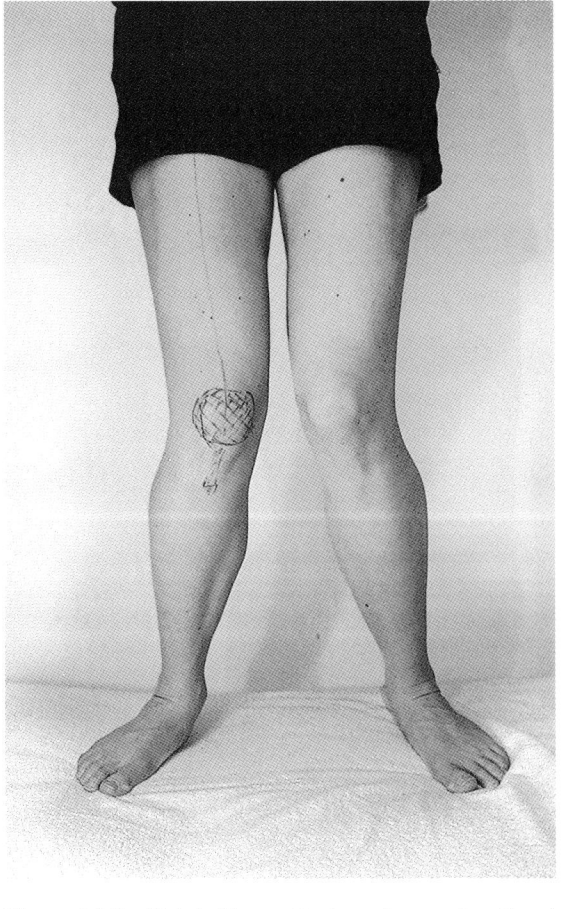

Figure 11.9   This half squat test produces a functional valgus at the knees increasing the angle and producing functional pronation at the feet, a cause of maltracking.

anteverted hips. The feet do not overpronate. The external rotators of the hip are weak.

Fault at the knee

(a) Problems are as described in general findings plus the patient's stance is with valgus knees, either because of too much fat around the thighs, a laterally placed tibial tubercle or narrowing of the medial compartment from osteoarthritis of the knee.

(b) There is tenderness over the tibio-collateral ligament on valgus stressing and palpation.

(c) The medial plica may be tender to palpation.

(d) There may or may not be anatomical overpronated feet, but the patient will overpronate in function, as the feet follow the effect of knees (see Fig. 11.9).

(e) Posterior tibialis is weak on resisted testing.

(f) Weiberg's 2+ patella, patella alta or patella beja may be present.

(g) Bayonette sign may be present.

See *Glossary* for various tests.

Fault at the feet

Problems are as described in general findings plus:

Group 1   Basic anatomical stance is normal but the feet are overpronated with weak posterior tibialis on resisted testing.

Group 2   Limited talar dorsiflexion (congenitally flattened talus or trauma to the talar dome) therefore in function, the foot must pronate to produce an apparent increase in functional range of dorsiflexion at the ankle and the knee may follow it into valgus.

Group 3   Tarsal coalition which may prevent the feet from adapting to rough ground so that the knees must make this adaption with valgus or varus movements.

Cause

The angle between the hip joint, quadriceps origin and the mid point of the patella lying normally between the femoral condyles, and the mid point of the patella and tibial tubercle, is increased beyond 15° (an increased Q angle) (see Figs 11.8 and 11.9). The patella therefore lies towards the lateral femoral condyle causing strain on the medial capsular structures plus decreased interchondral pressure between the medial patella facets and the medial femoral condyle, so disuse fimbrillation occurs over the medial patella facets. Chondral cartilage requires pressure between adjacent articular surfaces to squeeze synovial fluid into the nutrient canaliculi.

Investigations
Fault at the hip

None clinically required except to exclude other problems such as hip or bony lesions.

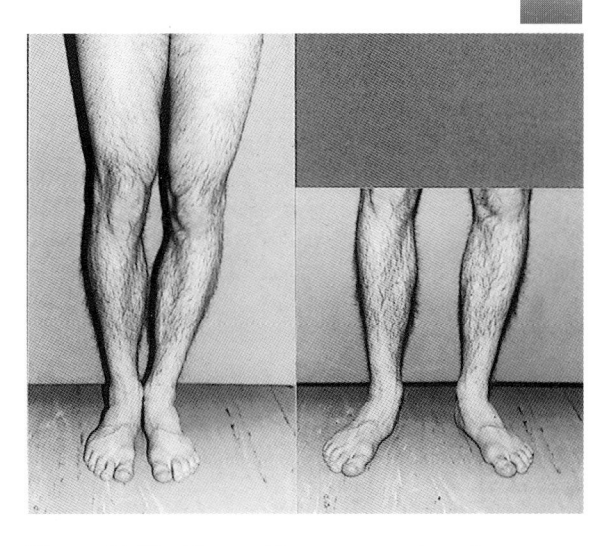

Figure 11.10   The problems start at these feet.

Fault at the knee

(a) X-ray with skyline views to assess Weiberg type and lateral X-ray to establish patella beja or alta.

(b) CT or MRI between 10 and 40° of knee flexion for maltracking.

Fault at the feet

Podiatric assessment of pronation (Fig. 11.10). Lateral X-ray of talar dome and check there are no tarsal coalitions for which CT may be required.

Treatment
General

May require capsular and ligamentous pains calming with electrical modalities and prevention of lateral patella tracking or rotation with McConnell taping or a patella brace with a patellar restraining ring and vastus medialis obliquus muscle exercises [14]. Check for weak posterior tibialis and rehabilitate if weak.

Fault at the hip

Strengthening and balancing exercises for external rotators of the hip. Walk and stand tall at the hip and pelvis, pulling the hips into external rotation by muscle tension. Concentrate on the knee staying over the first and second toes in one-legged half squats (see Fig. 11.8), and whilst cycling and going up stairs. Weak external hip rotators allow the pelvis to swing into adduction and the knee to follow into valgus. Put hands on the anterior superior iliac spine when doing a one-legged half squat, and do not let the pelvis rotate forwards and inwards (see Chapter 20). Orthotics may reduce functional pronation and thus reduce the work required from the hip rotators, but perhaps long-term development of strength in the external hip rotators is required.

Fault at the knee

(a) Manage the patient as in problems at the hip but also lose weight if the knees are fat, as is often seen in adolescents.

(b) Corrective orthotics in the shoes for overpronation, but note that a high arched foot can functionally swing too far into pronation and orthotics will reduce this range of movement and thus also its effect on the knee.

(c) Surface EMG biofeedback to vastus medialis obliquus may help establish function.

(d) Alteration of activities to use change of direction sports rather than continual running as this alters the angle of the loads on the knees, whereas running repeats the same angle of loading.

(e) Calm any ligamentous strains such as tibio-collateral or menisco-collateral ligament with electrotherapeutic modalities, NSAIDs or cortisone injection.

(f) Surgery if conservative treatment fails, such as a lateral release or tibial tubercle realignment.

> **Caveat** – The medial subcutaneous fat pad at the knee may be sore in the cold and on squeezing. It often changes colour with temperature and ultrasound may help. However, this problem can be confused with a knee problem.

Fault at the feet

Corrective orthotics are required as well as the corrective exercises for the cause from the hip and knee.

Group 1   Posterior tibialis strengthening and psoas may need strengthening to encourage knee lift during running, allowing the swing phase to complete before foot strike.

Group 2   A heel raise may help by producing a neutral foot in plantar flexion and thus an increase in functional dorsiflexion. Then encourage a shorter stride pattern. Prescribe high knee drills to encourage lift off of the foot at the mid stance phase rather than push through to toe off, at which stage the limited dorsiflexion of the foot induces a functional pronation, preventing effective push off. Use of orthotics, other than a heel raise, may help but can make the situation worse.

Group 3   May have to accept the problems and increment loads more slowly or consider a non-running sport.

Sports

(a) Change of direction sports cause less problems than running because the knee/patella positions alter, as opposed to being repeatedly maltracked, as in running.

(b) There are problems with swimming breaststroke and butterfly which encourage valgus at the knees.

(c) Horse riding may be helped by longer stirrups to reduce knee valgus.

(d) Hill running can cause problems if knee lift off is poor so the swing phase is not completed before foot strike thus landing in external rotation and pronation.

(e) Running on a camber may produce functional valgus.

(f) Step-ups can functionally produce valgus at the knee so the knee must be worked over the foot. Astride jumps if taken too wide increase functional knee valgus.

(g) Cycling must have play in the foot cleat so the knee is not locked into one position and forefoot varus must be corrected at the pedal with a wedge on the shoe or pedal. Vastus medialis obliquus use is encouraged by using a higher saddle and the knees should move in line over the pedals.

(h) Some runners, who land into the mid stance phase instead of heel strike, will run onto a soft pronating foot and the knee will suffer both overload and tracking problems. They work very hard to run, going nowhere fast, rather like running on a jelly! See *Problems of overload*.

Comment

This is the very common 'young adolescent girl's knee' and in children early orthotics after about 9 years of age may provide long-term correction and dramatically improve their athletic performance. However, orthotics are not the blanket answer as the three different types have different primary faults which must also be corrected. Not all clinical trials have divided the groups into possible differing mechanisms so that various clinical trials may not be cross comparable [15].

Subluxing patella

Findings

(a) This may present as the child who is always messing about because they often stumble, or may even fall, and when seen immediately after the incident, there is nothing wrong.
(b) Signs of maltracking are present (see *Maltracking of the patella*).
(c) Patella apprehension test is markedly positive.
(d) Tender medial patella facets.
(e) Weiberg's 2+ patella, patella alta or patella beja may be present.
(f) Bayonet sign may be present.
(g) High Beighton–Horan score is common.
(h) Clarke's sign may be positive.
(i) There is usually no underlying osteochondral lesion or synovial swelling.

See *Glossary* for diagnostic tests.

Cause

(a) Patello-femoral incongruency.
(b) Increased Q angle.
(c) Ligamentous laxity. Subluxation of the patella laterally is made more easy by ligamentous laxity and/or maltracking problems at the knee. Subconsciously the patient recognizes that when the knee is bent, and held into valgus, quadriceps contraction will move the patella laterally and thus dislocate the patella, so the quadriceps contraction is inhibited, causing a fall or stumble.

Investigations

None clinically required but scientifically may be analysed, as for maltracking of the patella.

Treatment

Stabilize the lateral patella tracking with McConnell strapping techniques [15], but this may prove too fiddly for active youngsters and a patella stabilizing brace will be more effective (see *Glossary*). Correction of maltracking at all levels, i.e. hip, knee and feet. Surgery is not very successful [16].

Sports

These people do struggle in almost all sports until the patella is braced (see *Maltracking of the patella*).

Comment

One is pleasantly surprised how well these people do with a simple relatively inexpensive neoprene patella stabilizer and strengthening exercises to the hips, combined with vastus medialis obliquus muscle work. Because ligamentous laxity is high, they usually require orthotics for their feet, let alone to correct the effect on the knees.

Medial plica syndrome

Findings

Maltracking of the knee (see *Maltracking of the patella*). There is a palpable tender medial plica.

Cause

The medial plica flicks over the articular corner of the medial femoral condyle and becomes thickened and painful.

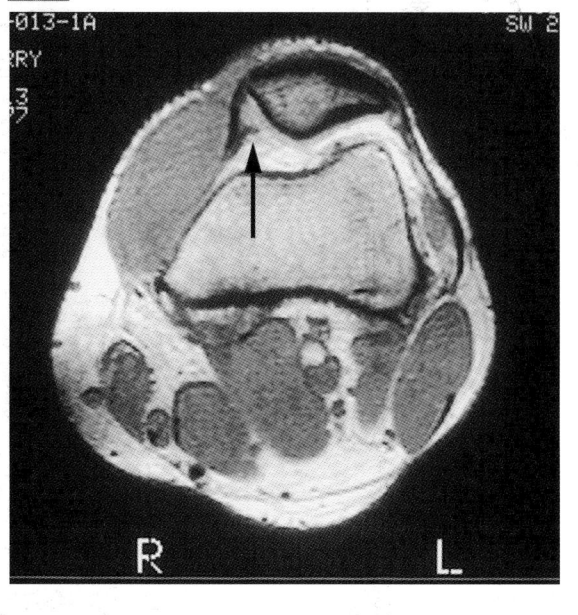

Figure 11.11 T1-weighted MRI showing a medial plica (arrow).

Investigations
None clinically required unless not responding to conservative management of tracking problems, then X-ray and MRI to exclude other problems. MRI can visualize the plica but whether it is diagnostic of pathology is debatable (Fig. 11.11).

Treatment
See *Maltracking of the patella*. Treat the inflammation of the plica with electrotherapeutic modalities or cortisone to the plica. Surgical division of the plica.

Sports
See *Maltracking of the patella*.

Comment
This is probably treated surgically too frequently, before correction of tracking problems have been achieved and, in my opinion, surgical plical resection and lateral release should only follow good adequate conservative management, *otherwise* a crescendo of repeat operations can follow.

C. Problems of overload

General findings

All have a history of pain on squatting, walking up or down stairs and hills, jumping, checking fast to stop, and kicking both with the striking and the supporting leg. Resisted quadriceps, active straight leg raise and/or bent knee extension are painful. May require a one-legged squat test or a step-down test to produce pain if lesion is mild.

Cause
Damage to the quadriceps, patella or patella tendon mechanism caused by the application of too much quadriceps work, both too long and too strong.

Treatment
(a) Overpronation produces a soft, mobile foot that does not reach supination in time to firm up for fore foot propulsion, thus the knee has to produce the impetus. The individual has a short stride and works really hard to produce a heavy laboured running style and consequent quadriceps mechanism overload. Correction of the foot will enable a longer stride and more propulsion from the forefoot and in some people this can totally correct the knee overload.
(b) Controlled reduction in quadriceps loads and then increment the loads by increasing repetitions at low loads for rehabilitation. Follow this by pyramids up to higher loads. Then use both the quadriceps ladders and the kicking ladders if required (see Chapter 20).
(c) Rarely surgery.

Lower patella pole syndrome

Findings

As *General findings*, plus:

Type 1 Palpable tenderness whilst the knee is bent or straight, that is located on the superficial surface, usually central, but often para central to the patella tendon origin.

Type 2 May be Hoffa's fat pad impingement, and is not tender with the knee bent and seems to be more related to the deep surface of the patella near the tendon origin.

Cause

Strain of the origin of the patella tendon. There is possibly some anomaly within this diagnosis, in that it responds to superficial treatment with physiotherapy or steroid injection, but MRI scanning of the more severe, recalcitrant cases shows fatty degeneration or disruption of the deep surface of the patella tendon.

Investigations

None clinically required unless failing to progress, then X-ray for avulsion of the lower pole and MRI scan for deep patella tendon disruption and patella tendon cyst. Real-time ultrasound will also display the cyst.

Caveat – In children X-ray for Sinding Larson Johannson syndrome (see Fig. 11.12).

Treatment

As described in *General findings*, plus:

Type 1 Treatment for inflammation with electro-therapeutic modalities, cortisone injection to the superficial tender areas, whilst the knee is bent. Massage techniques to organize chronic scar tissue.

Type 2 Cortisone beneath the lower border of the patella, to its inferior surface and Hoffa's

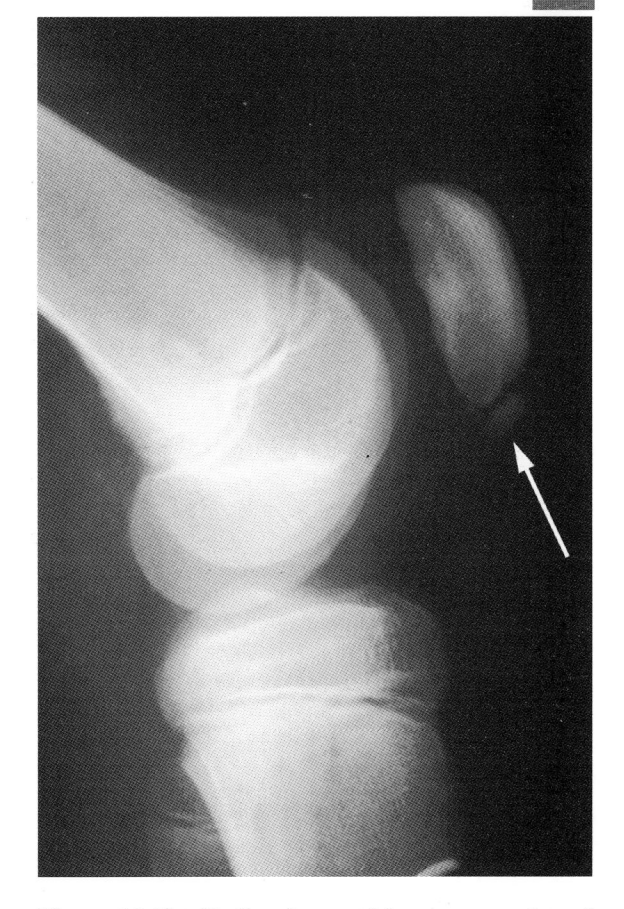

Figure 11.12 Sinding Larson Johansson apophyseal lesion (arrow).

fat pads, whilst the knee is straight. Physiotherapeutic modalities probably cannot reach this area.

Surgery to deep surface of patella tendon.

Sports

(a) All require to reduce the power of quadriceps activity as described in *General findings*.

(b) Particularly seen in jumpers – volleyball, basketball and weight training.

(c) The injury may take several months to settle and requires graduated loading, but in spite of this the patient often returns to sport too soon.

Comment

Physiotherapy modalities do not seem successful. Cortisone often produces a pain-free knee within days but rehabilitation will still take several weeks to months. I am not yet convinced by patella tendon braces. The deep surface of the tendon does seem to have the same degenerative yellow look as seen in Achilles tendons so it may be that following surgery there is increased circulation to the tendon that helps healing.

Sinding Larson Johannson syndrome

Findings

As described in *General findings*, but in a child before skeletal maturity is achieved, usually 10–15 years old. There is local tenderness over the lower patella pole on palpation and resisted quadriceps.

Cause

An apophysitis at the lower patella pole is caused by too much quadriceps loading.

Investigations

X-ray the knee to visualize the separate ossification centre (Fig. 11.12).

Treatment

Reduction in quadriceps loading by using low loads, high repetitions and, very occasionally, plaster of Paris for 2 weeks to rest the apophysis.

Sports

(a) Pain and limping must be the guide to monitoring the condition (see Chapter 20).
(b) Gymnastics. Use the ladder principles. Step 1: maintain training on parallel or asymmetric bars and balance routines, plus general abdominal and upper body conditioning. Step 2: walkovers. Step 3: when patient can run, increment the loads into vaulting but roll out the landings. Step 4: build into vaults using a landing pit. Step 5: plan sessions so as not to have vault and floor routines on the same day; finish session with vault or floor

routine but roll out landings. Step 6: as for step 5 but spot the landings.
(c) Kicking games (football or rugby) – move the player to a position where he kicks less, such as from fly half to wing three-quarter and do not take free or place kicks until better.
(d) Jumping sports. Reduce jumping until pain-free.

Comment

This responds, like any overload injury, to a reduction in load but an apophysis takes longer than expected to heal. Parents and coaches should be warned of this. In my experience ultrasound, interferential and laser do little to help.

Patella tendinopathy/tendinitis

Findings

As described in *General findings*, plus may also have a history of pain at rest, better, after movement which is from the paratenon or tendinitis; or a history of pain, better at rest, worse with loads which may be from a tendinopathy [17].

Cause

Inflammation of the paratenon or degeneration of the patella tendon, possibly following micro tears from quadriceps overload.

Investigations

If pain and tenderness is in the central tendon, look for a tendon cyst with diagnostic ultrasound or MRI (Fig. 11.13). MRI will show degenerative changes and possibly a tear in the deep surface at its origin from the lower pole.

Treatment

(a) Tendon cyst – curette out and then quadriceps rehabilitation (see Chapter 20).
(b) Peritendinitis – electrotherapeutic modalities to settle inflammation, peritendinous cortisone. Massage techniques to limit and organize adhesions and scar tissue. Rehabilitation to underlying tendon, via quadriceps ladders (see Chapter 20).

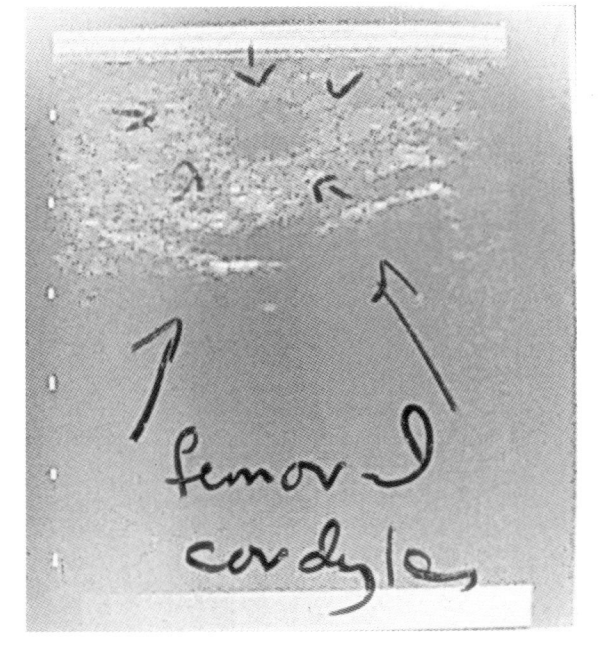

Figure 11.13 Ultrasound scan showing patella tendon cyst.

(c) Deep surface tendinopathy – controlled quadriceps rehabilitation. If not progressing, then surgical exploration of the deep surface.

Sports

Caused by powerful explosive quadriceps such as from volleyball, triple jump, high jump, etc., but also kicking where the support leg is often involved. Limit the number of games played and avoid taking the set piece kicks. They may require a considerable time to rehabilitate so early diagnosis and a reduction in training loads is most successful, but surgery may be required.

Comment

Central cysts are rare, but accompany mid tendon pain. Otherwise, the tendon can be as troublesome as the Achilles to settle in the long term. The cortisone breaks the pain cycle if it is caused by the peritendinitis so permitting rehabilitation of the tendon lesion underneath, but the loading of the tendon must be controlled. The timing of surgery, and precisely what it does, is open to debate, and it does not guarantee a rapid recovery.

Osgood–Schlatter disease

Findings

As described in *General findings*, plus: tenderness, sometimes local swelling, bony and/or soft tissue, over the tibial tubercle and it hurts to kneel on this area.

Cause

An overload of the tibial tubercle apophysis in children, especially during the growth spurt.

Investigations

Lateral X-ray of the knee shows apophyseal widening of the tibial tubercle and fragmented non-union in the skeletally mature (Fig. 11.14).

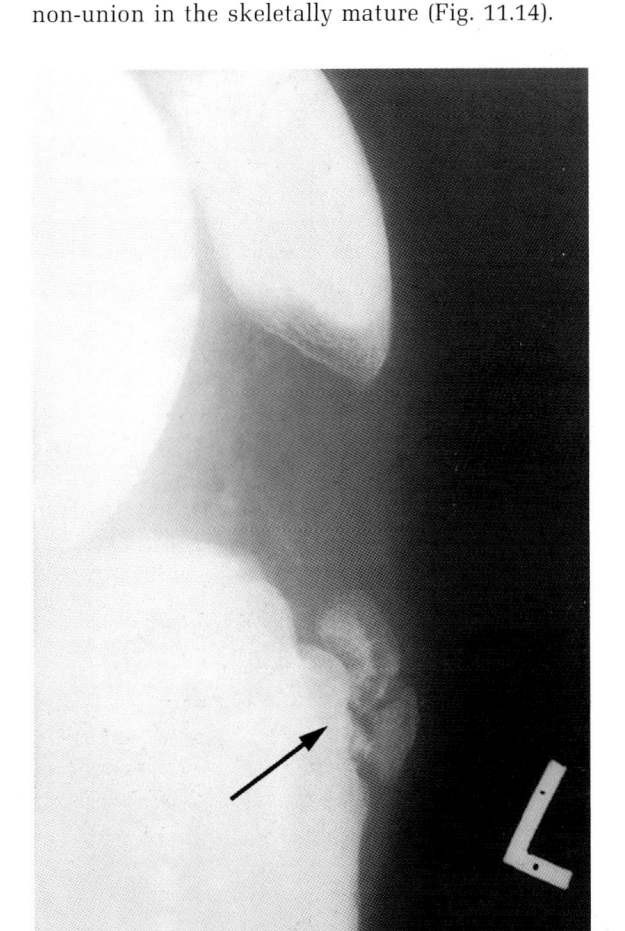

Figure 11.14 Fragmented non-union of the tibial tubercle. An 'Osgood–Schlatter' is in the growing apophysis.

Treatment

(a) As described in *General findings*, but especially this requires a reduction in quadriceps loads.

(b) Interferential to calm inflammation may help and occasionally plaster of Paris to rest an active child is required for about 2 weeks.

(c) Treat overpronation and posterior tibialis weakness if it exists.

> **Caveat** – This lesion can present in older teenagers or adults as a fragmented non-union of the apophysis and needs surgical removal of these fragments (see Fig. 11.14).

Sports

The child is often talented, playing school, club, county or junior international and several different games on the same day. Try to discover the child's sporting ambitions, not the parent's or coach's! Stop minor or less important sports and less important fixtures, and reduce the amount played. Stop the child from taking all the free and penalty kicks, and even move, for instance, the fly half to wing three-quarter. If the child aches after the game but is better by the next day, then this amount of exercise is within his tolerance. If the child limps during the game, or the next day is painful in normal life, then a reduction of exercise is required. Talented sportschildren need to be kept with their peers and there are no long-term side effects apart from a large tubercle, so judicial reduction in training of the quadriceps and the number of games played is the way forward.

Comment

Very common with these talented children, but also the child with overpronated feet who has to overload the knee to gain propulsion from this functional 'soft' foot. This second child needs orthotics and encouragement as their running skills will improve with orthotics.

Patello-femoral osteoarthritis

Findings

As described in *General findings*, plus:

(a) Clarke's sign is positive (see *Glossary*).
(b) May have a bulge test positive (see *Glossary*).
(c) Grating of the patello-femoral joint on passive and active compression.
(d) Patella facets are tender to palpation.
(e) May have long-standing maltracking of the patella from overpronation, and varus or valgus knees, from either anatomical or functional causes (see *Maltracking of the patella*).

Cause

Degenerative changes in the patello-femoral articulation, possibly from old trauma, maltracking or constant overload.

Investigations

(a) Lateral and skyline X-ray of the patella may display lipping and osteophytes (see Fig. 11.3) or CT scan for MRI is not quite so informative for the patello-femoral joint.
(b) Arthroscopy.

Treatment

(a) Settle inflammation with NSAIDs, and electrotherapeutic modalities such as shortwave diathermy and interferential.
(b) Correct maltracking at the feet and any functional valgus/varus at the knees. A patella brace may help.
(c) Reduce heavy loads but maintain quadriceps strength with static quadriceps exercises, particularly preventing patello-femoral movement, with straight leg raises or isometrics.
(d) When dynamic exercises are introduced use low loads, high repetitions and during quadriceps ladders the ski sit may be omitted (see Chapter 20).
(e) Avoid heavy impact activities and full knee bends.
(f) Arthroscopic trimming of fimbrillated chondral cartilage.

Sports

High loads, downhill running and jumping should be avoided. Low load, high repetition improves quadriceps and the joint. Doubles rather than singles at tennis. Be careful with full squats in weightlifting, field hockey, rowing, squash. Try using a higher saddle when cycling to limit the extent of knee flexion.

Comment

The articular cartilage reduces bony damage so conservative preservation of this cartilage should be exhausted before surgical trimming is contemplated. Quadriceps exercises should be maintained to tolerance as weak quadriceps exacerbate the problem and total rest is detrimental [18].

Stress/fatigue fracture of the patella

Findings

As described in *General findings*, plus:

(a) The stress fracture has a history of developing pain with quadriceps loads.
(b) It is tender to palpation over the mid patella between the upper and lower poles – usually on the medial or lateral side rather than central.
(c) The fatigue fracture breaks under muscular loads and without external trauma or without previous warning pains.
(d) Tender to palpation or a palpable gap if the fatigue fracture completes.
(e) A horizontal fracture of the patella.

Cause

A rare lesion caused by overload of the quadriceps mechanism centred on the patella, such as a sudden whipped extension of the knees as in the Fosbury flop to clear the bar or persistent overload with a bent knee.

Investigations

X-ray (Fig. 11.15), but bone scan if a stress fracture is suspected and X-ray is normal.

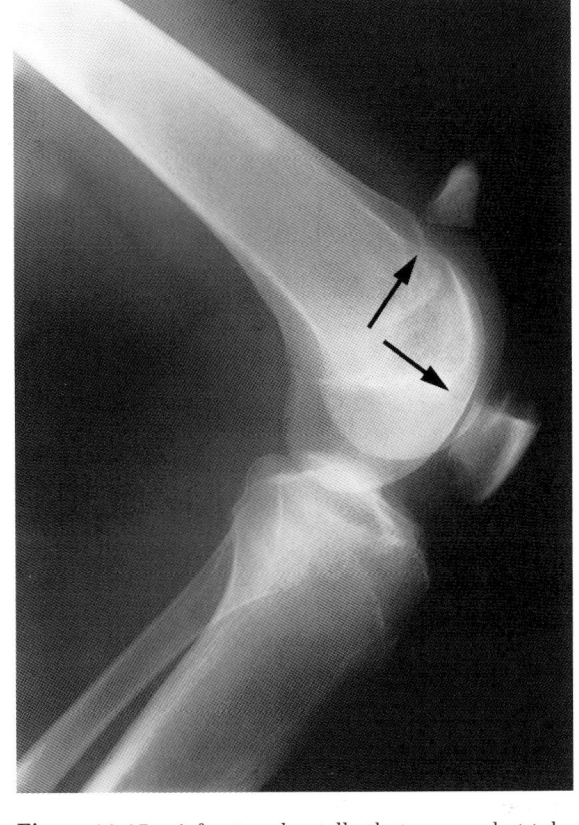

Figure 11.15 A fractured patella that occurred at take off at the high jump.

> **Caveat** – A vertical defect is probably a bipartite patella (Fig. 11.16) and note Haswell's lesion (see *Glossary*).

Treatment

(a) Reduction in quadriceps loads for the stress lesion until pain-free, then introduce the knee ladders but do not include ski sits (see Chapter 20).
(b) Immediate surgical repair of the fractured patella.

Sports

Although a case of mine with a positive bone scan returned, pain-free to field hockey, he fractured at take off on high jump 6–9 months later (see Fig. 11.15). Reported as occurring during the whip of

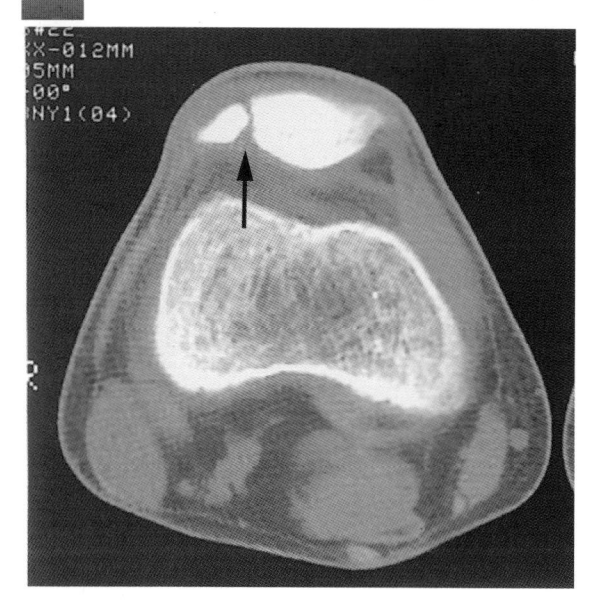

Figure 11.16 A bipartite patella.

legs into extension in Fosbury flop high jumping, and reported in a fast bowler at cricket and in skiing [19].

Comment

A rare injury. More common in adolescents [19]. Perhaps fatigue fractures have had previous minor symptoms that should not be ignored if palpation of the patella is tender and a bone scan would have helped diagnosis.

Rectus femoris tear

Acute pain in the thigh with a palpable lump in the mid thigh from the ruptured, contracted muscle end. Bruising may be present (see Chapter 10).

Quadriceps expansion

Findings

As described in *General findings*, plus: it is tender locally to palpation over the superior aspect of the patella, central, lateral or medial.

Cause

Micro tears of the quadriceps attachment to the patella but presumed graduation to full tear of insertional tendon may occur (see Chapter 10).

Investigations

None clinically required but if persistent, unresponsive pain, then MRI may localize the lesion; an X-ray may show Haswell's lesion (see Glossary) or a bipartite patella which may be more prone to problems with the quadriceps tendon insertion at the patella's fibrous union.

Treatment

(a) Modalities to calm inflammation and knee strapping to reduce loads (RICE).
(b) Electrotherapeutic modalities to settle inflammation together with cortisone injections.
(c) Modalities to release scar tissue such as frictions and cortisone.
(d) Quadriceps ladders (see Chapter 20).
(e) Surgical resuture.

Sports

(a) Mainly in weight training and weightlifting with deep knee bends. Beware anabolic steroid abuse.
(b) Occasionally from kicking or checking to stop with a deep knee bend.
(c) Hockey, squash, tennis and badminton produce problems by stopping fast with the knee bent as in stretching out over one leg to play a shot.

Comment

Most of these injuries settle with appropriate reduction in loads. Cortisone may break the pain cycle to enable rehabilitation to take place. I have only seen one come to surgery, who had a tear visible on MRI.

D. Extra-articular swelling

Pre-patellar bursa (housemaid's knee)

Findings
A pre-patellar fluctuant swelling with an underlying normal knee.

Cause
Trauma, usually frictional, between the patella and the ground. Usually seen in 'kneeling professions', but may be acute and produce a haembursitis.

Investigations
Clinically none required though aspiration, diagnostic ultrasound and MRI will display the lesion.

Treatment
(a) Knee pads for kneeling activities.
(b) Masterly inactivity. Just leave alone or ice application as required.
(c) Aspiration.
(d) Hydrocortisone and electrotherapeutic modalities to settle inflammation.

Sports
Rarely caused by sport but Canadian canoeists and three-position shooting may have problems that are prevented by the use of polystyrene padding, cut to shape, to kneel on.

Comment
Only treat if acute or painful, aspiration and intra-bursal steroids work rapidly, but the bursal swelling still tends to recur.

Deep infrapatellar bursa

Findings
As described in C, *Problems of overload*, general, plus: there is a tenderness around the tibial tuberosity, but behind and on either side of the patella tendon in the skeletally mature individual and this area may appear swollen.

Cause
Although a bursa can exist in kneelers between the skin and tibial tuberosity (pretibial bursa), a bursa which may become inflamed exists between the insertion of the patella tendon and the tibia, especially in those who have a large tubercle [20].

Investigations
None clinically required unless it fails to respond to a cortisone injection, then X-ray for a fragmented tibial tubercle (see Fig. 11.14).

Treatment
Electrotherapeutic modalities to settle inflammation, injection of cortisone into the bursa and surgery to the fragmented tibial tubercle if present and failing to respond to treatment. Rehabilitate through the quadriceps ladders (see Chapter 20).

Sports
No sport is particularly prone to this injury.

Comment
A rare problem that responds well to injection and not so well to electrotherapy.

Hoffa's syndrome

Findings
(a) History of recent increased amount of running, often after the first half marathon in fun runners training for a marathon.
(b) Pain at the anterior aspect of the knee with local tenderness to palpation either side of the patella tendon which may appear and be

described by the patient as swollen. This is better seen with the knee straight.

(c) May have tenderness over the lower patella pole when the knee is straight but not bent.

(d) The entry portals for arthroscopy pass through these fat pads, and may remain tender and sensitive for many weeks after surgery.

Cause

Not synovial swelling but oedema of the extra-articular fat pads in the front of the knee. These act as shock absorbers and may become painful and swollen after increased running.

Investigations

None clinically required though MRI may show arthroscopic entry portals.

Treatment

(a) Modalities to settle increased circulation and swelling such as ice.

(b) Electrotherapeutic modalities to settle inflammation, such as ultrasound.

(c) NSAIDs and rarely hydrocortisone.

Sports

Mainly long-distance running but some fast step and check games on hard pitches such as during hockey and squash may cause the problem to flare up.

Comment

Almost all settle with rest, NSAIDs and ultrasound, but cortisone injections may be required if time constraints demand.

E. Anterior knee pain as the presenting site

Anterior coronary ligament strain

Findings

McMurray's test (see *Glossary*) may be positive and full flexion weight bearing, such as the squat position is painful, with local tenderness to palpation over the tibial plateau antero-laterally or medially.

Cause

The coronary ligament that tethers the meniscus anteriorly is strained, usually by load bearing full flexion of the knee.

Caveat – Meniscal tears.

Investigations

None clinically relevant if signs do not immediately suggest a meniscal tear. If the pain fails to settle with treatment, then investigate with MRI for possible meniscal tear.

Treatment

Avoid full squat positions. Anti-inflammatory measures such as cortisone injections or electrotherapeutic.

Sports

Often has been caused in a fall or stumble, although usually can run or play through the pain, but full squats must be avoided.

Comment

A season of sport has been played just by the athlete avoiding full knee squats with this injury and it settled with time, but it can be quite responsive to cortisone injections, but, in my experience, it is unresponsive to electrotherapeutic or massage modalities.

Part 3
Medial knee pain

Tibio-collateral ligament

Findings

All have a history of forced abduction during a fall, twist, wrench or blocked adduction.

Cause

Abduction strain of the knee, straining or tearing the (medial collateral) tibio-collateral ligament. It may be part of a more major disruption such as O'Donaghue's triad (tibio-collateral ligament, anterior cruciate and meniscal tear) [21].

Grade 1

(a) No bruising.
(b) Passive abduction painful.
(c) Tender to palpation usually over the femoral attachment.
(d) Worse turning in bed and lying on the side with the bad leg uppermost.
(e) McMurray's manoeuvre may be may painful without the clunk.

Grade 2

As for grade 1, but local bruising and puffiness.

LEFT LEG (INSIDE)

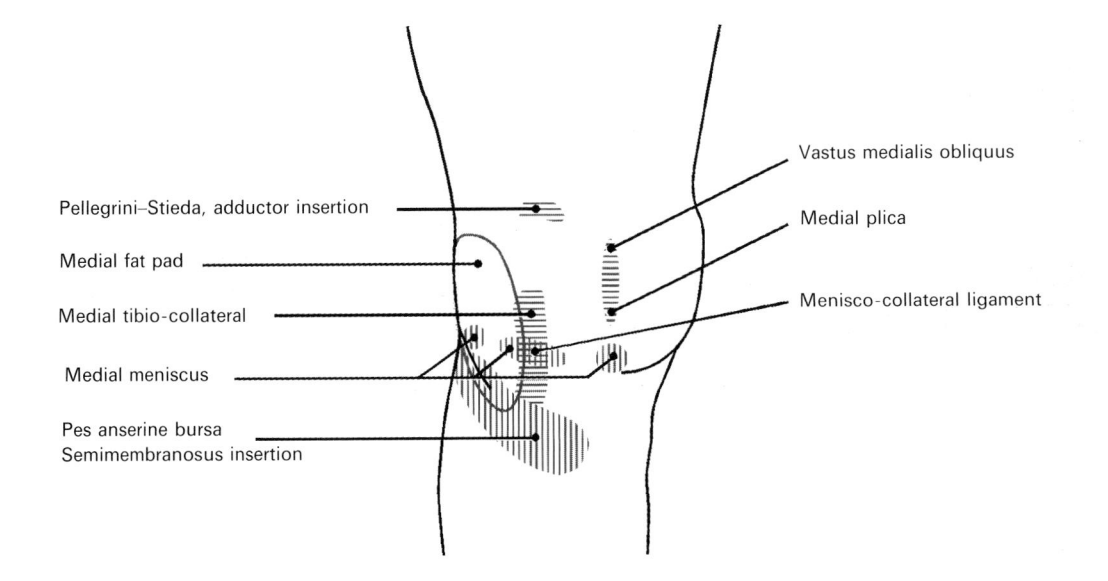

Grade 3

Bruising with passive abduction pain-free or relatively pain-free. There may be gapping of the knee joint even with the knee held straight and this requires crutches as the knee is unstable.

Chronic

The findings are similar to the grade 1, but without an acute episode. They usually have an anatomical or functional valgus at the knees and frequently overpronation at the feet.

> **Caveat** – If there is persistent pain over the tibio-collateral ligament, or indeed if the pain is getting worse, look for calcification or ossification of the ligament, the Pellegrini–Stieda syndrome, which must be rested. Active treatment encourages further calcification. The Pellegrini–Stieda syndrome may also complicate an adductor tendon tear (Fig. 11.17).

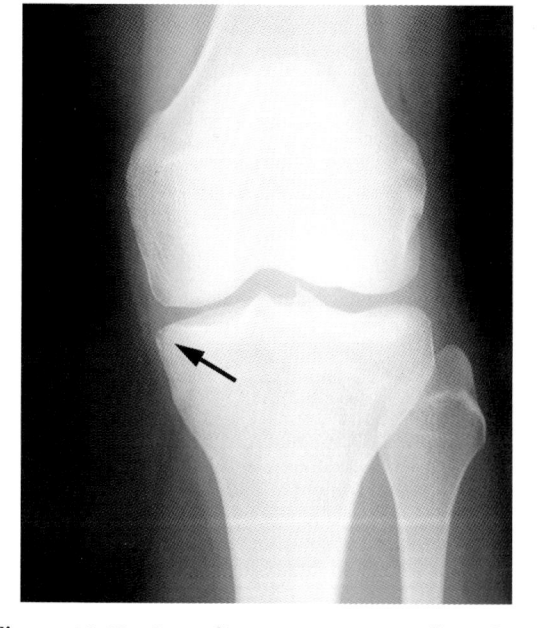

Figure 11.18 Segond's sign (arrow) small avulsion fracture line.

Investigations

(a) Plain X-rays – Segond's sign may be present medially (Fig. 11.18) plus stressed valgus X-rays, which may require injection of local anaesthetic to perform, show increased valgus gapping of the joint.

(b) MRI can display ligamentous damage, oedema and also whether internal derangement of the knee is present.

Treatment

Grade 1

(a) Limit oedema and inflammation with RICE for 48 hours – try a pillow between the knees when in bed to reduce abduction strains in the knee.

(b) Settle inflammation and organize scar tissue with electrotherapeutic modalities and massage, plus passive flexion/extension of the knees.

(c) Maintain static quadriceps exercises then add active knee flexion/extension.

(d) Closed chain knee exercises, with a brace or knee support.

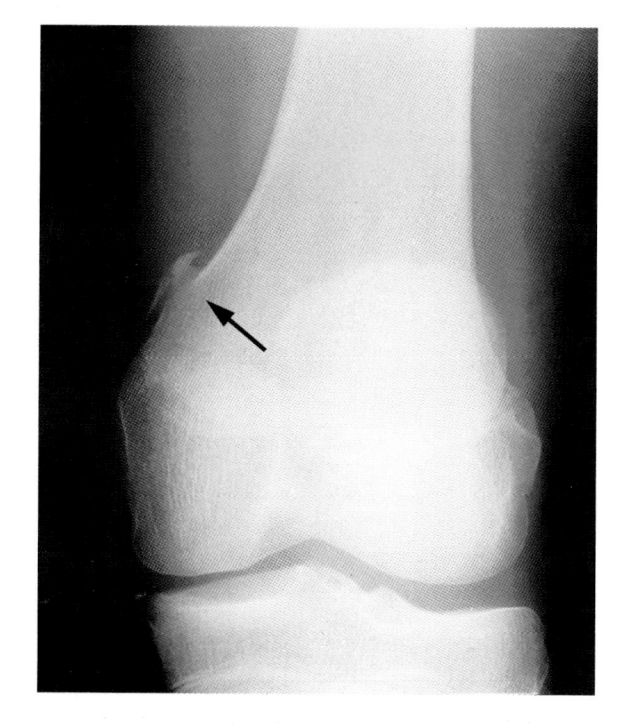

Figure 11.17 Pellegrini–Stieda (arrow).

(e) Cross-train non-impact, e.g. cycling, rowing or swimming, but not breaststroke.

(f) Knee ladders (see Chapter 20).

(g) Add side steps, figure of '8', cross-over steps, before match fit.

(h) Use support for 4–6 weeks for matches.

Grade 2

(a) Probably is a therapeutic balance between immobility to heal the ligament and mobility to maintain joint movement.

(b) A long length hinged knee brace, with lockable hinge range, is most effective.

(c) Maintain static quadriceps (note quadriceps and hamstrings can be worked against a brace so isometric exercise is done at varying angles of flexion). Straight leg raises and hamstring isometrics.

(d) Then as for grade 1 with, and then without, a brace.

Grade 3

Splint in the acute stage. Surgical repair and check for further damage – meniscus, cruciates and popliteal artery. Rehabilitate as described for grade 2.

Chronic

Treat as for grade 1 – but correct the cause of the valgus.

Sports

This is an important ligament for knee stability. Proprioception is improved by any support stimulating the skin for a few weeks, but a knee brace with hinge may be of mechanical value in sports where this is permitted. Problem sports include:

(a) Breaststroke – reduce the frog kick to a narrow wedge kick.

(b) Snow skiers who cannot parallel – edging and snow plough techniques overload the ligament.

(c) Twisting, turning and checking at any sport.

(d) Football – side foot kick and side foot tackle.

(e) Martial arts – side and round the head kicks.

Comment

This is a fairly common injury – do not confuse this with the tender deep fibres of the meniscocollateral ligament, which responds to injections and is tender to palpation along the joint line. The tibio-collateral ligament is tender on the bone of the femur and/or the tibia and should not be injected.

Menisco-collateral ligament

Findings

Sharp, intense pain, that may be constant, but usually comes with external rotation of tibia and a valgus knee. It is worse on turning over in bed, lying on the side with the bad knee uppermost and any twisting and turning, including getting into a car and driving with the knee externally rotated. There is no swelling but McMurray's test may be tender without the clunk (see Glossary). There is often loss of some degree of flexion and it is sore to palpation over the postero-medial joint line [1]. Check for overpronation.

Cause

Strain or nipping of the deep fibres of the tibio-collateral ligament, that attach to the peripheral margins of the medial meniscus, during external rotation and valgus forces, usually occurring in mid to old age.

Investigations

None clinically required.

Treatment

(a) Correct overpronation if present.

(b) Local cortisone to the tender area.

(c) Drive with the foot over the accelerator and toe into the brake, and get in and out of car with both legs together.

Sports

(a) Often a middle-aged person who has recently taken up running and has an overpronated foot.

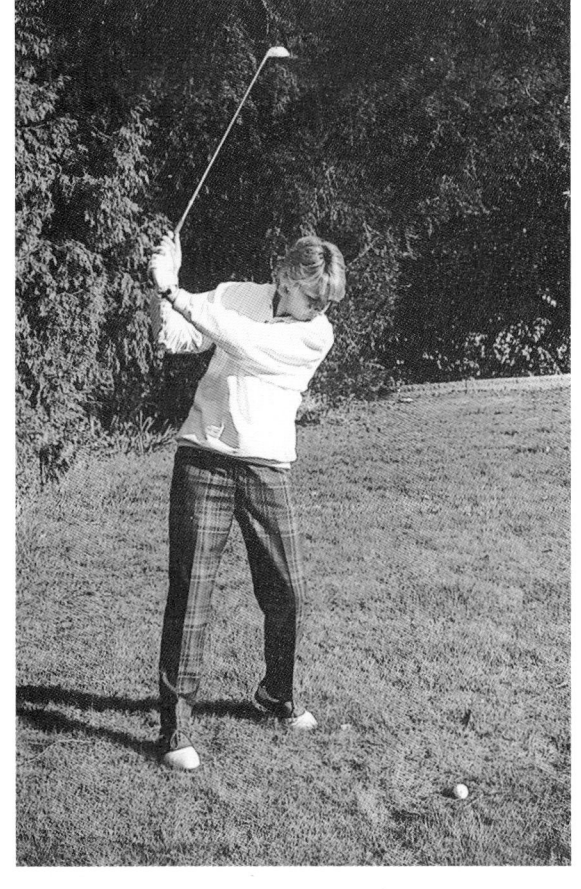

Figure 11.19 The reverse pivot pushes the weight on the left side, it should be on the right leg. This twist across the bent left knee can injure the menisco-collateral ligament (heel down) and the Achilles (heel up) as here.

(b) Windmilling style of running from a functional valgus.
(c) Breaststroke.
(d) Golf – reverse pivot, with the left heel on the ground (Fig. 11.19).

Comment
Although painful, cortisone gives dramatic relief. An overpronated foot will produce a recurrence if not corrected. Fairly frequently the presentation has pain over the joint line that is more posterior than this lesion but it seems to settle with corti-

sone but over a longer time, a few weeks, but there is no obvious meniscal damage.

Medial meniscal damage

Tenderness along the joint line can be indicative but if accompanied by intra-articular swelling is more probable as a diagnosis than menisco collateral ligament. (see *The swollen knee*).

Semimembranosus/pes anserine bursa

Findings
Type 1 A history of recent onset running, or increase in speed, in a shuffle runner who often stands with the ipsilateral foot externally rotated.
Type 2 A history of a knee injury that gradually changes its character during rehabilitation and moves or introduces a new pain over the semimembranosus bursa.

Both may or may not appear swollen and are tender to local palpation over the bursa or hamstring insertions. Resisted hamstrings with an externally rotated tibia and knee at 30–50° flexion are painful. Check for overpronation and a weak posterior tibialis.

Cause
The bursae under the semimembranosus, semitendinosus and gracilis become inflamed where these tendons cross the tibia towards their insertions.

Type 1 Running styles may be propulsive (bounding), pushing with the foot and calf muscle, or tractive (shuffle), with the hamstrings pulling the body up and over the foot. If the foot is externally rotated during shuffle running then the pressure over the pes anserine bursa increases and can cause inflammation.
Type 2 Hamstrings work co-actively to decelerate the swing phase and lock the knee ready for loading at impact. When the quadriceps are weak or the knee unstable the

hamstrings are worked harder to stabilize the knee at impact, producing a secondary compensatory injury in the semimembranosus bursa and hamstring insertions.

Investigations
Observe the running style.

Treatment
Type 1 Alter the running style to a more bounding style or correct the externally rotated foot. Anti-pronation orthotics may well help and the posterior tibialis must be rehabilitated if it is weak. High knee drills will strengthen the psoas and encourage a higher knee lift during running.

Type 2 Discuss the mechanism with the patient who must not lock up the knee or foot on impact, but learn to roll through the foot from heel strike to lift off. Try counting for rhythm (see Chapter 20).

For both, electrotherapeutic modalities to settle inflammation, such as ultrasound and laser, and friction and massage for any tenosynovitis. Cortisone injection will calm the bursitis.

Sports
(a) Usually running – see cause and treatment type 1.
(b) Golfers who increase 'coil' tension or take away by pressing the right foot into the ground may rarely produce this bursitis.

Comment
The protective mechanism is very common and unless recognized leads to a muddled pattern of knee pain during rehabilitation. Indeed some patients have been arthroscoped needlessly because this protective mechanism has not been recognized.

Medial patella facets

Tender to palpation under the medial side of patella (see *Maltracking of the patella* and *Dislocated patella*).

Vastus medialis obliquus

Pain to palpation over the medial superior border of the patella (see *Overload* and *Quadriceps expansion*).

Medial plica syndrome

Tender flickable medial plica over the anterior aspect of the medial femoral condyle, usually with other findings of maltracking (see *Maltracking of the patella*).

Pellegrini–Stieda syndrome

Persistent pain, or pain getting worse with treatment, after a medial ligament injury (see *Tibiocollateral ligament*).

Medial fat pad

A pad of subcutaneous fat that is often tender to squeeze or touch. It is often redder and worse in cold weather. The knee joint is normal. Ultrasound may help.

Part 4
Lateral knee pain

Lateral meniscal tear

Pain located over the lateral joint line, may have effusion (see *Swollen knee – Meniscal tear*).

Meniscal cyst

Findings
Painful or painless firm lump on the lateral side of the knee over the joint line, that is more prominent in extension than in flexion. May or may not have symptoms of a meniscal lesion (see *Swollen knee – Meniscal tear*).

Cause
Usually associated with an underlying radial tear of the lateral meniscus. It may rarely occur antero-laterally and is uncommon in the medial meniscus.

Investigations
None are clinically required as this can be pal-pated clinically, but MRI scan can be used to

LEFT LEG (OUTSIDE)

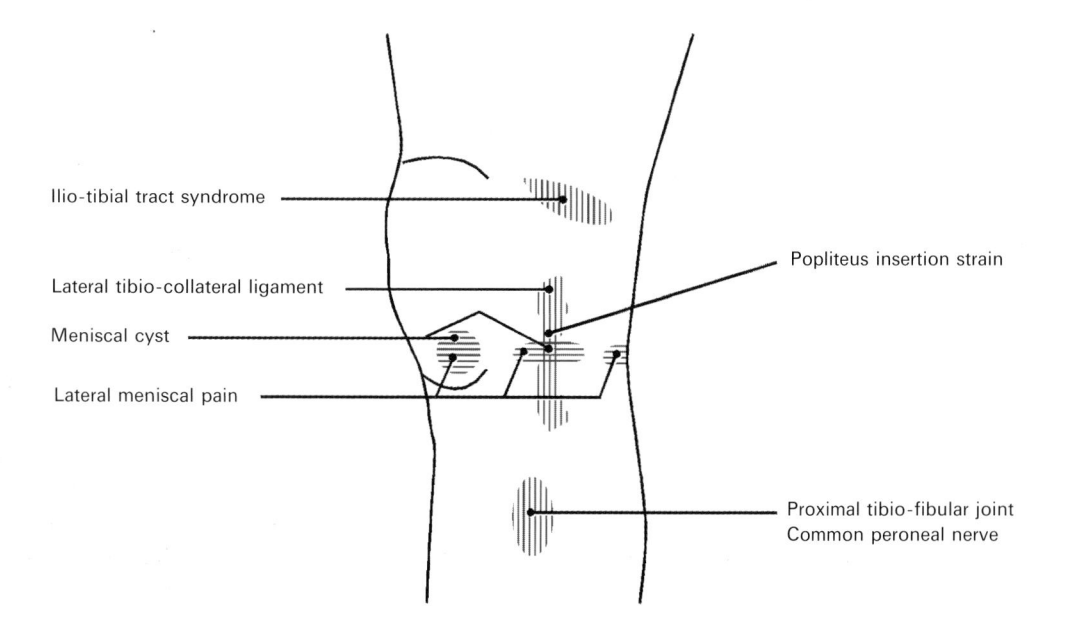

Ilio-tibial tract syndrome

Lateral tibio-collateral ligament

Meniscal cyst

Lateral meniscal pain

Popliteus insertion strain

Proximal tibio-fibular joint
Common peroneal nerve

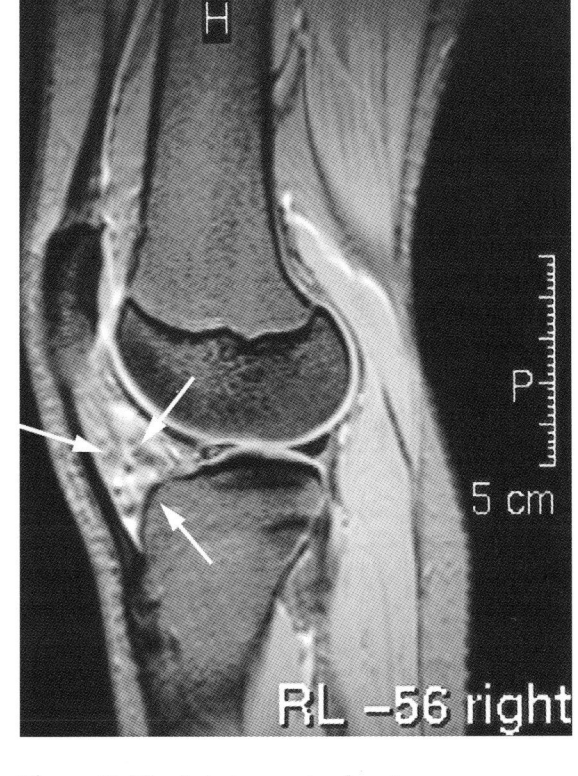

Figure 11.20   Anterior meniscal cyst.

demonstrate the cyst and underlying tear (Fig. 11.20), as can diagnostic ultrasound.

Treatment

No treatment is required if this is symptomless, but a trial of cortisone injection to the cyst if it is painful but there are no other symptoms may be of benefit. Arthroscopic surgery if there are other symptoms of a meniscal lesion such as catching and sticking or an effusion.

Sports

It does not influence performance unless there are meniscal symptoms.

Comment

It is probably worth a trial of cortisone as this may produce a painless swelling that the patient accepts, or even settles the cyst down entirely, but if this fails, surgery is required to remove the cyst and if possible repair the tear.

Lateral ligament sprain

Findings

(a) Acute. Pain or laxity to varus stress (see *Tibio-collateral ligament* and apply lateral for medial) except that a Pellegrini–Stieda complication is not associated with the lateral side.

(b) Chronic. Passive varus strain evokes pain over the lateral ligament, and the knee may have full passive flexion and extension, if the capsule is not involved. It is locally tender to palpation over the joint line, femoral condyle or its insertion at Guerny's tubercle on the tibia.

Cause

(a) Acute. Forced varus injury at the knee, which may have a rotational element and accompanying capsular or meniscal damage.

(b) Chronic. Congenital varus knee (bow legged) often with equino varus feet and camber running (see *Glossary*) will produce a varus load on the lower leg.

> **Caveat** – Look for any accompanying cruciate, meniscal or capsular damage in an acute injury as the lateral ligament can be a more frequent element of O'Donaghue's triad [1].

Investigations

None are clinically relevant for grade 1. X-ray (note Segond's sign) if grade 2 or 3 are suspected (see Glossary) (see Fig. 11.18). MRI may show a ligamentous tear with accompanying oedema but note that a small pocket of synovium, normally present, suggests a tear when it is in fact intact.

Treatment

(a) Initially to reduce the oedema and inflammation – RICE.

(b) Support with a hinged brace for preference and non-weight bearing with crutches.

(c) Electrotherapeutic modalities to settle inflammation and encourage healing, such as ultrasound, laser and interferential.

(d) Organize healing tissue with massage and by maintaining range of movement with non-weight bearing extension and flexion, both active and passive.

(e) Cross-train – non-impact such as cycling, rowing or swimming, but not breaststroke. Build to knee ladders (see Chapter 20).

(f) Surgical repair of grade 3 total rupture.

Sports

(a) Acute. Mainly an injury from contact sports though occasionally sudden checking and twisting with the foot locked, as on Astroturf, may cause the strain.

(b) Chronic. Usually running and straight line work, repeating the same strains over the ligament but without trauma, and thus change of direction sports are less of a problem; however, camber running will produce a varus load on the lower leg and stress the lateral ligament.

Comment

Not as common as the tibio-collateral ligament injuries.

Ilio-tibial tract syndrome

Findings

A normal knee, apart from local pain over the lateral femoral condyle, which is worse when the knee is moved back and forwards at 20–30° of flexion (Noble's sign). The patient may be bow legged and the ilio-tibial band tight with Ober's sign positive. The modified Thomas test may show a tight ilio-tibial tract (Figs 11.21 and 11.22) (see Glossary).

Cause

The ilio-tibial tract flicks backwards over the femoral condyle at about 20–30° of flexion causing irritation of the under surface of the ilio-tibial band and sometimes the bursa under this area.

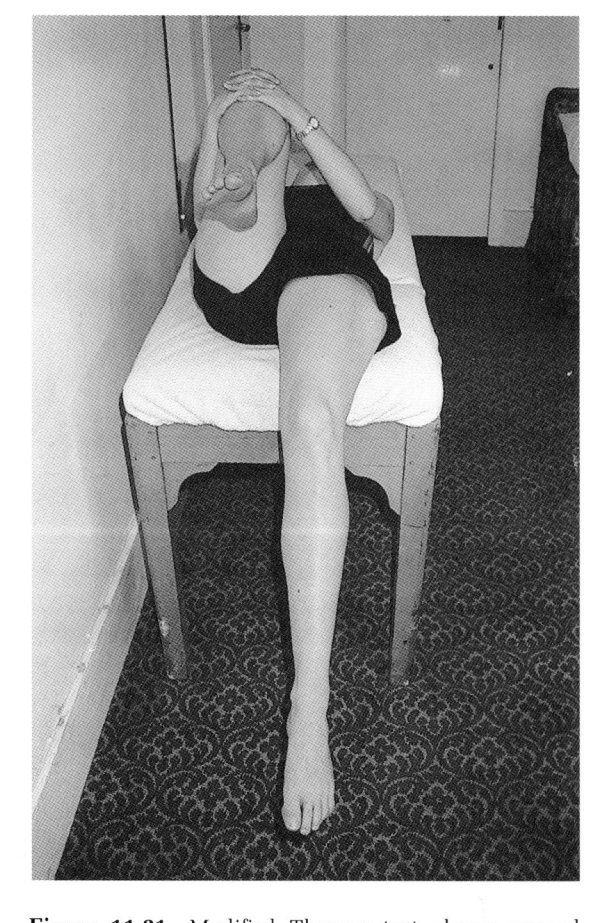

Figure 11.21 Modified Thomas test shows normal psoas and rectus femoris.

Investigations

None are clinically required in the presence of a positive Noble's sign unless the lesion is not responding to treatment, when an MRI scan may show the inflamed bursa on T2 or STIR sequences. The bursa is often seen by chance because a diagnosis is not made clinically and then a diagnostic MRI of the knee is ordered.

Treatment

(a) Settle soft tissue swelling such as RICE.

(b) Electrotherapeutic modalities to settle inflammation and organize scar tissue, such as ultrasound and laser.

(c) Massage to organize chronic scar tissue such as frictions.

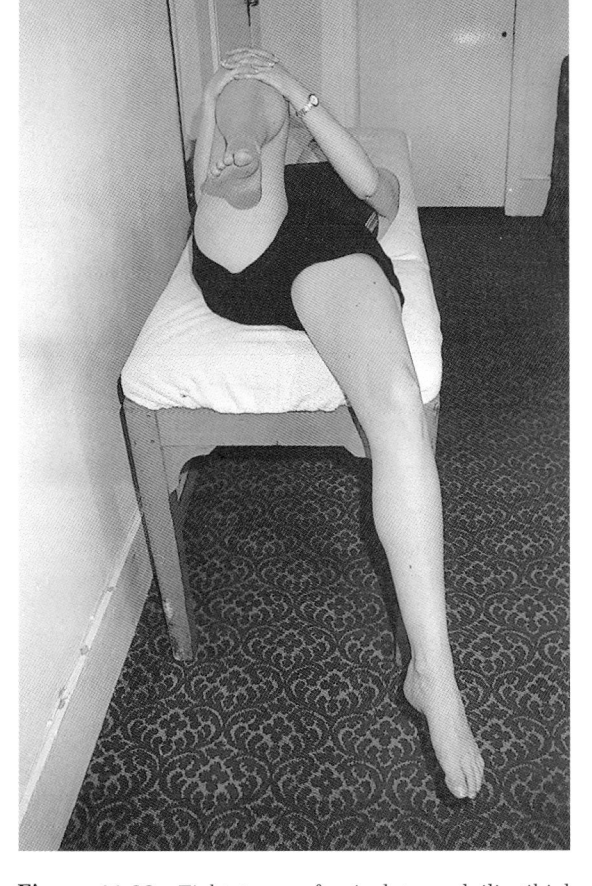

Figure 11.22 Tight tensor fascia lata and ilio-tibial band pulls leg into abduction.

(d) A lateral forefoot wedge may reduce supination at lift off and reduce pain.
(e) Injection of cortisone placed in the bursa.
(f) Surgery to the ilio-tibial band at the femoral condyle.

Sports

A rare finding in change of direction sports, being seen mainly in running and cycling. Check for camber running and downhill running or foot impact with the knee bent [22]. Check in runners for a supinated foot – this may require orthotic correction. A forefoot wedge in cycling may be curative but is less so in running. Cyclists must have 'play' in their cycle clips or cleats, especially if they cycle with an externally rotated foot which will be forced into neutral by the cleat.

Comment

I have seen too many patients who have been diagnostically arthroscoped because the ilio-tibial tract syndrome was missed. Although it responds well to physiotherapy and injection, surgery may be required to partially divide the ilio-tibial band.

Proximal tibio-fibular joint

Findings

(a) Usually a traumatic injury or from a heavy or awkward landing and examination of the knee joint is normal.
(b) Pain is located over the proximal tibio-fibular joint and is worse on walking, running and jumping. The pain may travel down the outside of the calf.
(c) Tender to local palpation of the joint and to translation of the tibio-fibular joint.

Cause

An uncommon capsulitis, acute or chronic, of the proximal tibio-fibular joint. Subluxation, antero-lateral dislocation, postero-medial dislocation and superior dislocation may occur.

Caveat – Consider the differentials of anterior compartment syndrome and spiral fracture of the fibula. The common peroneal nerve may suffer neuropraxia producing pain and pins and needles or even foot drop [23].

Investigations

X-ray to exclude fracture of the fibula and EMG of the common peroneal nerve if neuropraxia is suspected.

Treatment

(a) Rest and avoid crossing the legs such that local pressure is applied around the joint and nerve.

(b) Support taping or bandage may control the joint movement.

(c) Impact or even non-impact events may be curtailed by pain.

(d) Surgery may be required for dislocation.

Sports

Triple jump with its heavy pliometric work may produce stress across this joint. Taping and support may help but it may require a lay off from pliometrics. Otherwise it occurs by chance in sports where a bad landing or direct trauma can occur.

Comment

Fortunately a rare condition as rest is often the only long-term treatment.

Common peroneal nerve

Pins and needles and numbness over the antero-lateral shin or even foot drop, with tenderness around the superior fibular neck (see Chapter 12).

Biceps femoris bursa

Postero-lateral joint pain associated with the biceps femoris tendon (see *Posterior knee pain*).

Popliteus tendon insertion strain

Pain on palpation located over the femoral condylar notch for the popliteus (see *Posterior knee pain*).

Part 5
Posterior knee pain

General comments

Posterior knee pain is always difficult to diagnose accurately and investigations for intra-articular pathology are often required.

LEFT LEG (BACK)

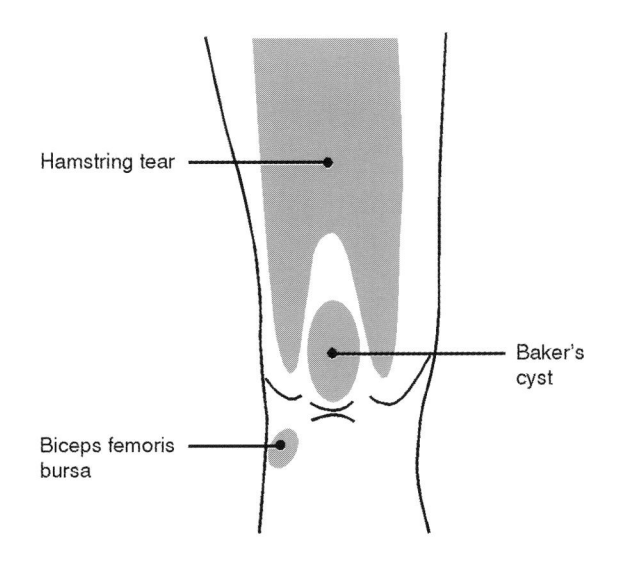

Hamstring tear

Baker's cyst

Biceps femoris bursa

Referred pain from the spine and back

Examination for posterior knee pain must include examination of the back; if examination of the knee proves negative, referred pain from the back must once again be considered (see Chapters 2, 5 and 9).

Popliteal (Baker's) cyst

Findings
The history is often of discomfort, fullness or tightness behind the knee rather than pain and this is worse on squatting. There is a palpable, non-pulsatile, often non-fluctuant swelling behind the knee. This can rupture acutely, giving a swollen calf, mimicking a deep vein thrombosis, or leak slowly, causing swelling of the calf or even the thigh (see Chapter 12). Fluid that is present in the knee may pocket in the cyst.

Cause
The cyst is part of the intracapsular space that can be occupied by an effusion, but a valve-like mechanism in the posterior aspect of the capsule allows fluid to collect posteriorly into the bursa but not escape back (Fig. 11.23).

Caveat – Popliteal aneurysm and effort-induced thrombosis.

Investigations
Mainly to establish the cause of a swollen knee and not to display the popliteal cyst, but MRI will display the cyst best of all and diagnostic ultrasound is most cost-efficient.

A Practical Guide to Sports Injuries

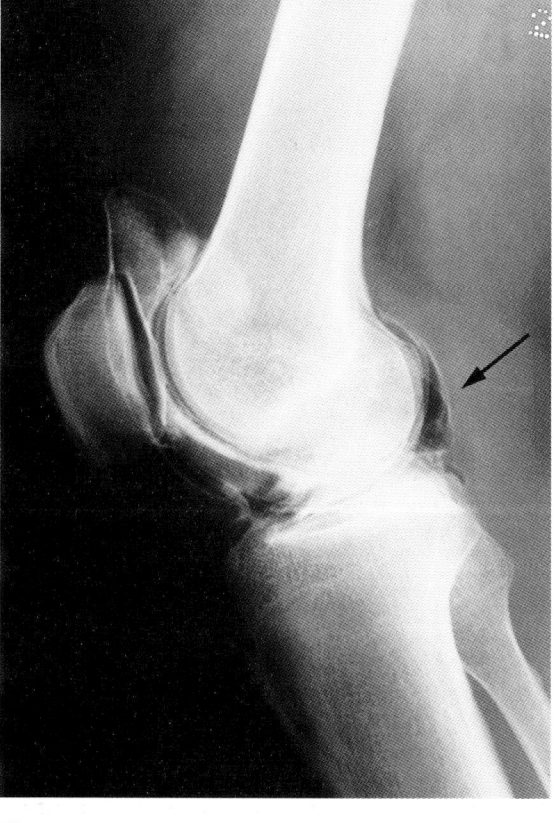

Figure 11.23 An arthrogram displays the posterior aspect of the joint from where a Baker's cyst can form (arrow).

Treatment
(a) Should be directed at the underlying cause of the swelling. For instance, if the fluid is secondary to early osteoarthritis, then an explanation of the cause of the posterior knee discomfort may be sufficient for the patient to tolerate the situation.
(b) Modalities to disperse synovial fluid, electrotherapeutic or injection of the knee with cortisone.
(c) Aspirate and inject the cyst with cortisone.
(d) Surgical removal.

Sports
Only full squats are affected because the cyst physically limits knee flexion, but general activity increases the amount of fluid and therefore the patient's awareness of the knee. The cause of the effusion governs the sporting activity.

Comment
Advice about the nature of the swelling and discomfort is all that is usually required with an osteoarthritic knee; however, injection of the anterior aspect of the knee may give temporary relief. Otherwise direct aspiration and injection of the cyst may be required.

Posterior horn meniscal tear

Often presents with a confusing history of intermittent pain especially with twisting movements or squatting with perhaps an effusion and poorly localizable pain – investigate with a diagnostic MRI (see *Swollen knee – Meniscal tear*).

Hamstring tear

A history of pain during activity, followed later by discomfort, stiffness and perhaps bruising behind the knee (see Chapter 9).

Popliteus muscle

Findings
Diffuse discomfort behind the knee, with sometimes tenderness at the insertion on the lateral aspect of the femur at the palpable notch. The figure of '4' sign (see *Glossary*) and resisted internal rotation may be painful (Fig. 11.24).

Cause
Strain of the popliteus muscle that runs from the back of the tibia to the lateral femoral condyle. The muscle may be injured at the posterior aspect of the knee and sometimes a tendon strain occurs at its insertion. It is usually strained in a twisting movement across the knee and very rarely the tendon is avulsed.

through games with discomfort and some limitation to performance whilst it settles.

Comment
I find this difficult to diagnose with certainty and MRI to exclude intra-articular pathology is often required.

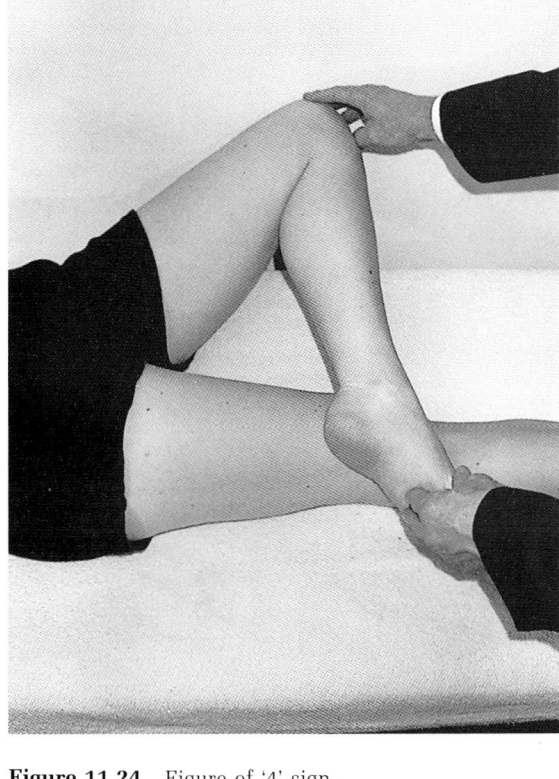

Figure 11.24   Figure of '4' sign.

Investigations
None clinically required unless failing to respond to treatment, then diagnostic ultrasound scan or MRI; however, both may be unhelpful.

Treatment
(a) Ice for the muscle is not advised due to the proximity of the popliteal neurovascular vessels but may help the insertion.
(b) Electrotherapeutic modalities and rarely cortisone to the insertion to settle inflammation.
(c) Massage to organize scar tissue at the insertion.
(d) Proprioceptive balancing (see Chapter 20).
(e) Hamstring ladder and knee ladder (see Chapter 20).

Sports
It is usually found in change of direction and contact sports, and many sportspeople play

Biceps femoris bursa

Findings
History of pain behind, and lateral to, the knee with sprinting or high heel (heel flick drills). Resisted hamstring testing with a bent knee may be painful and it is tender to palpation on the medial side of the biceps tendon near its insertion whilst examination of the rest of the knee is normal.

Cause
Uncommon irritation of the biceps femoris bursa at the head of the fibular, close to the insertion and in association with the fibular collateral ligament [24].

Investigations
None clinically required.

Treatment
Rest from running and/or a cortisone injection to the bursa.

Sports
Occurs in runners with short, fast, running cadence that encourages fast flexion at the knee. Encourage lengthening of the stride and increase drive from calf and forefoot.

Comment
Cortisone and alteration of the stride is usually effective. In my experience electrotherapeutic and massage techniques have not improved the healing time.

Intra-articular pathology

If in doubt about the cause of posterior knee pain then investigate further.

Popliteal artery entrapment syndrome

Cases of exercise-induced calf pain or pain behind the knee must have peripheral pulses checked and rechecked during calf activity, if possible, with a Doppler recorder. If any doubt about the arterial integrity, then refer to a vascular specialist (see Chapter 12, Part 2).

Further reading

1. Shelbourne, K. D. and Nitz, P. A. (1991) The O'Donaghue triad revisited. Combined knee injuries involving anterior cruciate and medial collateral ligament tears. *Am. J. Sports Med.* **19**, 474–477.
2. Maffulli, N. and King, J. B. (1998) Letter. Anterior cruciate ligament injury. *Br. J. Sports Med.* **32**, 266.
3. More, R. C, Karras, B. T, Neiman, R., *et al.* (1993) Hamstrings – an anterior cruciate ligament protagonist. *Am. J. Sports Med.* **21**, 231–237.
4. Shelton, W. R., Barrett, G. R. and Dukes, A. (1997) Early season anterior cruciate ligament tears. *Am. J. Sports Med.* **25**, 656–658.
5. Hull, M. L. (1997) Analysis of skiing accidents involving combined injuries to the medial collateral and anterior cruciate ligaments. *Am. J. Sports Med.* **25**, 5–40.
6. Ettlinger, C. F., Johnson, R. J. and Shealy, J. E. (1995) A method to help reduce the risk of serious knee sprains incurred in alpine skiing. *Am. J. Sports Med.* **23**, 531–537.
7. Webb, J. (1998) Rugby football and anterior cruciate ligament injury. *Br. J. Sports Med.* **32**, 2.
8. Stanitski, C. L. and Paletta, G. A. (1998) Articular cartilage injury with acute patellar dislocation in adolescents *Am. J. Sports Med.* **26**, 52–55.
9. Sallay, P. I., Poggi, J., Speer, K. P., *et al.* (1996) Acute dislocation of the patella. *Am. J. Sports Med.* **24**, 52–60.
10. Maenpaa, H. and Lehto, M. U. K. (1995) Surgery in acute patella dislocation – evaluation of the effect of injury mechanism and family occurrence on the outcome of treatment. *Br. J. Sports Med.* **29**, 239–241.
11. Boynton, M. D. and Tietjens, B. R. (1996) Long-term follow-up of the untreated isolated posterior cruciate ligament-deficient knee. *Am. J. Sports Med.* **24**, 306–310.
12. Videman, T. (1987) Experimental modals of osteoarthritis: the role of immobilization. *Clin. Biomech.* **2**, 223–229.
13. Henning, C. E., Yearout, K. M., Vequist, S. W., *et al.* (1991) Use of the fascia sheath coverage and exogenous fibrin clot in the treatment of complex meniscal tears. *Am. J. Sports Med.* **19**, 626–631.
14. Arroll, B., Ellis-Pegler, E., Edwards, N. A., Sutcliffe, G. (1997) Patello-femoral syndrome. *Am. J. Sports Med.* **25**, 207–212.
15. McConnell, J. (1986) The management of chondromalacia patella: a long-term solution. *Aust. J. Physiother.* **32**(4), 215–223.
16. Maenpaa, H. and Lehto, M. U. K. (1995) Surgery in acute patella dislocation evaluation of the effect of injury mechanism and family occurrence on the outcome of treatment. *Br. J. Sports Med.* **29**, 239–241.
17. Read, M. T. F. and Motto, S. (1992) Tendo Achilles pain: steroids and outcome. *Br. J. Sports Med.* **26**, 15–21.
18. Sallay, P. I., Poggi, J., Speer, K. P. and Garrett, W. E. (1996) Acute dislocation of the patella. *Am. J. Sports Med.* **24**, 52–60.
19. Teitz, C. C. and Harrington, R. M. (1992) Patella stress fracture. *Am. J. Sp. Med.* **20**, 761–765.
20. LaPrade, R. F. (1998) The anatomy of the deep infrapatellar bursa of the knee. *Am. J. Sports Med.* **26**, 129–132.
21. Millar, A. P. (1991) Meniscotibial ligament strains: a prospective survey. *Br. J. Sports Med.* **24**, 94–95.
22. Orchard, J. W., Fricker, P. A. Abud, A. A. and Mason, B. R. (1996) Biomechanics of ilio-tibial band friction syndrome in runners. *Am. J. Sports Med.* **24**, 375–380.
23. Gillham, N. R. and Villar, R. N., (1989) Posterio-lateral subluxation of the superior tibio-fibular joint. *Br. J. Sports Med.* **23**, 195.
24. LaPrade, R. F. and Hamilton, C. D. (1997) The fibular collateral ligament – biceps femoris bursa. *Am. J. Sports Med.* **25**, 439–443.

Bruckner, P. and Khan, K. (1993) *Clinical Sports Medicine.* McGraw-Hill, New York.

Hutson M. A. (ed.) (1990) *Sports Injuries: Recognition and Management.* Oxford Medical Publications, Oxford.

Reid, D. (1992) *Sports Injury Assessment and Rehabilitation.* Churchill Livingstone, Edinburgh.

12
Lower leg

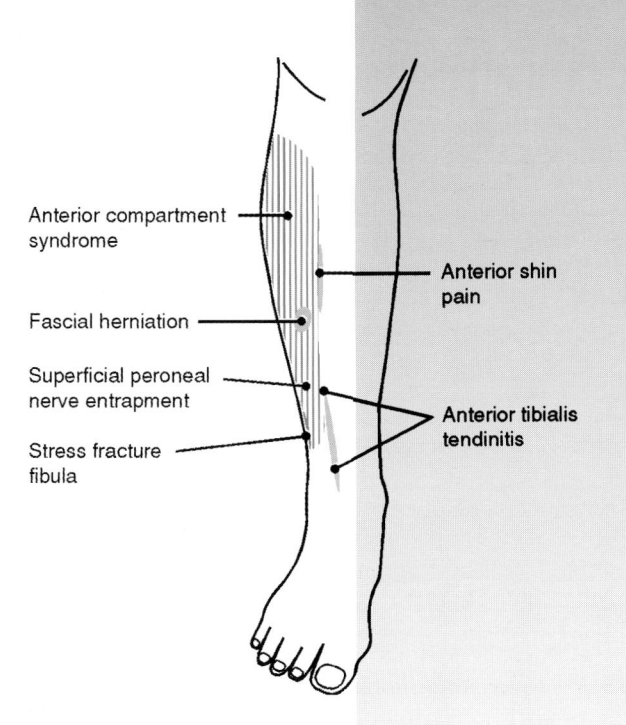

Anterior compartment
syndrome

Fascial herniation

Superficial peroneal
nerve entrapment

Stress fracture
fibula

**Anterior shin
pain**

**Anterior tibialis
tendinitis**

Part 1
Antero-lateral shin pain

Referred pain

Examine the back for evidence of referred pain from the L4/5 segment (see Chapters 2 and 5).

Stress fracture of the fibula

Findings
Pain on running; as it gets worse, the pain is also present on walking. There is typical localized tenderness to palpation so that tenderness to palpation in the area five fingers up from lateral maleolus in a 1–2 cm localized area is a stress fracture until proved otherwise.

Cause
A stress fracture 10–11 cm (five fingers) up from the tip of the lateral maleolus, produced in runners either from a supinated foot, bow legs or an internally rotated foot and tibia. Occasionally from a low knee style of running with a windmilling foot action with the above.

Investigations
An X-ray may show callus and a fracture line, but

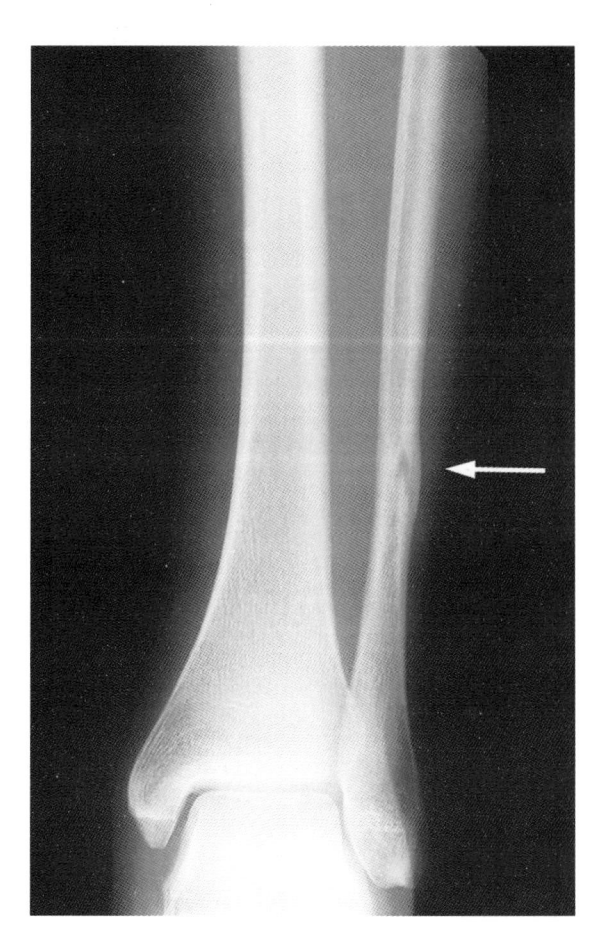

Figure 12.1 A fibula stress fracture is clearly seen (arrow).

may be normal and a bone scan will be positive if the X-ray is not diagnostic (Fig. 12.1).

Treatment
(a) Cross-training with no impact on legs for 6–8 weeks.
(b) Achilles rehabilitation ladder (see Chapter 20).

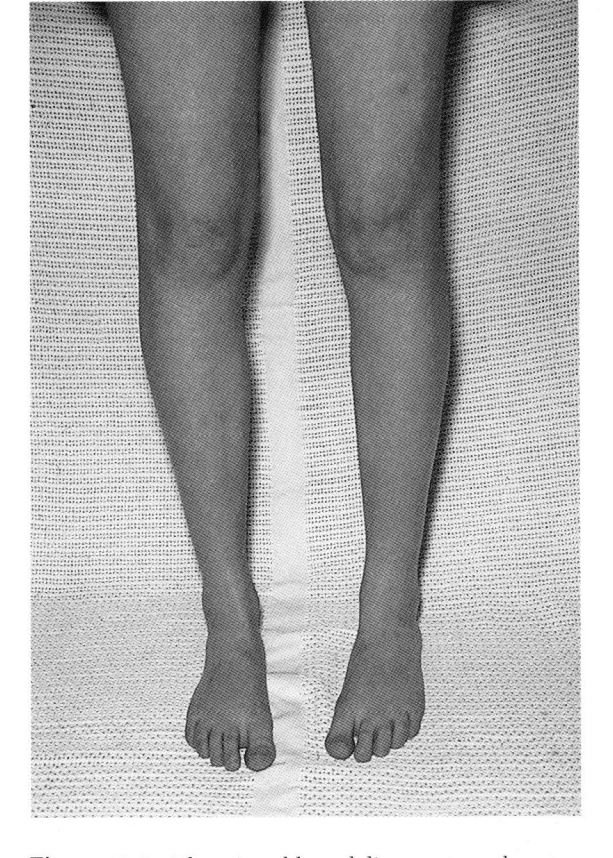

Figure 12.2 The miserable malalignment syndrome.

(c) Antisupination orthotics (see *Glossary*).
(d) Strengthen the hip external rotators and psoas.

Sports

Said to be a runner's injury. Generally with a supinated or cavoid foot but may also have an internally rotated foot, squinting patella and anteverted hip (the miserable malalignment syndrome) (Fig. 12.2). Either the incremental rate of loading must be reduced to permit adaptation or the anatomical/functional problems must be corrected. It also occurs in aerobics with astride jumps and jumping jacks onto a supinated foot, when landing on the balls of the feet.

Comment

Less common than a tibial stress fracture and pain

five fingers up from the tip of the lateral malleolus is a stress fracture until proved otherwise.

Anterior compartment syndrome

Findings

The history is as for the posterior compartment but relating to the anterior compartment (see *Posterior compartment*). The anterior compartment is often bulky and may be tender to palpation when the symptoms are acute.

Cause

See *Posterior compartment syndrome*, but affecting the anterior compartment between the tibia and fibula and interosseous membrane. The tibialis anterior, extensor hallucis and extensor digitorum longus muscles are involved.

Investigations

X-ray to exclude a stress fracture but a three-phase bone scan and anterior compartment pressure studies are more diagnostic.

> **Caveat** – All the differentials may have to be eliminated. Compartment pressure readings are interpreted differently depending upon continuous or interval monitoring and for some the rate of fall after exercise is important. Readings over 30 mmHg are probably relevant in the relaxation phase of muscle action; however, other authors measure the contraction phase, some considering 50 mmHg others, 85 mmHg, as abnormal (see *Glossary*).

Treatment

Reduction in loads and/or a surgical fascial split of the anterior sheath.

Sports

(a) Running where the shuffle type of runner often has worn a hole in the top of the shoe from the big toe pulling into dorsiflexion and rubbing into the shoe.
(b) Untrained cross-country skier from pulling the ski forwards with the foot.

(c) Sit-ups with the toes wedged under a bar to keep the feet down and provide leverage.

(d) Marching. Possibly from smaller individuals having to stride out with their feet, emphasizing dorsiflexion as part of a marching style.

Comment

Not that common in sport in spite of being well described, but perhaps more common in the armed forces. Correction of the cause is often successful but a fascial split returns the athlete to sport rapidly. Pressure studies done during the rest phase from injury may be negative. The compartment test exercise should copy the individual's exercise pattern [1]. The history is an important diagnostic indicator.

Tibialis anterior tendinitis

Pain on resisted tibialis anterior and local tenderness over the lower anterior compartment, especially if crepitus is present (see Chapter 13).

Anterior shin pain

Findings

Pain similar to the anterior compartment syndrome but with tenderness along the anterior tibial border rather than over the muscle (see *Anterior compartment*).

Cause

Stress changes on the lateral border of the tibia, either adaptive, occurring when the patient takes up running, or stress from the anterior compartment fascial attachment.

Investigations

(a) X-ray may show thickened, enlarged cortical bone which represents adaptive changes (Fig. 12.3).

(b) Three-phase bone scan may be hot in the blood phase and/or bone phase with linear increased uptake over the anterior tibia.

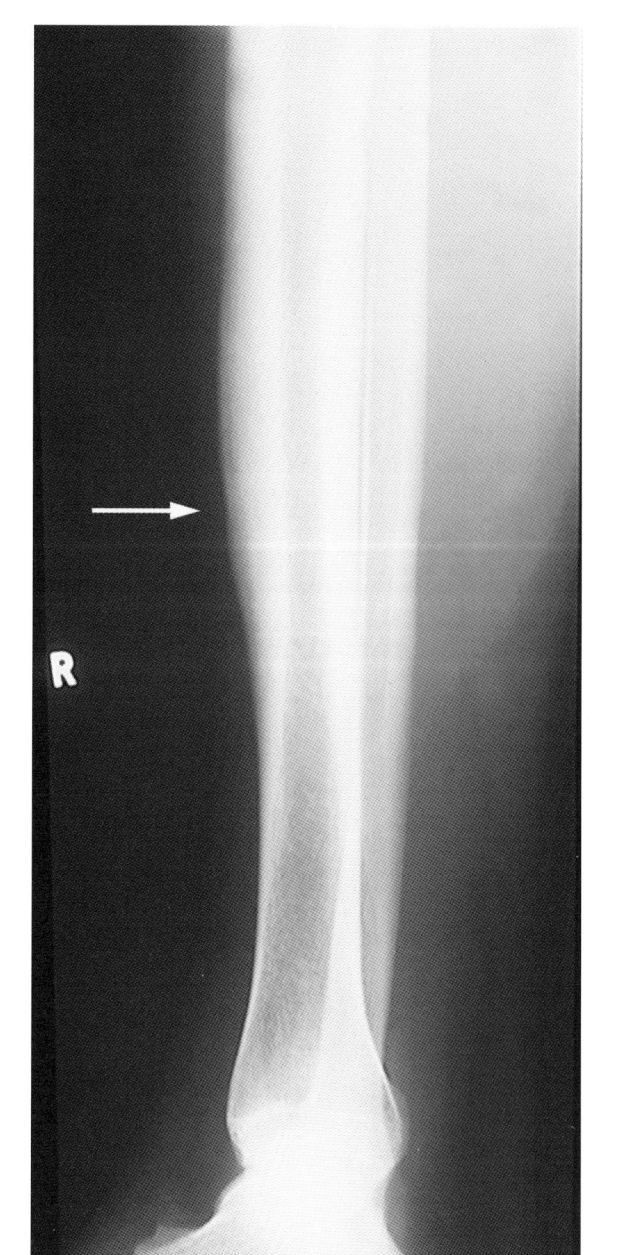

Figure 12.3 Thickened cortical bone on the anterior aspect of the tibia.

(c) Compartment pressure may also be raised or anterior shin pain may precede the compartment problems.

Treatment
Reduction in the rate of incremental loading and possibly a surgical fascial split, especially for patients whose bone scan shows hot in both blood and bone phases.

Sports
See *Anterior compartment syndrome*. In some sports, such as rowing, the athletes may run in the winter, and many oarsmen do not run well and have not had impact on their legs all summer. This can produce too rapid an incremental loading of the bones. The rowing ergo reduces the need for this type of training.

Comment
This is uncommon but does seem to be caused by both impact and also overuse of the anterior compartment.

Peroneal muscle strain

This is uncommon but may present as an ache in the shin and pain with resisted eversion. It is tender to palpation over the peroneal compartment. There may be crepitus with a tenovaginitis (see Chapter 13).

Muscle herniation (anterior compartment)

Findings
Painless or painful swelling which is worse on exercise, about 2–4 cm diameter, in the anterior compartment at about the mid point. Palpation may reveal a defect in the fascia, usually just below the mid point of the anterior compartment and, with exercise, a tense swelling develops.

Cause
A defect in the anterior compartment fascia, often close to the superficial peroneal nerve.

Investigations
(a) If painless, none are clinically required.

(b) If painful, probably none, as invariably compartment pressures often register as normal because the pressure releases through the hernia.

Treatment
None required if the lesion is painless, but if painful a surgical fascial split, with care for the superficial peroneal nerve.

Sports
See *Anterior compartment syndrome*.

Comment
Not common. The pit is often felt when the muscle is not in a flared state. Because the treatment is fascial split rather than repairing the defect, there is not much point measuring compartment pressures.

Common peroneal nerve entrapment

Findings
History of pain, numbness, and 'pins and needles' down the outside of the shin. The 'pins and needles' distinguishes this from other local causes. Sensation may be reduced over the anterior compartment and there is local pain on palpation of the posterior lateral surface of the neck of the fibula. The knee joint is normal and the patient may have bow legs.

Cause
Uncommon irritation of the common peroneal nerve as it swings around the upper fibular neck.

Caveat – Lumbar disc and problems with the proximal tibio-fibular joint. Spiral fracture of the fibula. Anterior compartment syndrome and superficial peroneal nerve entrapment.

Investigations
EMG if severe, but early neuropraxia may have a normal EMG.

Treatment

(a) Check for camber running (see Glossary) and rest from running, even possibly switch to change of direction sport.

(b) Avoid sitting knees crossed and compressing the nerve, especially with the foot pulled behind the ankle (secretaries).

(c) A lateral forefoot wedge may just reduce supination at forefoot lift off and ease the problem.

(d) Surgical release of the common peroneal nerve.

Sports

Mainly running and jumping, especially triple jump, when the knee may bow outwards on foot impact. Uncommon in change of direction sports.

Comment

Although cortisone helps the tarsal and carpal tunnel, I have not been impressed with results in this area. Rest and avoidance of the cause are best with perhaps some adverse neural tensioning, although most of my cases have come to surgery.

Superficial peroneal nerve entrapment

Findings

Pain over the lower anterior leg that can spread around the lateral maleolus and outer foot. May have 'pins and needles' and numbness. Worse with exercise and as the compartment pressure increases, but may come on sitting with crossed ankles, when pressure of the other leg onto the nerve causes pain. Very localized tenderness and re-creation of symptoms with palpation over the trigger area.

Cause

The peroneal nerve is compressed as it passes through the anterior compartment superficial fascia but there has often been external trauma.

> **Caveat** – Lumbar disc and common peroneal nerve.

Investigations

None clinically required. EMG is probably valueless but may exclude a root lesion.

Treatment

Avoid further external trauma and avoid causes such as crossed ankles, irritating the nerve further. Cortisone to the trigger area may help, but surgical release may be required.

Sports

See *Anterior compartment syndrome*. A stirrup may catch across this nerve with odd riding positions.

Comment

I have seen this usually from office workers, sitting with crossed ankles, rather than from sport.

Part 2
Calf pain and medial shin pain

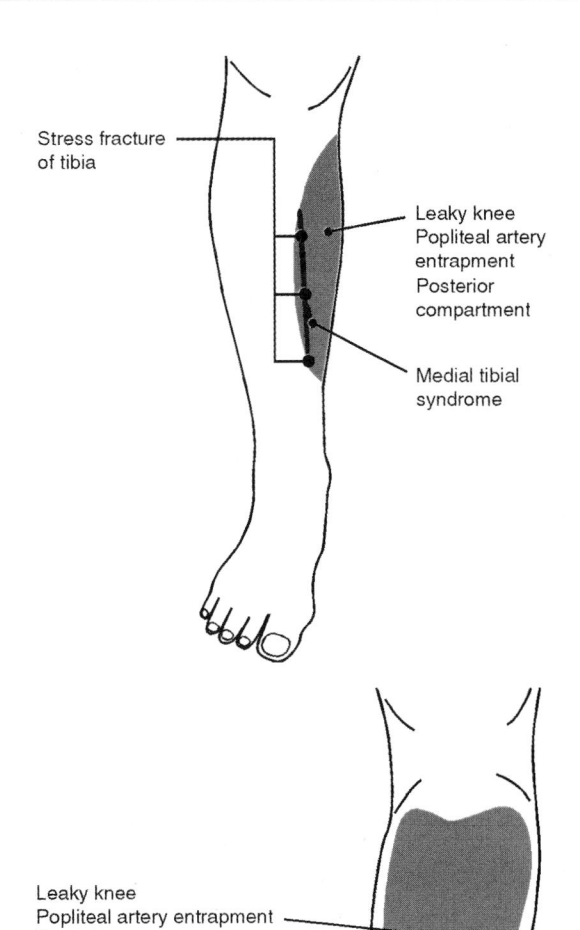

Referred pain

Always examine the back for evidence of referred pain from the L5 S1 segment (see Chapters 2 and 5).

Torn gastrocnemius

Findings

Presents with a history of acute pain in the calf and this is the classical 'who hit me with a ball in the back of the leg' story. It then becomes acutely swollen and may bruise extensively. There is pain and tenderness over the medial gastrocnemius or aponeurosis and a haematoma may be present. The healing or less severely damaged muscle has persistent discomfort, usually over the medial gastrocnemius, although the lateral gastrocnemius can be involved. There is pain on walking, jogging, going up stairs and on tip toe.

Cause

Usually an acute episode of torn medial gastrocnemius, but it is often a tear of the gastrocnemius/

soleus aponeurosis. The normal jump mechanism is for the quadriceps to contract first and when the knee is almost straight, plantar flexion from the gastrocnemius to follow. If this mechanism is reversed, plantar flexion, when the knee is bent, or, when standing on tip toe with a bent knee, and then the knee straightens, a tear may occur.

> **Caveat** – A calcified haematoma may remain in chronic cases.

Investigations
Diagnostic ultrasound for haematoma, but the more chronic cases may lead to difficulty of diagnosis, for an MRI is normal and investigations are used to exclude other diagnoses, when an arthrogram will display a leaky knee syndrome, and Doppler ultrasound both the deep vein thrombosis and effort-induced thrombosis.

Treatment
(a) RICE and crutches.
(b) Early aspiration of haematoma under ultrasound control. This may require repeating weekly for a while (Fig. 12.4).
(c) Heel raise.

(d) Massage techniques such as effluage to remove tissue debris and swelling.
(e) Electrotherapeutic modalities to settle inflammation and hasten healing such as laser and ultrasound.
(f) Gastrocnemius and soleal stretching to prevent scar contraction.
(g) Achilles ladders (see Chapter 20).

Sports
Particularly prone in sports where acceleration occurs from the plantar flexed foot and a bent knee; squash, tennis or a quick single to leg off a backward defensive shot at cricket.

Comment
Aspiration of the haematoma quickens the rate of healing. Full pedantic rehabilitation is required to prevent scar tissue and repeat injuries occurring. Chronic calf strain requires pedantic rehabilitation, taking time over the early ladder stages, through to running and pliometrics.

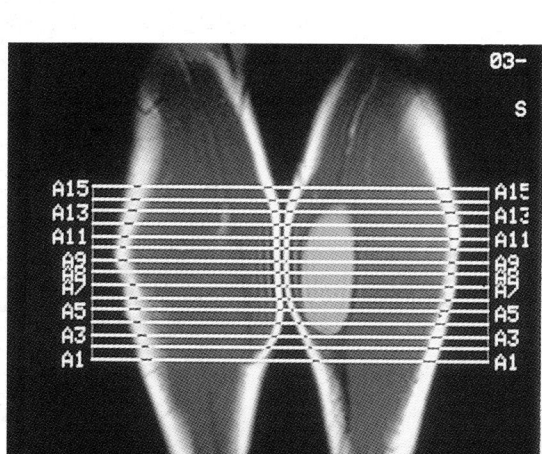

Figure 12.4 Weighted MRI shows a clearly defined haematoma. This is more easily displayed and aspirated with ultrasound control.

Stress fracture of the tibia

Findings

It is uncommon in change of direction sports and has a history of impact-induced pain, usually running, but if severe may be on walking or even at rest. The tenderness is on the medial border of the tibia and is localized to 1–2 cm, and is classically palpated at:

(a) The junction of the lower third and mid third of the tibia.
(b) The junction of the upper third and mid third of the tibia.
(c) The mid shaft of the tibia.

There may be bony swelling and localized soft tissue swelling, and, if severe, with pain on tapping the tibial shaft. This lesion is often accompanied by anatomical or functional overpronation of the foot.

Cause

Repetition of the same load produces cortical subperiosteal stress fractures, either from valgus stress or, most commonly, valgus and external rotatory stress across the tibia. This external rotation and valgus pressure may be increased by increased external rotation of the tibia and an externally rotated foot with anatomical or functional overpronation of the foot, valgus knees and anteverted hips. Weak posterior tibialis strength is often found with this injury. Broken heel cups and cut-away arches in running shoes will over precipitate these strains in the tibia.

Investigations

(a) None actually necessary as clinically palpation of the tender spot in these three locations is diagnostic and 'marketable' to the patient.
(b) X-ray can show chronic callus or a lytic area of the stress fracture.
(c) The bone scan is good for displaying an early lesion, especially if the diagnosis is in doubt.
(d) MRI will show the oedema of a very acute lesion, but is not as accurate for a cortical lesion when more chronic.

(e) CT scan will assess the extent of the lesion, especially for mid shaft stress fractures.

> **Caveat** – A subperiosteal haematoma from a stress fracture can look like an osteosarcoma on X-ray. The mid shaft fracture is usually horizontal, often bilateral and more common in dancers where it has been known to fracture entirely (Fig. 12.5).

Treatment

Rest from impact for 6–8 weeks but cross-train by cycling, rowing, swimming, etc. Correct the biomechanical cause if relevant and start the Achilles top ladder after 6–8 weeks. (See Chapter 20 for ways to increase pace and distance.)

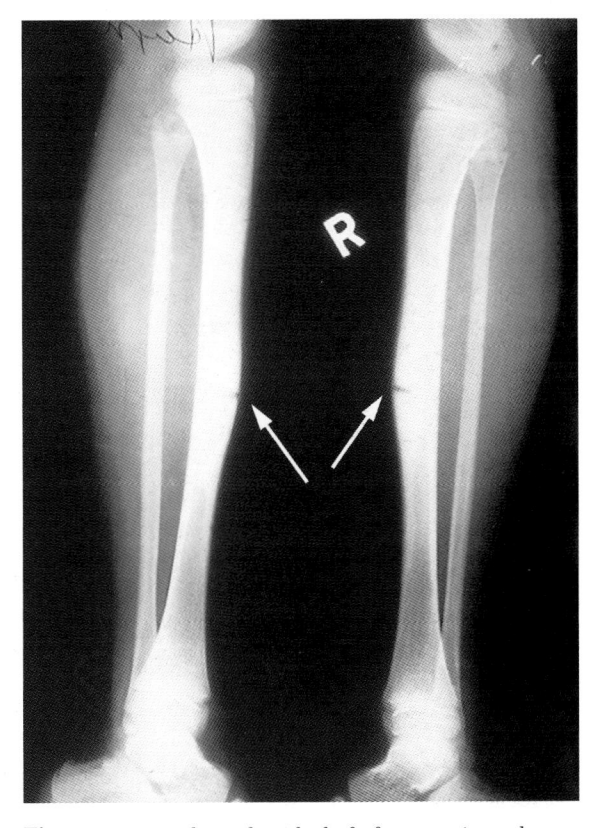

Figure 12.5 Bilateral mid shaft fracture in a dancer (Mr. Justin Howe).

Sports

(a) Athletics. A classical distance running injury, usually caused by biomechanical problems; however, increasing pace and distance at the same time together may precipitate the problem. Switching to lightweight cut-away arch running shoes may precipitate over-pronation in the well-established runner (see *Glossary*; Figs 22.21 and 22.22) and the shoe cup can break down, ceasing to prevent excess calcano valgus and overpronation, a mechanism that is made worse by camber running (see *Glossary*). Running into the mid stance phase, as opposed to heel strike, causes the foot to impact into pronation and thus stress the tibia, and the treatment is to encourage heel strike and a longer stride, but note that these patients may require time to strengthen their calf muscles to cope with this new style of running. Hill running and windmilling action can prevent the foot reaching heel strike thus shortening the swing phase and thus impacting at mid stance.

(b) Aerobics. Astride jumps (Jumping Jacks) and astride bench jumps force genu valgus and may cause a stress fracture.

Comment

This is an extremely common injury, especially seen in runners, though because many other sports do their training by running, it appears in a number of sports. Almost all patients have anatomical or functional genu valgus or overpronation of the foot.

Medial tibial syndrome

Findings

This is impact initiated, but the patient may have good biomechanical function with large calves. The palpable tenderness extends over several centimetres to almost all the medial border of the tibia and there may also be a stress fracture present as well. There may also be anatomical or functional overpronation.

Cause

This is not well understood, but fortunately is not that common. It may be the same mechanism as for a stress fracture, and possibly reflects a gradual adaptation to the loads; however, the loads are just too high, causing periosteal stress from the fascia of the posterior compartment or the elongated muscle enthesis from the posterior tibialis.

Investigations

Three-phase bone scan is taken with an immediate blood flow phase and a delayed blood phase, 2–5 minutes, followed by the bone phase, 2 hours after injection. The blood phase being positive indicates the fascia and muscle attachments are inflamed, whilst the bone scan will show an extensive linear increase in uptake along the tibial border. Pressure studies for posterior compartment syndrome may be of value – if they are raised, then fasciotomy will help.

Treatment

(a) Blood-phase positive – try a fascial split.
(b) Bone-phase positive – try tibial drilling.
(c) Like all overload problems, a reduction in loads and then incremental loading, when pain-free, can be successful but takes time.
(d) Correct overpronation.

Sports

Running or dancing, but also in other sports when running is used for training.

Comment

Often difficult to handle and most patients are too impatient, as it takes several months to settle under a conservative regimen, and so they proceed to surgery which can also have a delayed recovery rate.

Posterior compartment syndrome

Findings

(a) Acute. Follows a history of trauma with a tense swelling of the calf, which may be rapidly increasing. There is increasing pain even without activity and on compression of the muscle. Eventually the peripheral pulses, dorsalis pedis and posterior tibial, disappear.

(b) Exercise induced. The onset of exercise is usually pain-free with increasing pain as the exercise continues and the pain settles when the activity stops. When the syndrome is established the pain may persist for some days after activity. There is no clinical evidence of stress fracture nor of a medial tibial syndrome, both of which have bony tenderness on palpation.

Cause

It is thought that the muscles swelling within their fascial confines increases the compartmental pressure and gradually reduces the blood supply producing muscle anoxia. Superficial compartment: gastrocnemius, soleus and plantaris. Deep compartment: flexor digitorum longus, posterior tibialis, and flexor hallucis, plus the posterior tibialis, although some define this as a separate compartment. Can be produced by acute post-traumatic bleeding or chronically by muscle exercise, usually in runners, causing localized anoxia due to a block of the venous return and/or arterial perfusion.

> **Caveat** – As the syndrome becomes established or the athlete continues to run through the pain, so the cessation of activity may not reduce the pain, which can persist for 2–3 days. A rare differential is popliteal artery entrapment syndrome.

Investigations

(a) Acute. Ultrasound Doppler to assess arterial flow.

(b) Exercise induced. Compartment pressure studies with a split needle catheter (see *Glossary*).

Treatment

(a) Acute. Emergency release of the fascia.

(b) Exercise induced:

- RICE and massage such as effluage to reduce the swelling.
- A reduction of speed and mileage during running.
- Correction of overpronation may unload the posterior compartment and ease the anoxic effect.
- Surgery to release the fascia of both deep and superficial compartments.

Sports

This is a running problem from 1 mile upwards, and often also in a ball player or sprinter who has taken up distance running, and is still using a fore-foot strike or strong calf thrust. Alteration to a heel strike and shorter stride length may help. Other repetition activity sports like aerobics and trampolining can be problematical. Speed work in runners may produce some problems. Check for increased pronation.

Comment

Posterior compartment syndrome often requires surgery – usually of the deep compartment. Some cases will be diagnosed on the history, as compartment studies are not always diagnostically accurate for the pressure measurements may well be normal, especially if the athlete has had a few weeks' rest (as the problem occurs incrementally). The test exercise should mimic the exercise that produces the problem [1]. Pressure studies may record 50–85 mmHg as abnormal during the contraction phase of exercise, whilst others accept 30 mmHg and above in the relaxation phase as abnormal.

Posterior tibialis tendinitis or muscle strain

Findings

Tenderness over the medial deep compartment close to the tibia and worse on resisted testing of posterior tibialis. This ache may be the earliest problem with functional overpronation, but it usually does not present alone but accompanies the tenderness of posterior tibialis tenovaginitis around the ankle or foot (see Chapter 13). It may also present as part of the medial tibial syndrome (see *Lower leg*).

Cause

An overload of the posterior tibialis muscle which may be strained, secondary to overpronation, or it may be a type of compartment syndrome.

Treatment

Correction of technique and corrective orthotics is curative (see *Glossary* and Chapter 13).

Sports

This is part of the group of anatomical or functional overpronators (see *Glossary*). It is unlikely to be camber or hill running induced and much more likely to be caused by a sudden increase in mileage, pace, bend running or dancing. However, walking and edging the foot along the side of a hill for a long while can strain the muscle.

Comment

Probably the medial tibial stress syndromes, stress fractures and posterior tibial muscle strains have the similar cause of functional overpronation plus an increase in loading rate to which the tissues cannot adapt.

Leaky knee syndrome

Findings

(a) Usually follows a history of swollen knee, or Baker's cyst, which may then settle as the synovial fluid leaks out.
(b) Semi-acute swelling of the calf, but, unlike a muscle tear, painless until the volume of fluid causes discomfort.
(c) There are no dilated superficial veins as with a thrombosis.
(d) Homan's sign is negative and it is not tender to palpation.

Cause

The capsule of the knee is not intact so the synovial fluid leaks out. This occurs with a swollen knee or Baker's cyst. Note this fluid can be pumped upwards by muscle action or joint movement into the quadriceps if the tear is in the superior pouch, giving swelling of the thigh.

> **Caveat** – May also be deep vein thrombosis, haematoma in the calf or effort-induced thrombosis.

Investigations

Doppler ultrasound to exclude deep vein thrombosis. An arthrogram will display the fluid leak into the calf or thigh.

Treatment

Elevate when at rest and use effluage massaging techniques. A compression support over the calf may help and the problem is usually self healing over time, only rarely requiring surgery.

Sports

Continue as desired.

Comment

This problem is usually misdiagnosed as one of its more serious differentials.

Effort-induced thrombosis

Findings

An index of suspicion is required to differentiate this from a leaky knee, which has a history of a Baker's cyst and a swollen calf, and as the leaky knee syndrome appears so the Baker's cyst settles because the fluid has leaked from the knee. This presents with a swollen calf with no history of trauma or tear and may occur during travel on a long journey from sitting in a cramped position. Homan's sign is positive and the calf is tender to palpation.

Cause

Paget–von Schroetter syndrome. Possibly from a tear of the internal wall of a vein and sitting for a long time whilst traveling, local trauma or systemic causes of increased vascular coagularity. It is common in the upper limbs.

Investigations
Ultrasound Doppler studies and a venogram.

Treatment
Anticoagulate.

Sports
Reported in joggers, skiers, soccer players and kick boxers, but probably not sport related.

Comment
Rare but sometimes presents following very long journeys with travelling teams.

Deep vein thrombosis

Swelling of the calf which is often uncomfortable and tender to palpation or squeezing. The superficial veins may be dilated and Homan's test is positive. Refer urgently for vascular opinion.

Reflex sympathetic dystrophy

May occur after trauma, fracture or a sudden forced stretch of the neurovascular bundle causing sympathetic nerve effects.

Stage 1
Raised circulation. Oedema. Hot dry skin. Livid colour. Burning, everlasting pain. Worse to touch. Often stocking distribution.

Treatment
Intravascular sympathetic blockade with guanethidine. Sympathetic ganglion block. Peripheral nerve block. Epidural or spinal block with indwelling catheter. Elevate and treat with NSAIDs. Patient may gently exercise but no massage. Neuroleptics are required.

Stage 2
Pale cold cyanotic skin. Vasospasm. Sweating.

Atrophy of skin and muscle. Contraction of the joint.

Treatment
Treat pain as in stage 1. Therapy is less effective.

Stage 3
Irreversible atrophy of bone, muscle and connective tissue. Joint contractures. Skin is cold, pale and dry. X-ray shows osteoporosis, particularly around the joint. Pain. At rest this may ease – movement causes terrible pain. Sympathetic blockade may not work.

Treatment
Epidural or sympathetic plexus block to try and obtain movement. TENS. Neuroleptics.

Comment
This may be seen in sportspeople after trauma, but I did see a gymnast who was stretching her hamstring on someone's shoulder when the foot slipped and this forced stretch produced a reflex sympathetic dystrophy over the next few days. Fortunately she responded to therapy for stage 1 and 2. See Fig. 12.6.

Popliteal artery entrapment syndrome

Findings
Intermittent claudication in active young or middle-aged people which is often unilateral. There are diminished pedal pulses with calf activity or held passive dorsiflexion of the foot, and cramps appear with exercise which paradoxically may be worse walking than running. It is worse in endurance events rather than stop/start events.

Cause
A rare anatomical variation of popliteal artery entrapment by cysts or fibrous bands on the medial head of the gastrocnemius, often defined into four types depending on the nature of the obstructing band.

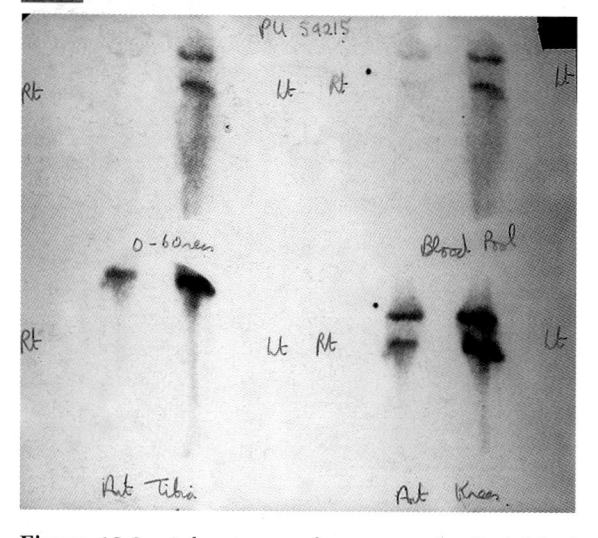

Figure 12.6   A bone scan shows severely diminished uptake of the right leg in the second stage of reflex sympathetic dystrophy in a gymnast.

Caveat – May also be atherosclerotic claudication, venous claudication or posterior compartment compression syndrome of the calf.

Investigations

Ultrasound Doppler studies during exercise plus angiography or spiral MRI.

Treatment

In the early stages reduce activity but if this does not improve the situation then surgery to correct the extra-articular obstruction.

Sports

None are contributory.

Comment

Fortunately rare; history and a high index of suspicion are required.

This could be called the 'skiving syndrome' as the player avoids hard endurance runs and effort on the pitch but appears to play comfortably in short bursts. Most coaches feel they are 'skivers'.

Further reading

1.   Padhair, N. and King, J. B. (1996) Exercise induced leg pain – chronic compartment syndrome. Is the increase in intra-compartment pressure exercise specific? *Br. J. Sports Med.* **30**, 360–362.
2..   Gorard, D. A. (1990) Effort thrombosis in an American football player. *Br. J. Sports Med.* **24**, 15.

Bruckner, P. and Khan, K. (1993) *Clinical Sports Medicine.* McGraw-Hill, New York.

Hutson M. A. (ed.) (1996) *Sports Injuries: Recognition and Management*, 2nd edn. Oxford Medical Publications, Oxford.

Reid, D. (1992) *Sports Injury Assessment and Rehabilitation.* Churchill Livingstone, Edinburgh.

13

Ankle

Part 1
General ankle pain

Referred pain

Ankle pain may be referred from the back, and common peroneal and superficial peroneal nerves, which will often have a history of 'pins and needles', hyperaesthesia and numbness (see Chapters 2, 5 and 12).

Capsulitis of the talar joint

Findings
(a) There is a history of trauma to the ankle followed by synovial swelling of the ankle joint, infilling the posterior aspect of the joint bilaterally producing a ballottement on examination.
(b) Passive ankle flexion, extension and talar translation hurt because trauma will disturb the ligaments and tendons, and there will be signs and symptoms from these as well.
(c) Inflammatory disease will have systemic stigmata.

Cause
Sprain of the talar joint, often as part of a ligamentous disruption of the talar joint or inflammatory joint disease.

Caveat – If there is no history of trauma consider the diagnoses of gout, osteoarthritis, rheumatoid (adult and juvenile) arthritis, spondylarthropathies, reactive arthropathies and infective arthropathies.

Investigations
X-ray for fractures or joint disease and the appropriate blood tests if required.

Treatment
(a) RICE and crutches.
(b) Electrotherapeutic modalities to settle inflammation, such as interferential and pulsed shortwave diathermy.
(c) NSAIDs.
(d) Diagnostic aspiration of the joint which must be sent for culture and crystal microscopy.
(e) Injection of cortisone to settle capsular inflammation via either the anterior or posterior approach.
(f) Isometrics to the posterior tibialis and peroneals to maintain strength.
(g) Balancing or wobble board for proprioceptive skills.
(h) Non-impact cross-training, such as swimming, cycling or rowing routines.
(i) Achilles ladders when impact is permitted (see Chapter 20).

Sports
Following injury, most ankles will require supporting for 4–6 weeks after reaching match fitness.

Comment
As this is a traumatic inflammatory lesion, early cortisone enables faster pain relief and therefore earlier rehabilitation to follow, but take an aspirate before the injection if possible. If the cause is not diagnosed, then a bone scan is the watershed

investigation to separate bony from soft tissue causes.

Osteoarthritis of the talar joint

Findings
Examination shows a swollen joint which may be bony, soft tissue and sometimes synovial fluid. There is pain on weight bearing, and with passive flexion, extension and translation of the ankle joint. The range of dorsiflexion and plantar flexion is often restricted physically with a hard end feel, and posterior tibialis and peroneal muscles are often weak.

Cause
Osteoarthritis of the talar joint which often later may be associated with subtalar and mid tarsal osteoarthritis. The osteoarthritis often follows a Pott's fracture or gross long-standing over-pronation.

Investigations
X-ray is usually sufficient and cost-effective but sometimes CT or MRI scan will define early changes.

Treatment
(a) Electrotherapeutic modalities to settle soft tissue inflammation and pain, such as inter-ferential and pulsed shortwave diathermy.
(b) NSAIDs.
(c) Intra-articular injection of cortisone for relief of the capsular pain.
(d) Heel raise to increase functional dorsiflexion which may allow pain-free walking.
(e) May require a firm supportive orthotic if sub-talar and mid tarsal joints are also involved.
(f) Surgery to arthrodese the joint or joints (a triple arthrodesis).

> **Caveat** – Limited dorsiflexion of the ankle is helped by pronating through the foot. Therefore blocking pronation with an orthotic may make osteoarthritis of the talar joint worse, and a heel raise may be a better solution unless the subtalar and mid tarsal joints are involved which require supporting.

Sports
(a) Avoid impact sports to limit further degeneration if possible.
(b) Limited dorsiflexion may also require a change of technique for non-impact sports such as skiing where a heel raise will increase the functional range of dorsiflexion.
(c) Swimming, rowing or cycling for aerobic fitness, but the seat height may have to be adjusted to accommodate the range of ankle movements.

Comment
Osteoarthritis severely alters activities, and individual adjustments in technique and playing aspirations need to be discussed thoroughly with the patient.

Osteochondral defect

Findings
A history of ankle injury without fracture in which the bruising and swelling often occurs on both the medial and lateral sides. The most usual presentation is of long-standing ankle pain failing to settle after treatment of ligamentous and capsular injury (see *Capsulitis of the talar joint*). Weight bearing to some degree is painful and swelling of the joint may be present. There is variably pain on dorsi- or plantar flexion but translatory pain is invariably present. The injury may produce a loose body.

Cause
Often is a sequela of severe sprain of the ankle but may represent a compression stress fracture. Osteochondral lesions are usually in the talar dome and only rarely in the tibial plafond. They can be graded through 1–5 (Fig. 13.1).

Investigations
(a) Antero-posterior and lateral X-ray is often negative.
(b) Bone scan is the watershed diagnosis, a positive scan is invariably from an osteochondral defect (Figs 13.2–13.4).
(c) CT or MRI scan if the bone scan is positive to display the site and grade of the lesion.

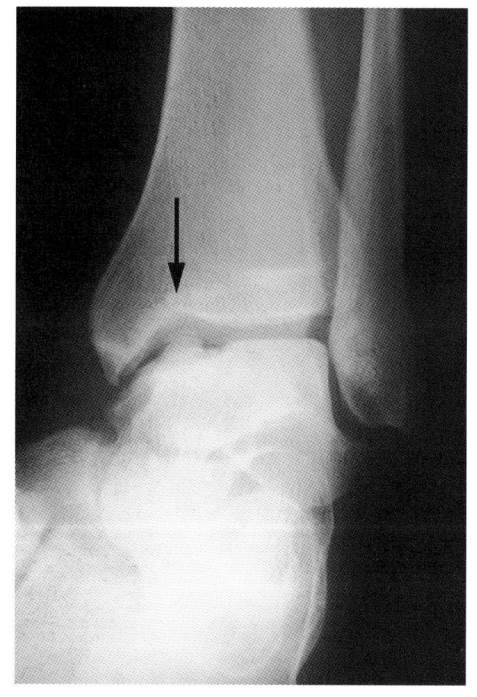

Figure 13.1   X-ray showing osteochondral lesion of the talus.

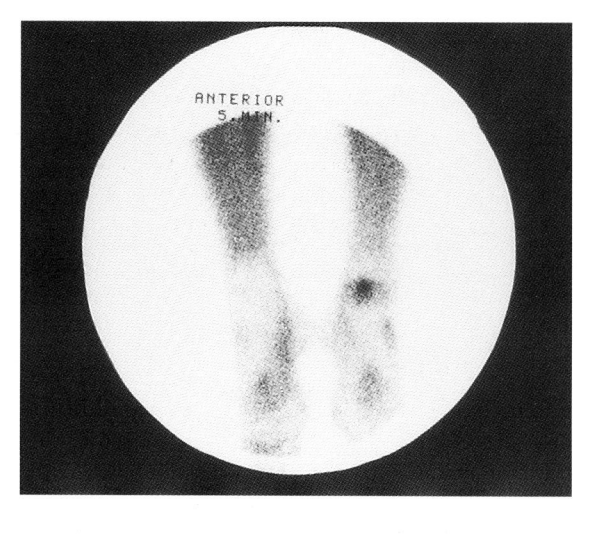

Figure 13.3   A hot bone scan of the patient in Fig. 13.2.

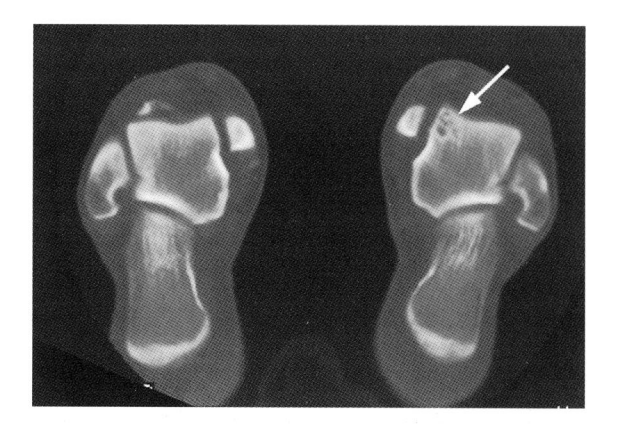

Figure 13.4   A CT scan shows the osteochondral defect in the talar dome of the patient in Fig. 13.2.

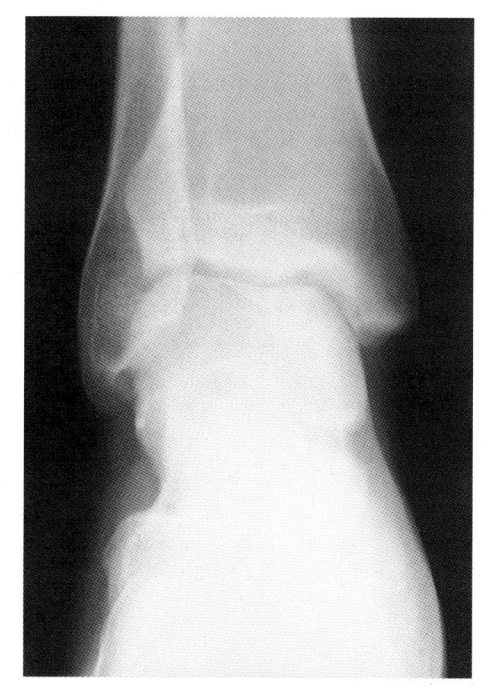

Figure 13.2   A normal X-ray of a patient with ankle pain.

Treatment

Grade 1–2   Reduce impact and allow time to heal.

Grade 3–5   Surgery.

Sports

Train non-impact by cycling, rowing, swimming or other non-impact gym equipment, and maintain balance and calf strength. Build via the Achilles ladders, when impact is free of pain (see Chapter 20).

Comment

Management of chronic ankles is helped by a bone scan. If the bone scan is positive look for a bony lesion and if negative, stress X-ray. If the ankle is stable mobilize the ankle, possibly with manipulation under anaesthetic, and inject hydrocortisone to the posterior aspect of the joint.

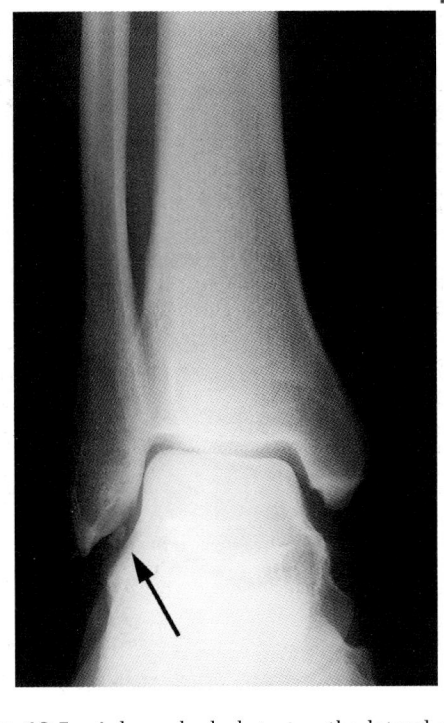

Figure 13.5   A loose body between the lateral maleolus and talus (arrow).

Loose body

Findings

A history of intermittent catching pain that can come or go abruptly and may be combined with other symptoms from an osteochondral defect, talar joint capsulitis or footballer's ankle.

Cause

Osseous or chondral fragment within the talar joint following trauma.

Investigations

(a) X-ray is often the most accurate (Fig. 13.5).
(b) CT scan can be effective but can miss the lesion.
(c) MRI is not good at showing cortical bone and non-visualization of a loose body does not exclude the diagnosis. However, all can miss the loose body but may show the defect from where it came.
(d) Arthroscopy.

Treatment

Surgery to remove the loose body.

Sports

Rehabilitate via the Achilles ladder (see Chapter 20) and increase non-impact cross-training for future protection of the joint.

Comment

The intermittent history of catching pain is almost pathognomonic.

Footballer's ankle

Findings

A history of rest pain, better with activity. Inspection and palpation shows thickened, swollen, soft tissue around the ankle with no synovial swelling unless a loose body is in the joint or the capsule is inflamed. There is a stiff, limited joint range.

Cause

Chronic minor trauma to the ankle from both sprains and direct blows from being kicked which heals with thickened soft tissue, osteophytes, calcification and loose fragments.

Investigations

X-ray shows extracapsular soft tissue swelling and calcification (Fig. 13.6).

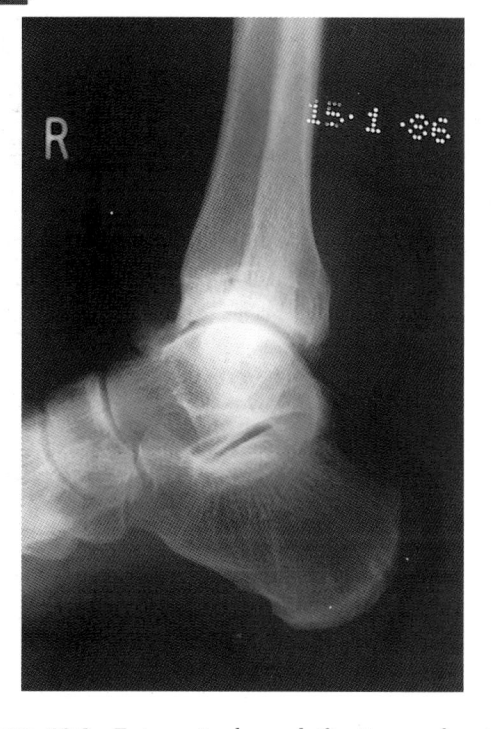

Figure 13.6 Extra-articular calcification and osteophytes and early joint space narrowing in a footballer's ankle.

Treatment
(a) Electrotherapeutic modalities to settle inflammation, such as ultrasound and laser.
(b) Massage and mobilizations to release scar tissue such as frictional massage.
(c) Ankle mobilizations and electrotherapeutic modalities to warm and mobilize scar tissue, such as interferential, pulsed shortwave diathermy and ultrasound.
(d) Proprioceptive rehabilitation.
(e) Achilles ladders (see Chapter 20).

Sports
Invariably soccer but the patient can play with this ankle, but may prefer strapping and an ankle support plus shin pads with ankle flaps. NSAIDs may help during the game.

Comment
Physiotherapy and mobilization help and an injection is rarely required.

Syndesmal strain

Findings
Usually a severe ankle injury with patients attending accident centres but not severe enough to be picked up at the acute stage as a fractured ankle. There is often a history of acute trauma that at the time had medial and lateral bruising, and a capsulitis of the ankle, but the X-ray showed no apparent fracture. This ankle sprain takes longer to heal and often presents as a chronic ankle pain that attends a soft tissue or sports clinic with a history of a severe acute injury in the past and now pushing off into acceleration is painful. Initially all stress movements may be positive but in the chronic case the syndesmal stress test or external rotation stress test is positive [1] (see *Glossary*).

Cause
Severe ankle injury where the medial malleolus and ligaments have withstood the force, but the distal tibio-fibular and interosseous ligaments are disrupted.

> **Caveat** – May have a proximal fibular fracture.

Investigations
X-ray – note ectopic calcification in the interosseous ligament may be present (Fig. 13.7) [2].

Treatment
(a) Plaster of Paris or ankle brace for stability.
(b) Electrotherapeutic modalities to settle inflammation, such as ultrasound, laser and interferential.
(c) Massage techniques to organize scar tissue.
(d) Proprioceptive rehabilitation.
(e) Achilles ladders (see Chapter 22).
(f) Surgery if unstable or a widened distal tibio-fibular syndesmosis.

Sports
None particularly relevant.

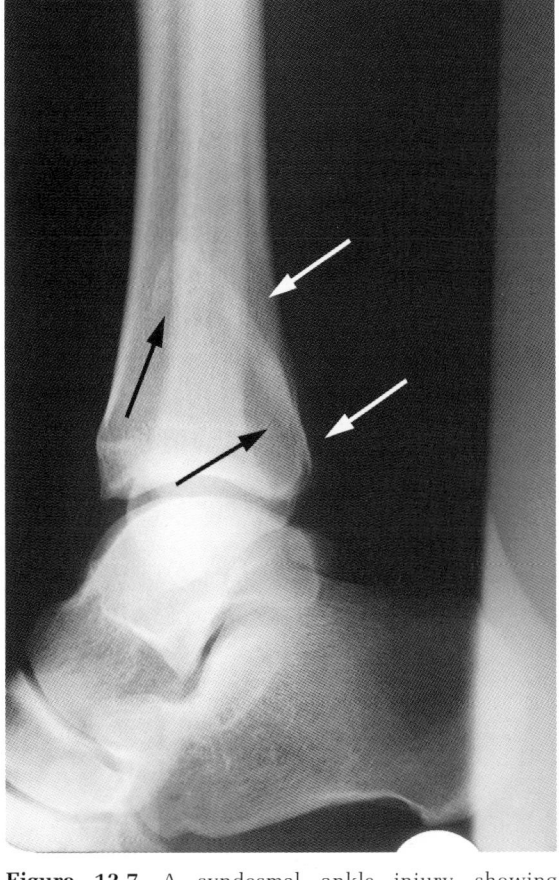

Figure 13.7 A syndesmal ankle injury showing calcification in the osseous ligament and behind the tibia.

Comment

Usually the trauma produces an ankle fracture, so the syndesmal strain is uncommon and will therefore present as a chronic ankle. Stability of the ankle governs the management as to whether

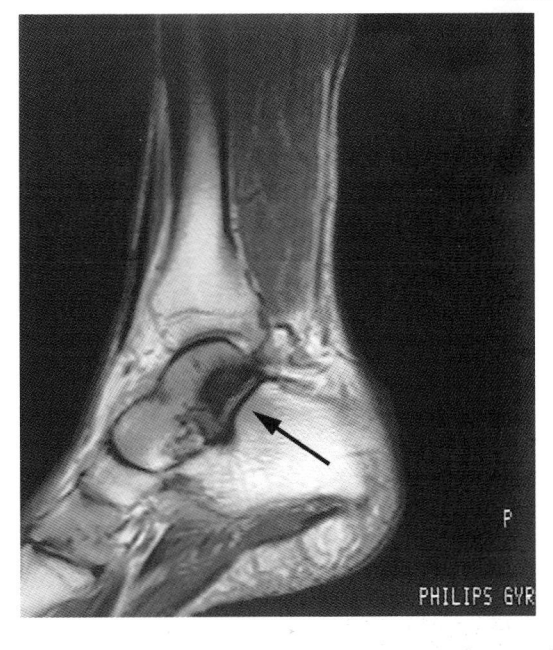

Figure 13.8 T1-weighted MRI showing decreased signal in the talus and around the subtalar joint from avascular necrosis.

surgical screwing is required. The syndesmal lesion takes longer to heal and may leave ectopic calcification and a persistent low-grade discomfort [1–3].

Avascular necrosis

Usually from non-sporting causes, alcohol in particular, but may be after trauma and in scuba diving the 'bends' must be considered (see *Glossary*) (Fig. 13.8).

Part 2
Anterior ankle pain

Tibialis anterior tendinitis

Findings

Pain that may travel up into the tibialis anterior muscle and down to its insertion at the medial cuneiform and first metatarsal. There may be palpable crepitus and there is tenderness to palpation over the tibialis tendon. The pain is worse with resisted dorsiflexion of the foot.

Cause

(a) A tendinopathy or tenovaginitis of the tibialis anterior muscle. It may be at the insertion or under the anterior retinaculum of the ankle joint and occasionally low over the musculo-tendinous junction. It is not a common injury.

(b) The mechanisms are similar to the anterior compartment syndrome, but usually this is a more acute overload (see Chapter 12).

(c) This injury often appears later in a foot or ankle problem because the patient is wary of impact onto the unstable or damaged foot, and the tibialis anterior, long extensors, posterior tibialis and peroneals all lock up at impact to stabilize the foot. The tibialis anterior and

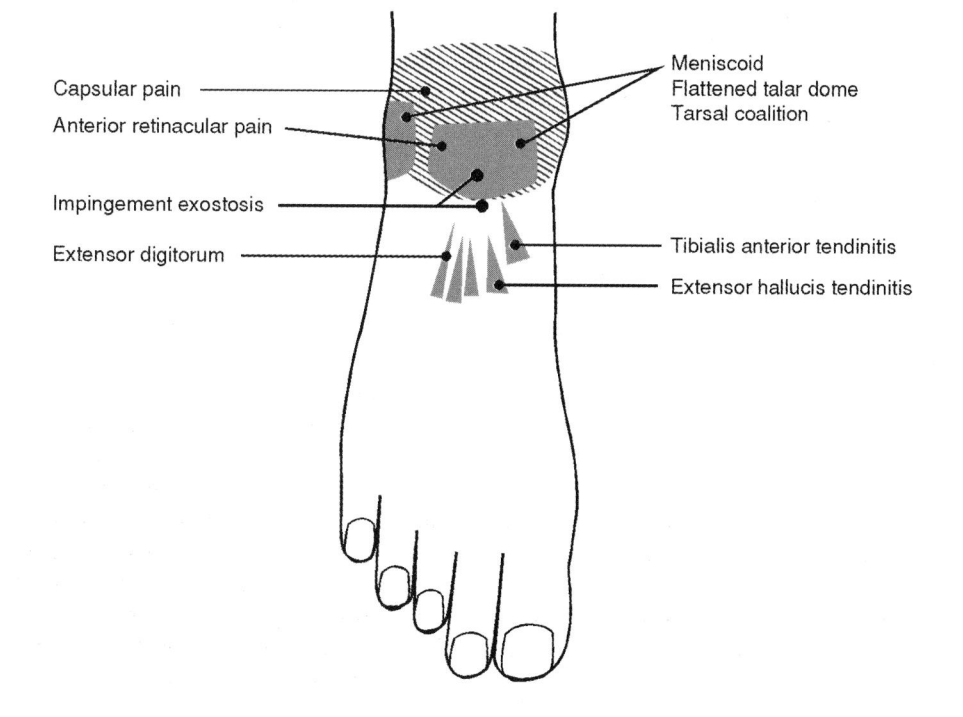

Capsular pain

Anterior retinacular pain

Impingement exostosis

Extensor digitorum

Meniscoid
Flattened talar dome
Tarsal coalition

Tibialis anterior tendinitis

Extensor hallucis tendinitis

extensor digitorum are not accustomed to this work, and suffer an overload and rubbing injury as they stand out and lock into the shoes.

(d) Occasionally it is caused by the shoe with the laces tied up too tightly and rubbing against the insertion.

Investigations
None clinically required.

Treatment
(a) RICE.
(b) Electrotherapeutic modalities to calm inflammation, such as ultrasound and laser.
(c) Massage techniques to release adhesions, such as frictions.
(d) Steroid to the synovial sheath of the retinaculum or enthesis to settle inflammation and reduce adhesions.
(e) Use padding either side of the tendon which will take the shoe pressure off the tendon where it bows out across the dorsum of the foot.

Sports
(a) Avoid inclined or ordinary sit-ups with the feet under a bar or held by a colleague for leverage.
(b) Occurs also in cross country skiing when the foot dorsiflexion is overused to accelerate the ski forward.
(c) Also in 'shuffle runners' who do not thrust from the forefoot to achieve lift off, and thus have to raise the toes and feet faster to clear the ground.
(d) Step aerobics and hill running can produce the problem.

Comment
Not common in sport but quite frequent as part of a protective mechanism. A major help is to lengthen the stride and relax the foot during the lift off and carry phase, and work on psoas strength to improve the knee carry. Responds well to most therapeutic modalities but the insertion and retinaculum probably improve faster with cortisone.

Extensor hallucis tendinitis

See *Extensor digitorum longus tendinitis* but note weak painless muscle may be L5 nerve palsy.

Extensor digitorum longus tendinitis

Findings
Pain in the anterior compartment of lower leg and/or the anterior retinaculum at the dorsum of the foot which is tender to palpation and worse with resisted toe extensors. The skin over the tendons may be red and sore.

Cause
Overuse of extensors of the toes or rubbing of the tendons by the shoes. These muscles are used either to protect an unstable foot or ankle when they lock up together with the calf, posterior tibialis and peroneals, or when they try and do the work of posterior tibialis. They can be overused by shuffle runners who dorsiflex the foot and toes in the swing phase. See *Tibialis anterior tendinitis* and *Anterior retinacular pain*.

Treatment
As for *Tibialis anterior tendinitis* but applied to the extensor tendons.

Sports
As for tibialis anterior tendinitis.

Comment
Some of these runners will wear a hole in the top of their running shoe from the big toe nail, pulling up into the shoe during the swing phase of running. These runners are made worse by tight lacing. Padding either side of the affected tendon will remove the lace-up pressure. This can be sufficient as it is very difficult to change this particular running style. An orthotic might help as this lock up mechanism is used to prevent overpronation in an externally rotated foot.

Impingement exostoses

Findings

Pain is worse after active and passive dorsiflexion movements of the ankle, and landing from jumps and vaults into dorsiflexion of the ankle hurts. There is local tenderness to palpation.

Cause

Exostosis from impingement of anterior tibia onto distal talus and talo navicular [4] from forced dorsiflexion.

Investigations

Lateral X-ray of ankle and foot (Fig. 13.9).

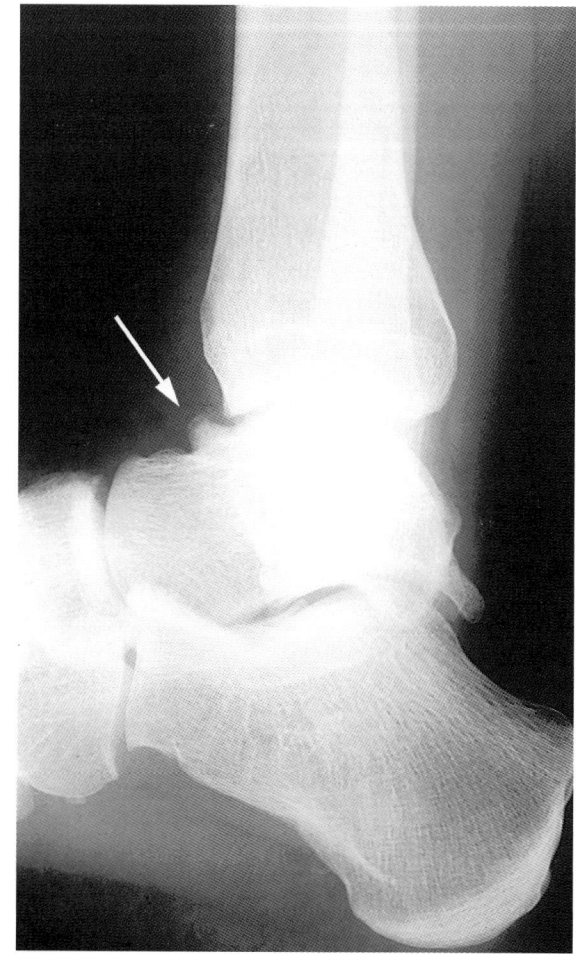

Figure 13.9   An impingement exostosis in a gymnast (arrow).

Treatment

Reduction in dorsiflexion activities until the pain is tolerable; rarely surgical removal although this is advised for the navicular fragment in highly symptomatic cases [4].

Sports

Particularly gymnastics where over-rotating front landings or under-rotating backward landings produces increased dorsiflexion at the ankle. The coach may help lift rotations or use a landing pit whilst the injury is sore. Adjustment of mat height, higher for forward landings, lower for backward, may be possible in practice. A heel raise may help by producing a slightly plantar flexed, neutral position and thus a greater range of functional dorsiflexion. This injury may be part of the footballer's ankle (see *Footballer's ankle*).

Comment

These exostoses develop over time, often without problems, when they are seen by chance on an X-ray, but they may be acutely traumatized and can fracture which is when the pain appears. Management is to see them through this phase, limiting training to the pain-free elements such as asymmetrical bars, with no dismounts, and limit the number of causative landings per training session.

Meniscoid

Findings

A persistent pain after an ankle injury, that is worse on active and passive dorsiflexion of the talar joint and tender to local palpation at the anterior, superior lateral or superior medial corners of the talus.

Cause

A name given to a leish of vessels and connective tissue that lies over the front of the talar joint and is contiguous with the synovium of the talar joint. It becomes hypertrophied and inflamed after injury or chronic impingement.

Caveat – Osteochondral lesion and impingement exostosis.

Investigations
None clinically required until failure of a trial of therapy, when a bone scan may be hot in the blood phase.

Treatment
Injection of hydrocortisone into the meniscoid and if this fails surgical debridement [5].

Sports
May be undertaken as there is no long-term damage, but it will hurt afterwards.

Comment
Although surgery has been discussed none of my cases have come to surgery, as all have responded well to one or two cortisone injections and correction of foot biomechanics.

Anterior retinacular pain

Findings
Puffy red, tender to palpation over the anterior retinaculum.

Cause
Compression of the anterior retinaculum by a boot or shoe whilst the extensor hallucis or extensor digitorum longus or tibialis anterior are being used.

Investigations
None clinically required.

Treatment
Release pressure of the shoe as this is often produced by tying the laces into the eyehole that is highest and widest, therefore do not lace shoes up to top eyelet holes. Soft padding under the tongue of the shoe. Electrotherapeutic modalities to settle inflammation, such as ultrasound and laser. NSAIDs.

Sports
See *Tibialis anterior tendinitis*.

Comment
Modern shoes are being cut higher. The top eyelet holes are being placed further round the side of the shoes and rubbing is occurring more frequently over the retinaculum.

Tarsal coalition

Bony or fibrous fusion of the talus, calcaneum or cuboid limits mid-foot movement and requires more range from the talar joint (see Chapter 14).

Flattened talar dome

This problem may limit ankle dorsiflexion and produce impingements, meniscoid or capsular pains (see Chapter 15).

Sprained ankle: lateral bruising

See *Acute lateral ligament sprain* and *Chronic lateral ligament sprain*, and if the bruising appears more towards the toes, see *Calcaneo-cuboid ligament sprain* (see Chapter 15).

Ankle sprain: lateral and medial bruising

Findings
(a) A history of an inversion sprain accompanied by plantar flexion, with rapid swelling which may or may not bruise.
(b) Tender to palpation over the anterior talo-fibular, middle talo-fibular ligament or calcaneo-fibular ligament.
(c) Talar translation is painful, as is passive plantar flexion. If anterior translation is painful, it suggests a combined lesion with

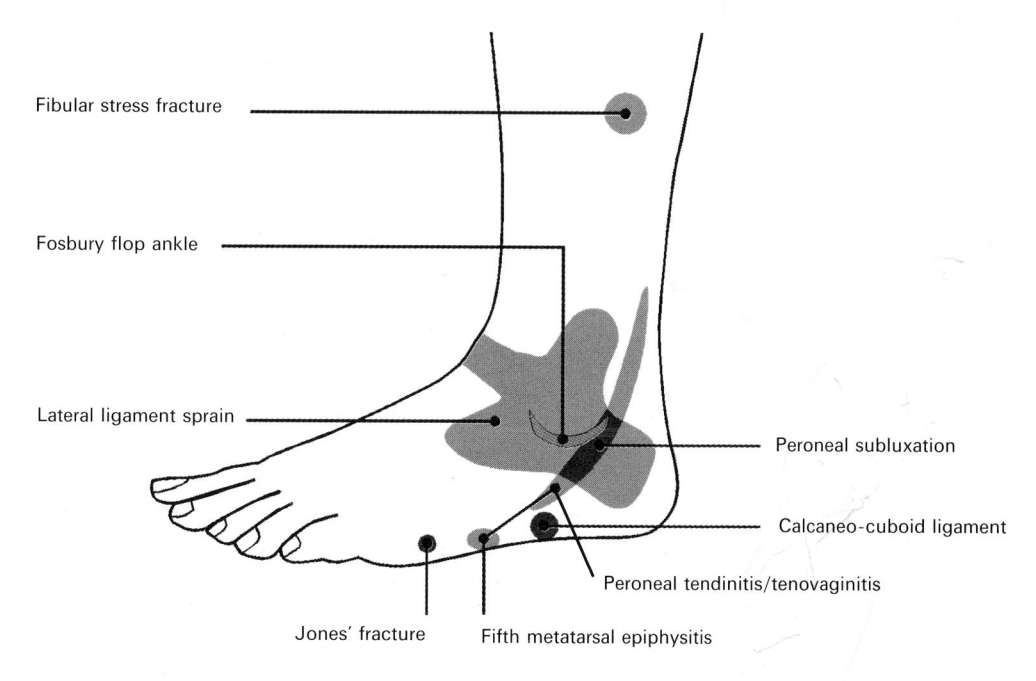

Fibular stress fracture

Fosbury flop ankle

Lateral ligament sprain

Peroneal subluxation

Calcaneo-cuboid ligament

Peroneal tendinitis/tenovaginitis

Jones' fracture   Fifth metatarsal epiphysitis

capsulitis or posterior tibio-fibular ligament damage has occurred.

(d) Possible capsular signs from the ankle joint, extension and flexion hurt.

(e) Calcaneo-tibial compression test is positive (see Glossary).

(f) Bruising is lateral, posterior and medial.

(g) There is often an effusion of the ankle joint.

Cause

The ankle ligaments are sprained in inversion and forced plantar flexion, so that the posterior capsule and posterior tibio-fibular ligaments are damaged, plus the tissues at the posterior aspect of the ankle joint are compressed and traumatized. There may also be a traumatic capsulitis present.

Investigations

X-ray because clinically this lesion is more difficult to distinguish from a fracture and therefore is worth an X-ray.

Treatment

(a) As for unilateral swelling but electrotherapy also for the ankle joint, such as interferential and shortwave diathermy.

(b) Cortisone injection of the back of the ankle joint and posterior calcaneo-tibial space when the tissue oedema has settled. The injection may require repeating.

Sports

These problems are common during training or returning to the sport after the injury.

(a) Kicking, especially with the foot-plantar-flexed as in the drive and volley. This problem persists after the acute phase has settled until the injury has healed entirely. Strapping to limit plantar flexion may help.

(b) A sudden stop to change direction as in field hockey or squash which forces the posterior aspect of the calcaneum upwards against the tibia is painful.

(c) The accelerated plantar flexion of jumping is painful.

(d) Dancing on 'points' causes problems.

Comment

All may require injection at the posterior aspect of the ankle to reduce inflammation and speed recovery, and this type takes more time to heal than unilateral bruising, often becoming a chronic ankle.

Acute lateral ligament sprain

Findings

(a) A history of an inversion sprain with rapid swelling which may or may not bruise laterally or just pain and no swelling if mild.

(b) Tender to palpation over the anterior talo-fibular, middle talo-fibular ligament or calcaneo-fibular ligament.

(c) Distraction of the ankle joint by passive inversion and plantar flexion tests the anterior talo-fibular ligament and passive inversion and dorsiflexion tests the calcaneo-fibular ligament.

(d) Compression of the talus against the fibula is pain-free.

(e) If anterior translation is painful, it suggests a combined lesion with capsulitis or posterior tibio-fibular ligament damage has occurred.

(f) Bruising is lateral and concentrated around the ankle and mid foot.

Cause

An inversion sprain of the foot with sprain, partial tear or tear of the ankle ligaments, particularly the anterior talo-fibular in plantar flexion and the posterior calcaneo-fibular ligament during dorsiflexion.

Investigations

Not clinically required if the patient can weight bear or compression (not distraction) of the talus on the fibula or tibia is pain-free, as a fracture usually hurts in these circumstances. X-ray to exclude fracture if there is a history of trauma as opposed to an inversion sprain, and if compression is painful, but see *Fosbury flop ankle*.

Treatment

(a) RICE for 48 hours plus non-weight bearing crutches.

(b) Compression can be specifically applied beneath and behind the lateral maleolus with orthopaedic felt.

(c) NSAIDs.

(d) Electrotherapeutic modalities to settle inflammation, such as laser and ultrasound.

(e) Massage techniques to remove tissue debris and to organize fibrocytes, such as effluage and frictions.

(f) Non-weight bearing flexion, extension and plus inversion, eversion exercises.

(g) Weight bear as soon as possible with support but note that the first few paces hurt but then eases up as the patient continues to walk. Pain returns when standing still or resting.

(h) Support initially with a pressure pad beneath the fibular and over the calcaneum and use an adjustable elastic bandage, tubigrip, elasticated anklet or ankle brace [6].

(i) Cross-training should be non-weight bearing, such as swimming, rowing or cycling, and raising or lowering the saddle will encourage ankle range of movements.

(j) Proprioception should be trained by one-legged balancing exercises at home whilst doing hair, cleaning teeth, answering the phone, etc. Balancing with the eyes shut and a wobble board whilst at the physiotherapy department or at home.

(k) Walk with 'rhythm' by counting 1–9 to make the damaged ankle perform normally.

(l) Isometrics to maintain the strength of the posterior tibialis and peroneal muscles.

(m) Follow the Achilles ladders and, after sprinting, add in the kicking ladder, figure of '8' cutting drills and side step routines (see Chapter 20).

(n) Surgery is required if the ankle is unstable, but this is usually assessed later [7].

Sports

Change of direction sports should not have too high a sole on the shoe because this leads to ankle instability. Use a support for about 6 weeks after returning to games. Evidence from basketball is that prophylactic ankle braces or taping is of value in preventing injury to the ankle. Straight line sports must follow the Achilles ladders, whilst change of direction sports must add sideways movements such as side steps and cutting manoeuvres (see Chapter 20).

Comment

This is a very common injury for which it is important to give home proprioceptive exercises so that rehabilitation is done frequently, as too many feel 20 minutes three times per week on a wobble board is all that is required but it is too little. The major problems are instability with weak peroneals or later a chronic stiff ankle that has not been rehabilitated properly. Major ankle damage usually has synovial swelling and bilateral bruising. There is evidence that prophylactic strapping is of benefit [6].

Chronic lateral ligament sprain

Findings

Type 1 Painful or painless inversion, weak peronei and poor balance.

Type 2 Inversion range increased and pain-free. The peronei may be either strong or weak.

Type 3 Tender to palpation over the relevant lateral ligament with a thickened appearance of the soft tissues. Inversion is limited and painful.

Cause

All have a history of previous inversion injury of the ankle or repetitive injuries.

Type 1 Weak peronei and proprioceptive dysfunction.

Type 2 Unstable ankle joint from a partial tear of the lateral ligaments.

Type 3 Adhered scar tissue from poor rehabilitation, producing a stiff ankle joint.

Caveat – Osteochondral fracture of the talus and meniscoid of the ankle.

Investigations

(a) X-ray of the ankle for osteoarthritis, osteophytes, footballer's ankle and osteochondral lesions.

(b) Stress the talus and mid foot into inversion and X-ray for talar tilt or talar translation in type 2 (Fig. 13.10).

(c) If (b) above is normal then bone scan. If the bone scan is hot in the bone phase then look for an osteochondral lesion (see Figs 13.3 and 13.4). A meniscoid and chronic ligament damage may be hot in the blood phase or not at all.

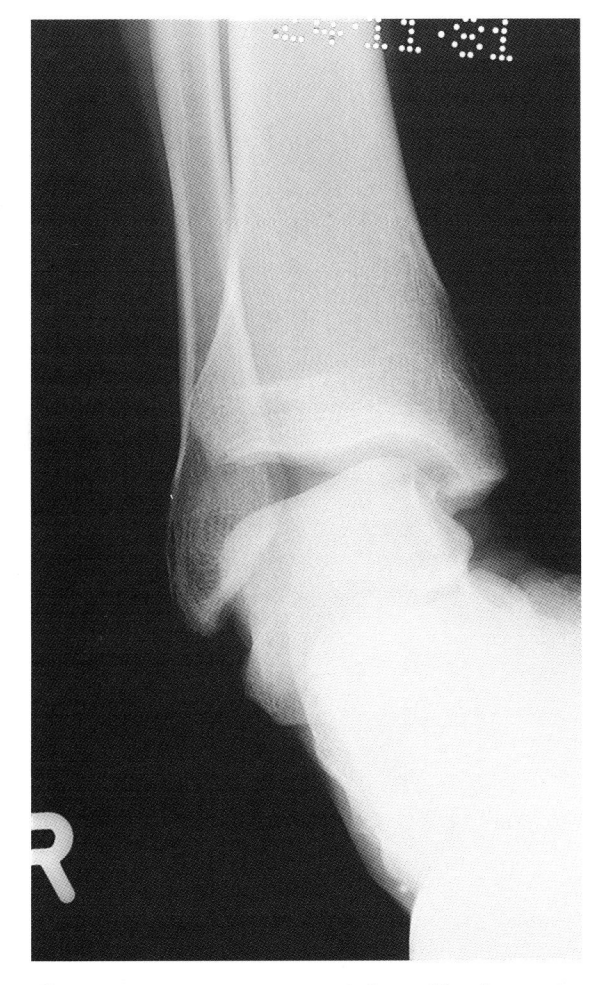

Figure 13.10 Stress views of the ankle show talar tilting due to torn and lengthened lateral ligaments.

Treatment

Type 1   Balancing on a wobble board and proprioceptive exercises to be done during the rest of the day (see *Lateral ligament sprains*). Peroneal isometrics and then the Achilles ladders.

Type 2   Strapping or preferably bracing of the ankle. Surgery if still unstable [6], then the Achilles ladder.

Type 3   Manipulations and mobilizations of ankle. Cortisone injections to the joint via the posterior approach, frictions to the scar tissue and if no progress then manipulation under anaesthetic followed by immediate rehabilitation via the Achilles ladders (see Chapter 20).

Sports

Change of direction sports need support for 6–8 weeks but if unstable then should play in a support brace for longer, if not always, although surgery might have to be considered. Rehabilitation includes figure of '8', side steps, cross over steps and court drills for racket games (see Chapter 20).

Comment

The bone scan and stress X-rays are the watershed investigations in chronic ankles – the bone scan to rule out possible osteochondral lesions, the stress X-rays to rule out partial tears. If both are negative then manipulation under anaesthetic becomes the treatment of choice.

Calcaneo-cuboid ligament sprain

Pain on stressing the mid tarsal joint with tenderness over the calcaneo-cuboid joint line (see Chapter 15).

Peroneal tenovaginitis

Findings

Tenderness over the peroneal tendon and possibly proximal tip of the fifth metatarsal. Resisted eversion is painful and passive inversion may be painful. There may be pain around the back of the lateral maleolus and peroneal muscle pain (see Chapter 12).

Cause

Strain of the tendon from an over-supinated foot (see *Peroneal subluxation*). It is not as common as one would expect, for it seems that an acute inversion is not resisted by the peronei to an extent that damage occurs and therefore the injury damages the ankle ligaments. The tendinitis tends to occur with over-corrected antipronated orthotics, or walking to edge the outside of the foot, as in hill walking along a mountain side, or broken heel cups in a supinated foot. Occasionally a high cut shoe will rub the peroneal retinaculum and sheath, producing a tenovaginitis.

Investigations

None are clinically required. MRI only if rupture of the tendon is suspected.

Treatment

(a) RICE.
(b) Electrotherapeutic modalities to settle inflammation, such as ultrasound and laser.
(c) Massage techniques to prevent adhesions in the tenovaginitis, such as frictions.
(d) Cortisone to the sheath.
(e) Correct orthotics or shoes.
(f) Peroneal isometrics.
(g) Proprioceptive balancing.

Sports

Check the heel cups of the shoes are stable (see Glossary). Worn heels from heel strike can increase the amount of supination. Use strapping or an ankle brace if fell walking with a lot of edging or running on rough ground.

Comment

This is an uncommon injury – it is more common for the muscles to become weak or dysfunctional rather than develop a tendinitis. Note, during rehabilitation of the ankle ligaments, peroneal muscle pain may occur in the lateral compartment of the lower leg.

Peroneal subluxation

Findings

History of a click or flick plus or minus pain over the lateral maleolus and a feeling of insecurity of the ankle. Subluxation of the tendon is reproduced with resisted eversion of the foot, and can be seen and palpated as it jumps forward onto the lateral maleolus.

Cause

The peroneal tendon subluxes anteriorly from the groove behind the lateral maleolus.

Investigations

None clinically required.

Treatment

Minor episodes may be restrained with padding and strapping over the fibula which functionally deepens the peroneal groove. Perhaps orthotics to correct over supination may help. If this cannot control the tendon then surgery to deepen the peroneal groove is required [8].

Sports

(a) Rehabilitate through the Achilles ladders but after a sprint add figure of '8' and shuttle run drills. Side step and karioke drills should be started as early as possible (see Chapter 20).
(b) Karate. Some kicks with the outside of the foot may cause problems.

Comment

Not common and if minor worth a try with conservative padding before considering surgery.

Flat foot impingement syndrome

Findings

A pronated foot with calcaneo-valgus that is often severe. Pain is experienced anterior and inferior to the fibula which is worse on passive eversion and dorsiflexion.

Cause

Excessively pronated foot, especially from calcaneo-valgus. The fibula impinges onto the calcaneum or anterior talus. Sometimes a pes planus will also suffer this problem but a pes planus is a normal variant whereas overpronation is pathological.

Investigations

None clinically required.

Treatment

Local steroid to the area will give rapid relief but correction of the overpronation with an orthotic and proprioceptive exercises is required for long-term control.

Sports

Check the heel cups of the shoes have not broken thus increasing pronation. Camber running or edging in hill walking may precipitate the problem (see *Glossary*).

Comment

This may well be the presenting area of pain in a chronically pronated foot and usually occurs when activity is increased.

Fosbury flop ankle

Findings

Pain on compression of the fibula and talus, not on distraction.

Cause

Impingement between the lateral surface of the talus and fibula. If the take off foot of the Fosbury flop high jumper is planted with too much external rotation then the fibula is driven into the talus causing impingement and bruising of the articular surfaces.

Investigations

None clinically required in a high jumper with the above clinical signs; however, if in doubt an MRI STIR sequence for bone bruising and to exclude other diagnoses.

Treatment

Alter the technique to reduce rotation of the take off foot. Electrotherapeutic modalities to settle intra-articular inflammation, such as interferential and shortwave diathermy.

Sports

Fosbury flop style of high jumping requires a reduced external rotation of the foot at plant and take off.

Comment

This was more common when jumpers tried to get more rotation in their jump but coaches now seem aware of the problem.

Subtalar joint

See *Sinus tarsi* below.

Sinus tarsi

Lateral ankle pain without any other cause and possibly worse on subtalar inversion and eversion (see Chapter 14).

Part 4
Medial ankle pain

Sprained lateral ankle

An inversion, plantar-flexed sprain will affect the capsule of the ankle and produce bruising and swelling around the medial side as well, but the dominant physical signs are from the lateral ligaments (see Part 3, *Ankle pain – Bilateral bruising*).

Deltoid ligament sprain

Findings
A history of fairly major trauma to the ankle with tenderness over the deltoid ligaments and on passive eversion of the foot. If there is bruising, check compression of the talus onto the tibial malleolus is pain-free as compression pain indicates bone damage may be present.

Cause
Eversion injury to the ankle from rough ground, a blocked side foot kick or direct trauma. This requires a fair degree of force just below that required to produce a Pott's fracture to damage the strong deltoid ligament.

Investigations
With bruising, X-ray as this is a strong ligament and avulsion or frank Pott's fracture may be present.

Treatment
Treat any fracture as the priority, but for ligamentous damage alone cast brace to rest and maintain immobility over 7–10 days. Then crutches and non-weight bear, gradually introducing weight bearing. Maintain active dorsi- and plantar flexion, and add electrotherapeutic modalities to settle inflammation plus massage techniques to reduce and control scar tissue. Manage then as

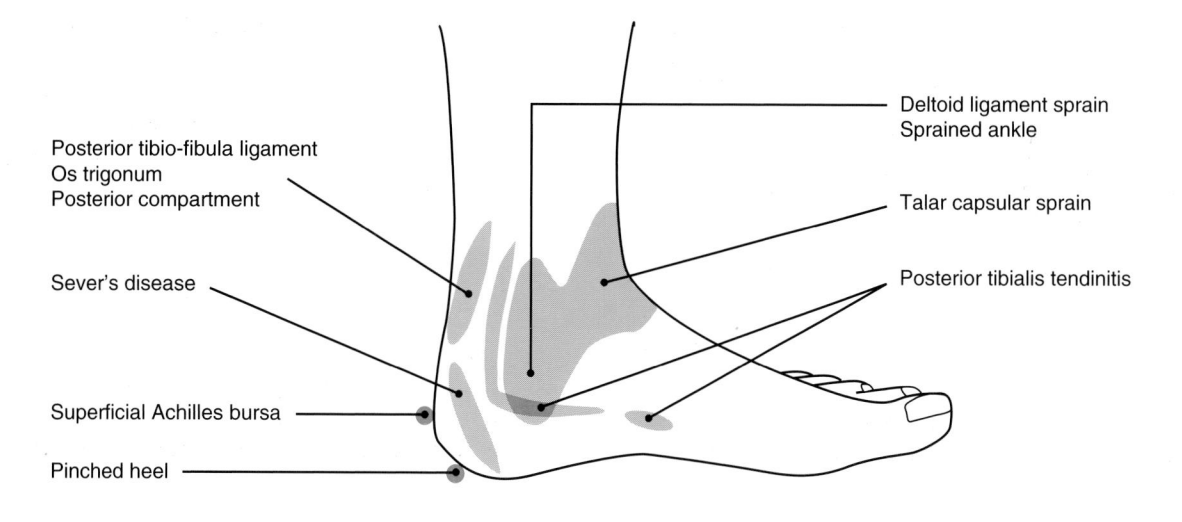

Posterior tibio-fibula ligament
Os trigonum
Posterior compartment

Sever's disease

Superficial Achilles bursa

Pinched heel

Deltoid ligament sprain
Sprained ankle

Talar capsular sprain

Posterior tibialis tendinitis

for the lateral ligament. A chronic deltoid sprain may require a cortisone injection to release scar tissue and aid mobilization.

Sports
Deltoid ligament sprains at a low-grade, repetitive level are part of the footballer's ankle (see *Footballer's ankle*).

Comment
In the acute phase it is important to exclude a possible fracture; however, the chronic deltoid ligament pain often does not settle with physiotherapy and will require a cortisone injection.

Posterior tibialis tenovaginitis

Findings
A history of medial calf pain which may extend around the medial maleolus to the navicular tubercle or even under the transverse arch of the foot. Swelling over the line of the posterior tibialis may be present that is tender to touch and crepitus may be felt posterior to the ankle. It may be tender to palpation over the navicular tubercle and under the transverse arch. Resisted posterior tibialis is painful and weak (Fig. 13.11). A weak, painless posterior tibialis is dysfunctional (rarely ruptured unless there is marked swelling of the

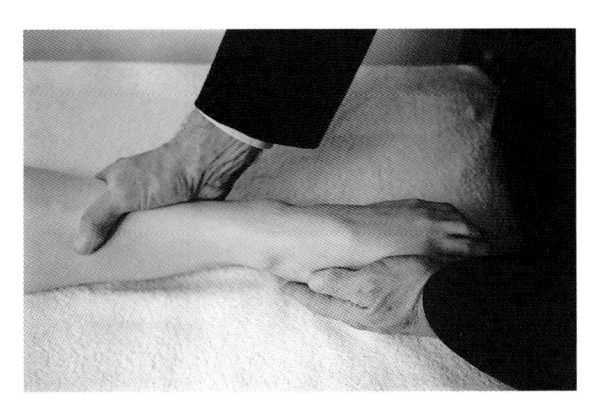

Figure 13.11 Resisted posterior tibialis. The foot and toes must be plantar-flexed to prevent tibialis anterior helping this movement.

sheath) and follows failed ankle rehabilitation or chronic overpronation.

Cause
The chronic pronated foot does not have posterior tibialis tendinitis as in this case the posterior tibialis has an inhibitory weakness rather than pain, thus posterior tibialis tendinitis occurs to prevent functional overpronation. It may therefore occur following Achilles injury when the patient externally rotates the foot to achieve propulsion from the posterior tibialis thus avoiding stressing the Achilles. The same happens if the patient runs with externally rotated feet or strives for ankle propulsion from pronated feet. Semi-acute collapse of the longitudinal arch or the avoidance of weight over the first two rays of the forefoot provokes protective posterior tibialis activity and overload especially in dancers on points.

There may be a tenovaginitis or even a rupture of the tendon.

> **Caveat** – Stress fracture of the tibia, tarsal tunnel and accessory navicular (Fig. 13.12).

Investigations
(a) None clinically required.
(b) X-ray for accessory navicular (see *Glossary*) especially in children with local tenderness (see Fig. 13.12).
(c) MRI for posterior tibialis tendinitis and rupture if failing to rehabilitate or there is no evidence of posterior tibialis function returning when the pain eases (see Fig. 13.13).
(d) Fbc, ESR, Rh factor and antinuclear antibodies, as this is a problem often accompanying systemic inflammatory disease.

Treatment
(a) Strapping or bracing for support.
(b) RICE – beware of the posterior tibial nerve with ice.
(c) Correct any technique that promotes functional pronation. Check the heel cups have not broken in the running shoes (see *Glossary*).

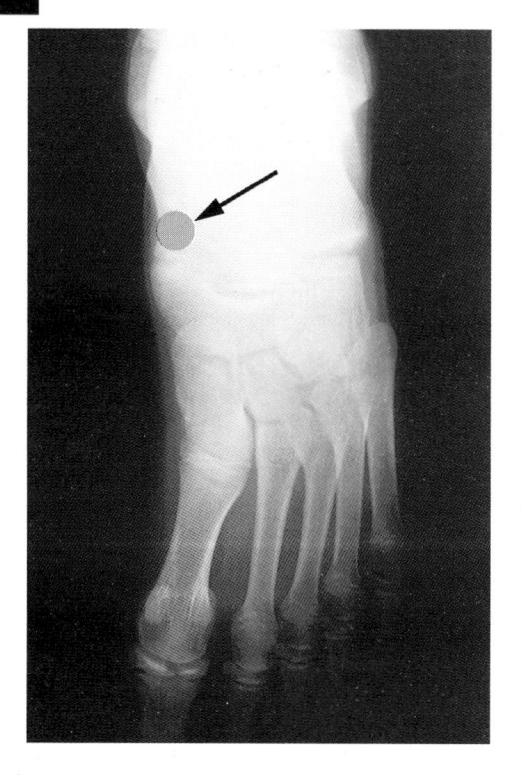

Figure 13.12   The accessory navicular forms the navicular tubercle and is joined by a fibrous band to the navicular (arrow).

(d) Correct any functional genu valgus (see Chapter 11).

(e) Corrective orthotics or orthotics to reduce functional pronation.

(f) Electrotherapeutic modalities to settle inflammation and reduce adhesions, such as ultrasound and laser.

(g) Massage techniques to reduce adhesions, such as frictions.

(h) Cortisone to tenovaginitis or the navicular insertion.

(i) Posterior tibialis isometrics.

(j) Achilles ladders (see Chapter 20).

(k) Surgery for any rupture.

Sports

(a) Change of direction sports are more of a problem and require ankle braces until better.

(b) Running. Beware of camber running and rough ground. Uphill running, bend running, sprint start drills and windmilling style of running can all produce this problem, and the treatment should include high knee drills to encourage a longer gait, swing phase, and in fact psoas and rectus femoris are often weak. Correct externally rotated foot style of

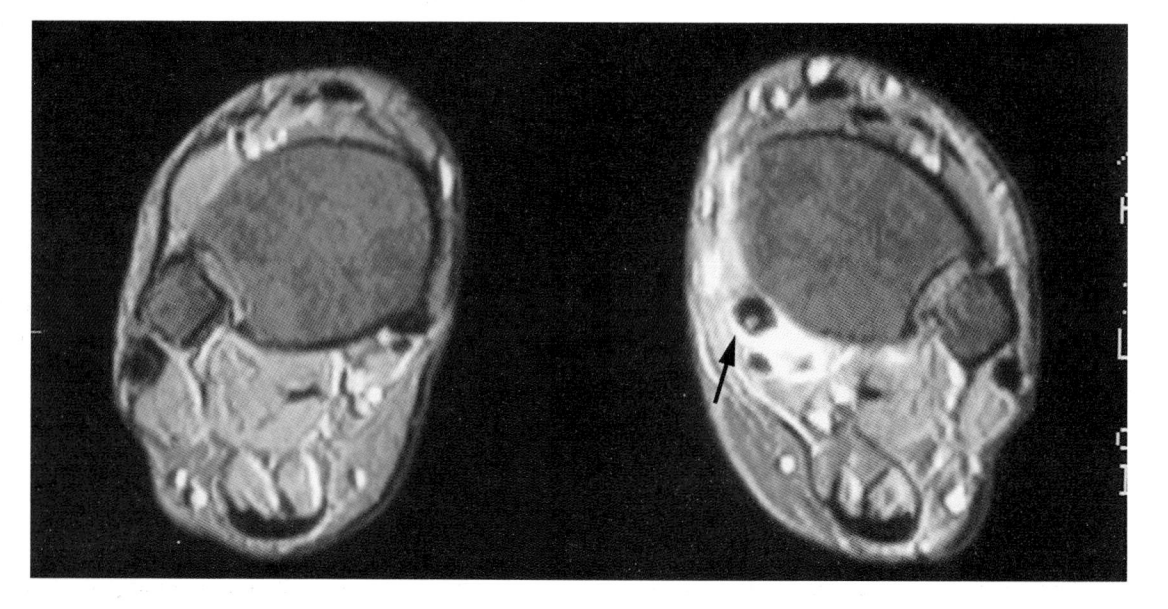

Figure 13.13   T2-weighted MRI scan shows oedema around the posterior tibialis and an intratendinous lesion (arrow).

running or block functional pronation with orthotics and stop hill running until recovered.

(c) See *Maltracking of the patella* and *Tibiocollateral ligament pain* in the knee (see Chapter 11).

(d) Fell walking. Edging the outside of the boot for a long time when walking along slopes.

(e) Rolling over plies at ballet. Dancers without full turn out should be permitted to reduce turn out. They are never going to make professional ballet dancers so they should be permitted to dance and enjoy themselves, without hurting themselves. Correct technique for demi-point work.

Comment

Posterior tibialis problems epitomize sports medicine, where the anatomy promotes overpronation and an inhibitory weakness or the technique causes a functional overpronation with overuse of the posterior tibialis trying to correct the problem. The orthotic 'corrects' the anatomy of the first and minimizes the skill fault in the second to help new skill learning. Running must be taught, it is a skill. These faults may then be transferred onto the knees causing presenting knee pain rather than foot pain. Tenovaginitis improves dramatically with cortisone to the sheath allowing rehabilitation of the muscle tendon, which is often inhibited by pain. The presence of an accessory navicular suggests the injury will take longer to recover.

Flexor hallucis tenovaginitis

Findings

Pain at the posterior medial aspect of ankle at the musculo-tendinous junction and sometimes the medial aspect of the heel and arch of the foot (see Chapter 14). Resisted great toe flexion is painful and weaker, and rarely may be ruptured. In this case, resisted toe flexion is weak and painless unless an adhesive tenovaginitis has developed around the rupture when pain is present and hides the diagnosis.

Cause

Strain of the flexor hallucis from sprinting or bounding, but it is most commonly seen in dancers, especially ballet from point work.

Investigations

Clinically none required unless failing to progress when an MRI will display the tendon and vaginitis or a rupture.

Treatment

(a) Electrotherapeutic modalities to settle inflammation, such as ultrasound and laser.
(b) NSAIDs.
(c) Cortisone to the vaginitis.
(d) Massage techniques to reduce adhesions, such as frictions.
(e) Passive toe flexion and extensions to reduce adhesions.
(f) Isometric toe curls against the other foot.
(g) Block starts, initially with hands on a desk, then hands lower on a bench and finally block starts.
(h) Achilles ladders (see Chapter 20).
(i) Surgery if a rupture is present, usually in ballet dancers.

Sports

(a) Ballet. Rest from points and large jumps.
(b) Running. The insertion of a forefoot bar may help gradually increment increased stride length and bounds by reducing the push from the toes. As this bar is lowered so the toes will come more into use, until the forefoot bar is removed for normal drills.

Comment

Not common except in dancers, but it may occur with plantar fasciitis that is medially placed or indeed may be the actual cause of pain of some types of so called plantar fasciitis.

Tarsal tunnel syndrome

Findings

Pain over the medial ankle radiating to the sole of the foot, which may radiate up into the calf. It might wake the patient at night, and have 'pins and needles', numbness, and paraesthesia worse with walking or dorsiflexion of the foot. Tinel's sign (see *Glossary*) over the posterior tibial nerve is positive and two-point discrimination may be lost in the foot. Weakness of the intrinsic muscles of the foot may be present. A fusiform swelling may be palpated over the nerve. Over-pronation is present.

Cause

Compression of the posterior tibial nerve around the inferior border of medial maleolus within the tarsal tunnel almost invariably found in a calcaneo-valgus pronated foot.

Caveat – Referred root pain or other causes of neural pain, check pulses and diabetes.

Investigations

(a) X-ray of foot and ankle to assess bony and arthritic state.
(b) EMG may show abnormalities of the medial and lateral plantar nerves.
(c) Blood for systemic inflammatory disease and diabetes.

Treatment

(a) Correct pronatory malfunction (see *Glossary*).
(b) NSAIDs.
(c) Perineural steroids if severe.
(d) May require surgical arthrodesis of hind foot if this is deformed and unstable.

Sports

Rarely seen as pronatory problems occur and are treated before problems are severe enough to cause tarsal tunnel symptoms. Presents more in those with a chronic subtalar problem who take up activities. Skiing boots with cable adjustment may cause compression [9].

Comment

Not common and usually caused by gross foot deformity at the rear foot. Orthosis and shoe heel cup strengthening are treatments of choice.

Part 5
Posterior ankle pain

The posterior structures of the ankle are shown in Fig. 13.14.

Achilles peritendinitis

Findings

A history of rest pain, better with activity [10], therefore the pain is worse first thing in the morning, better on walking, and sitting makes the pain worse, but it clears with walking. Runners can 'run off' the pain. The foot attitude

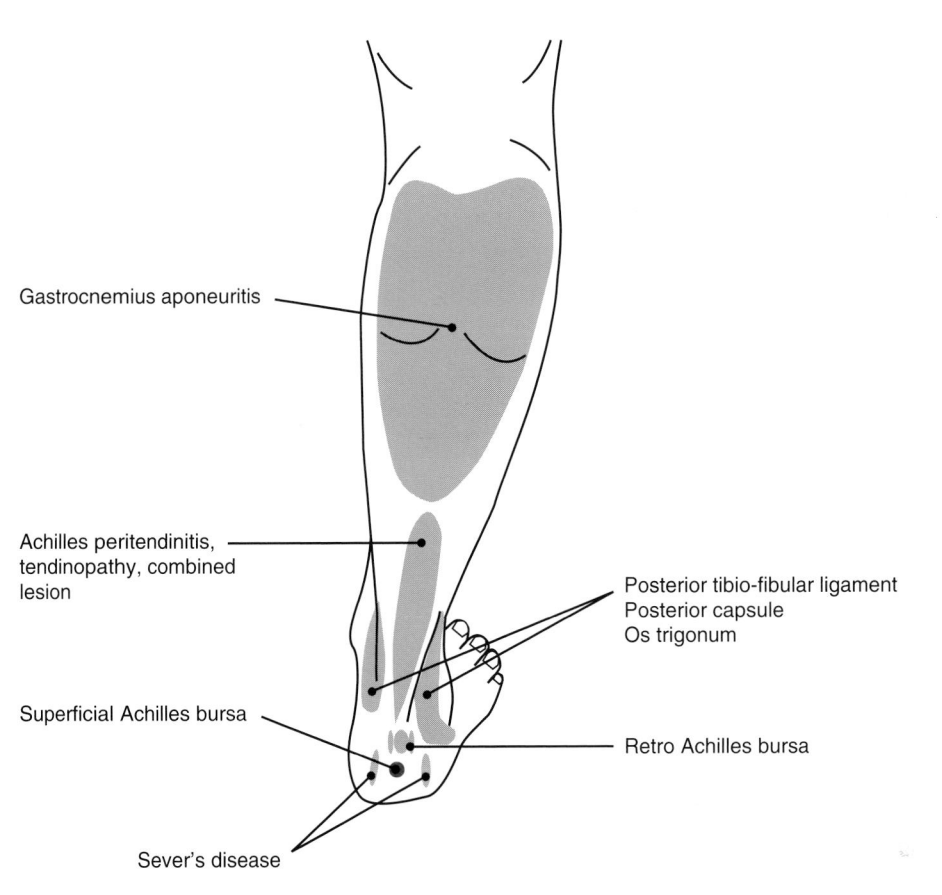

Gastrocnemius aponeuritis

Achilles peritendinitis, tendinopathy, combined lesion

Posterior tibio-fibular ligament
Posterior capsule
Os trigonum

Superficial Achilles bursa

Retro Achilles bursa

Sever's disease

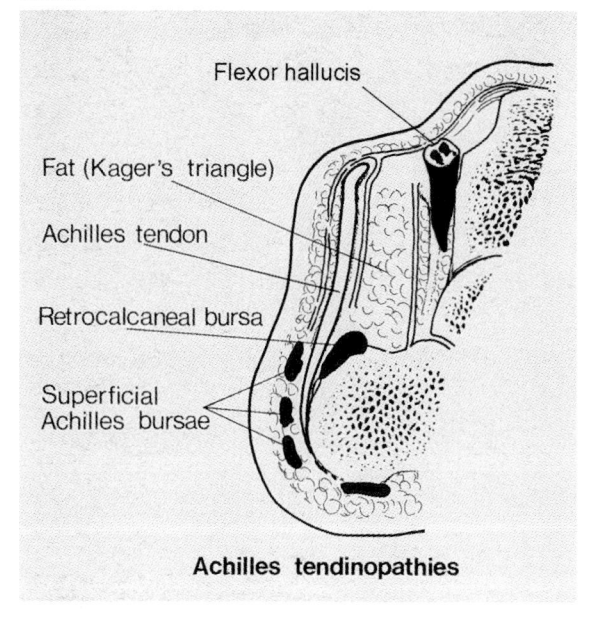

Flexor hallucis

Fat (Kager's triangle)

Achilles tendon

Retrocalcaneal bursa

Superficial
Achilles bursae

Achilles tendinopathies

Figure 13.14   Diagram of the posterior structures of the ankle.

is normal as is Simmonds'/Thomson's test (see *Glossary*) Calf stretching, rising onto the toes and hopping are painful. The tendon is tender to touch and may have crepitus in the acute stage. The tendon may appear puffy and swollen.

Cause
Inflammation of the paratenon from rubbing by the Achilles tag of a shoe or boot, or being part of a combined lesion (see *Combined Achilles lesion*). Following surgery to the Achilles tendon.

Investigations
None clinically required if the history is typical of rest pain, better with activity unless a trial of treatment fails to make progress, in which case diagnostic ultrasound or MRI will help to display if it is part of a combined lesion.

Treatment
(a) Settle the inflammation with peritendinous cortisone, NSAIDs and electrotherapeutic modalities, such as ultrasound and laser.
(b) Prevent adhesions forming with massage techniques, such as cross-frictions.

(c) Achilles ladder but only the bottom ladder to be attempted before review by the physician, with no hopping until then.
(d) Top Achilles ladder (see Chapter 20).

> **Caveat** – Once the history of rest pain has gone but pain still persists then check for an associated tendinopathy to form a combined lesion.

Sports
Check for Achilles heel tag rub; note, the apparent cut-away heel tag may still be too high, so cut away the tag or release the tension on the Achilles with cuts at the side of the heel tag. Do not lace the shoes into the lace holes that extend backwards around the ankle (see *Glossary* and *Achilles tendinopathy*).

Comment
Unlike depomedrone and triamcinolone, hydrocortisone acetate causes little subcutaneous atrophy, and mobility and rest pain morbidity is dramatically improved in 1–2 weeks [10, 11]. It may require self frictions with NSAID gel for maintenance. Peritendinous injections do not appear to increase the rupture rate [11] and if the needle is placed in a tendon extreme pressure is required to inject, so withdraw the needle whilst maintaining injection pressure until the injection flows. A 'Bent' needle may help the technique [12].

Achilles tendinopathy

Findings
A history of pain increasing with activity and better at rest. Active and passive stretch of gastrocnemius is painful and limited (knee straight, dorsiflexed ankle) or soleus tender and limited (with knee bent, dorsiflex ankle). Resisted plantar flexion incrementing through to one leg heel raise or hop is painful depending on the extent of the lesion. Passive whipped plantar flexion, the calcaneo-tibial compression test is pain-free (Fig. 13.15). There may be swelling in the tendon and the swelling moves with the

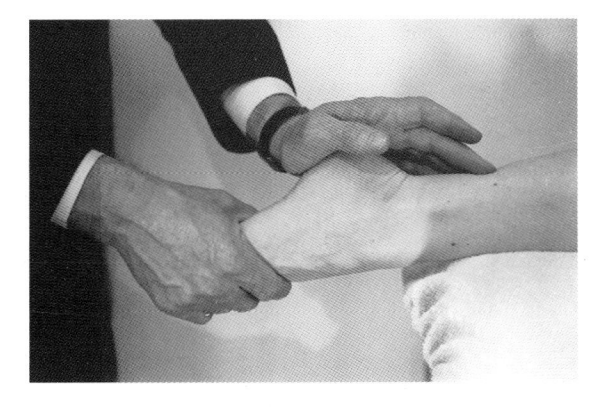

Figure 13.15 The calcaneo-tibial compression test whipping the foot into plantar flexion.

tendon. It is locally tender to compression. The attitude and Simmonds'/Thomson's test are normal (see *Glossary*).

Cause
Partial tear (Fig. 13.16), myeloid, myxoid, hyaline degeneration of collagen fibres (Fig. 13.17) or cystic degeneration (Fig. 13.18). Possibly attritional from vibrating shock of impact, overpronation or discoordination between the quadriceps

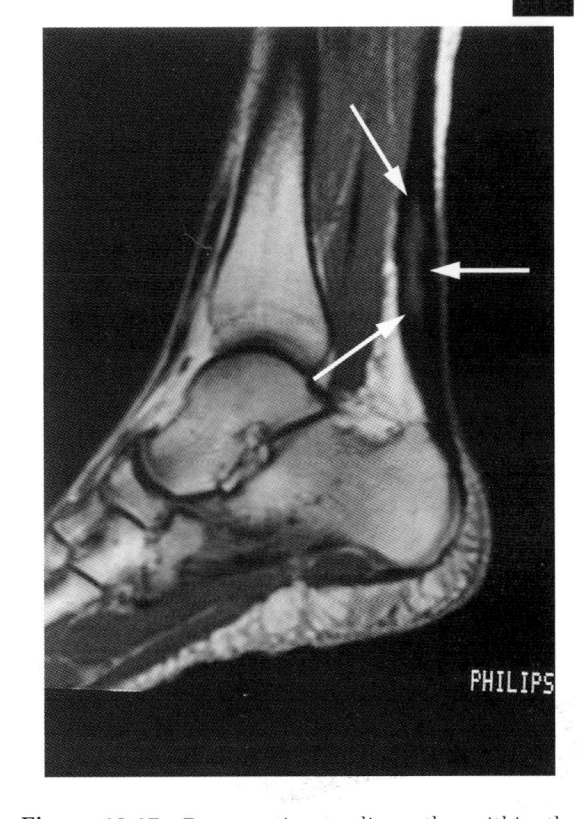

Figure 13.17 Degenerative tendinopathy within the Achilles tendon seen on T1-weighted MRI.

and calf muscle. EMG studies suggest that the quadriceps straightens the knee before the calf plantar flexes the foot and movements that stress this mechanism or that encourage plantar flexion whilst the knee is bent may promote Achilles attrition.

Investigations
None clinically required initially but diagnostic ultrasound scan and MRI scan can expose the extent of the lesion and display degenerate cysts.

Treatment
(a) Heel raise in the shoes to reduce the load on the Achilles tendon.
(b) Orthotics if overpronation is contributing to a side to side distortion during movement.
(c) Achilles ladder (see Chapter 20).

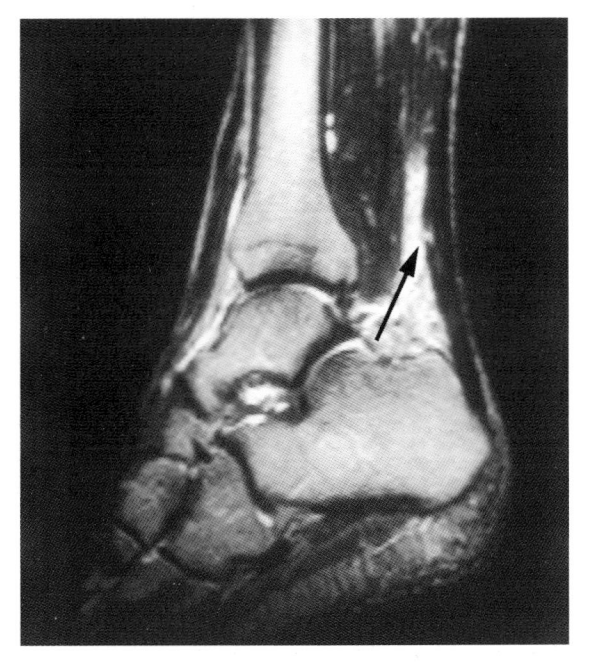

Figure 13.16 Partial tear of the Achilles (arrow).

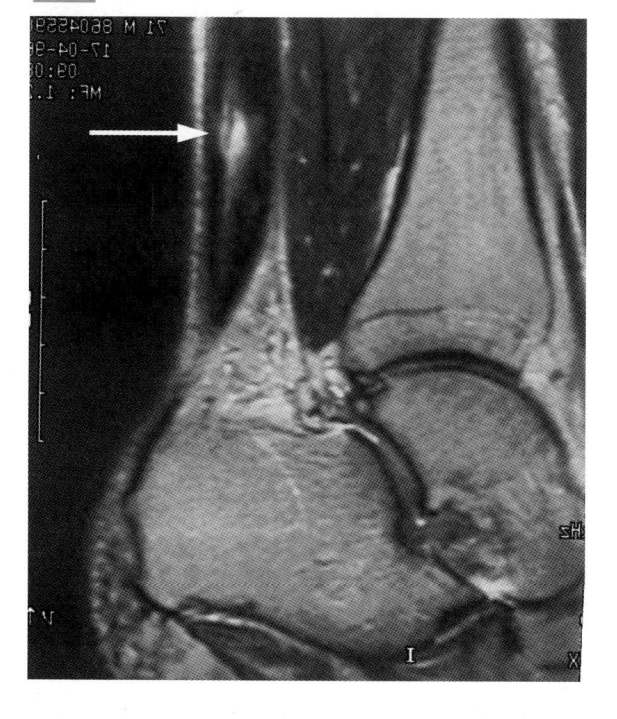

Figure 13.18 T2-weighted MRI shows cystic degeneration (arrow).

(d) A cyst, sometimes called 'red degeneration', which can be seen on scanning should be curetted out.

(e) Surgery to longitudinally split the tendon fibres and encourage vascular neogenesis.

Sports

(a) Athletics. A sudden increase in speed or distance may be too much for the tendon. Camber running encourages lateral movement of the calcaneum and bowing of the tendon. Repetition sprints with too little recovery time can fatigue the quadriceps causing an upset in calf/quadriceps coordination. Uphill running may produce overload of the Achilles.

(b) Hill walking and climbing. When climbing using the forefoot, the heel may drop too low increasing the forces on the Achilles; however, by using 'high heels', i.e. finding a rock to support the heel or zig-zag up using the sides of the foot, this problem is prevented.

(c) Cricket. Very often Achilles tears occur with the back foot shot played to mid wicket and a call for a quick single, so the weight is on the ball of the back foot when the knee straightens for the run, upsetting the calf/quadriceps coordination.

(d) All sports. Sudden acceleration from a bent knee position and a dorsiflexed foot.

Comment

It is the tendinopathy, a degenerative lesion, that delays healing and this damage may cause later rupture. Whether surgery with longitudinal splitting encourages invasion of new blood vessels to repair tissue, or whether post surgery the patient accepts a longer rehabilitation is still debatable. Certainly a patient with a tendinopathy can go all the way up the Achilles ladders, play four games and break down again so it is difficult to project when full recovery has occurred. Vitamin C encourages the formation of collagen from fibroblasts *in vitro*; however, collagen neogenesis is still the problem *in vivo*.

Combined Achilles lesion

Findings

A history of both a peritendinitis and tendinopathy with elements of rest pain and exercise induced pain (see *Achilles peritendinitis* and *Achilles tendinopathy*). Therefore exercise pain will still be present once the rest pain has settled with treatment.

Cause

An Achilles tendinopathy with surrounding peritendinitis.

Investigations

Diagnostic ultrasound to show thickening of the tendon and possibly the tendinopathy. MRI will display the paratendinitis on STIR and T2 and other fat suppressed sequences, and the tendinopathy on T1-weighted sequences (Fig. 13.19).

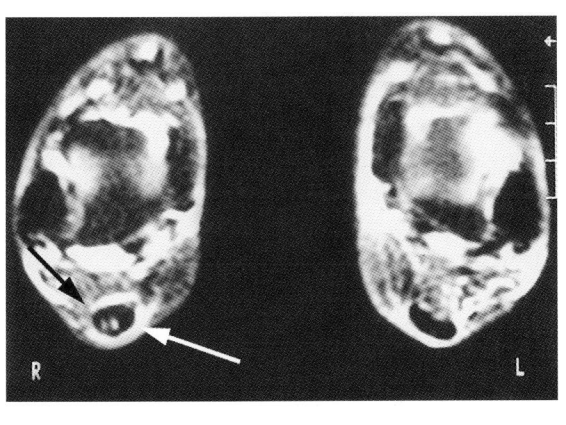

Figure 13.19 T2-weighted MRI showing a combined lesion with increased signal around the tendon from the peritendinitis and two areas of degeneration within the tendon.

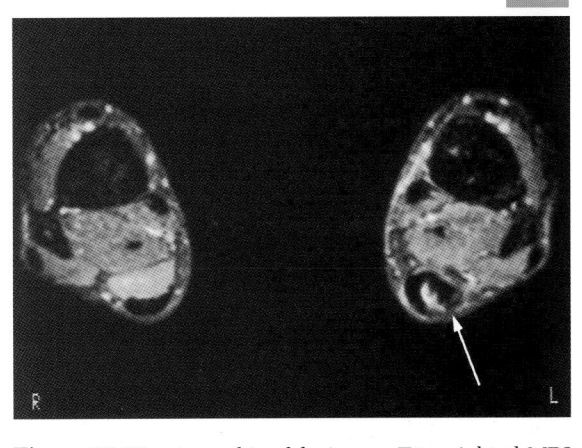

Figure 13.20 A combined lesion on T1-weighted MRI with nearly full thickness tendinopathy.

Treatment

The paratenon is an inflammatory lesion and responds to anti-inflammatory therapy, whereas the tendinopathy is a degenerative lesion and does not respond to anti-inflammatory therapy, therefore treatment with anti-inflammatory methods will help the peritendinous element. Electrotherapeutic and massage techniques to settle inflammation and prevent adhesions, or cortisone to the paratenon if required, but only whilst a history of morning and rest pain remains. The peritendinitis element usually settles in 1–2 weeks with this treatment, and the history converts to no morning and rest pain, and the exercise pain becomes dominant. Then start the Achilles ladders and stretching for the tendinopathy (see *Achilles tendinopathy*). Self massage, physiotherapy or ultrasound to the peritendon during rehabilitation will limit adhesions. Possible longitudinal splitting of the tendon for the non-progressing lesion and surgical strip of the paratenon if it becomes chronic and stenotic.

Sports

See *Achilles tendinopathy*.

Comment

This is the most common lesion of achillodynia. The pain of the paratenon will stop rehabilitation and produce a pain morbidity with daily activities so that when this is treated rehabilitation can be tolerated. Do not allow rehabilitation until clinical review 1–2 weeks after any cortisone injection, so that the extent of any underlying tendinopathy (Fig. 13.20) and therefore the type of rehabilitation can be assessed.

Retro Achilles bursa

Findings

There may be a history of pain at night and in the morning, initially feeling better with activity, but increasing the activity induces pain. There is painful reduced active and passive dorsiflexion of the ankle. Active plantar flexion is painful and there may be palpable tenderness over the bursa, which may be slightly swollen.

Cause

Inflammation in the bursa between the Achilles insertion (mid one-third of the calcaneum) and upper one-third of calcaneum and the overlying Achilles tendon (see Fig. 13.14), possibly from calcaneo-valgus or an overlying Achilles lesion. It may be part of Haglund's syndrome.

Caveat – Retro Achilles bursae are associated with seronegative or seropositive arthropathies.

Investigations

If a recurrence or not settling then do full blood count, ESR, auto-immune profile, HLA-B27 and Rh factor.

Treatment

(a) Hydrocortisone acetate to the bursa.
(b) Electrotherapeutic modalities to settle inflammation, such as ultrasound and laser.
(c) Treat any accompanying features of Haglund's syndrome.
(d) Treat any systemic cause.
(e) Remove or alter a tight heel cup or 'Achilles tag' from the shoes.
(f) Use a gel second skin.

Sports

See *Achilles tendinopathy*.

Comment

More common than expected and a surprising number are associated with systemic inflammatory problems.

Superficial Achilles bursa

Findings

Pain is located over the bursa which is locally tender to palpation and the pain may be worse in the morning, better on the move, then worse with increased activity. Active and passive dorsiflexion of the foot is painful. Resisted plantar flexion is pain-free. The pain is worse in shoes and the bursa may be red and swollen. It may be part of Haglund's syndrome.

Cause

Inflammation in the bursa between the posterior aspect of the calcaneum and the skin which is generally rubbed by the shoe (see Fig. 13.14).

Investigations

None clinically required.

Treatment

(a) Electrotherapeutic modalities to settle inflammation, such as ultrasound and laser.
(b) Cortisone injection into the bursa.
(c) Correct heel rub from the shoes by fitting grips at the side of the heel to hold the shoe but stop rubbing of the posterior aspect. Skin gels, slick plaster with soap or two pairs of socks that prevent rubbing between the shoe and skin.
(d) Check if calcaneo-valgus needs correcting.
(e) Check heel cups are not too hard or cut at an angle.
(f) See *Haglund's syndrome*.

Sports

Make certain shoes fit and are correct for the sport.

Comment

Steroid will settle the bursitis rapidly but the cause must then be corrected. Silicone gels are very effective to prevent rub.

Haglund's syndrome [13]

Findings

Large, thickened superficial Achilles bursa, known as a 'pump bump', caused by shoe rub. There is also an inflamed retro Achilles bursa (see *Retro Achilles bursa* and *Superficial Achilles bursa*).

Cause

A combination of retro and superficial Achilles bursae produced by a protuberant superior boss of the calcaneum rubbing against the shoe and Achilles tendon.

Investigations

Weight bearing X-ray to record the angle of calcaneum and assess the relevance of the superior calcaneal boss in causing pressure on the overlying structures.

Treatment
(a) Treat as for superficial and retro Achilles bursae.
(b) Use soft heel cups and even sandals to prevent local rubbing.
(c) Surgical removal of the calcaneal boss.

Sports
Obviously this syndrome is better with a sport that uses no shoes or sandals unless surgical correction is considered.

Comment
Fortunately rare. It is still better to adjust the shoes rather than the individual if at all possible.

Ruptured Achilles

Findings
(a) Prone lying foot attitude is vertical, whereas the normal foot has a degree of plantar flexion (Fig. 13.21).
(b) During prone lying, knee bent the ruptured Achilles foot lies horizontal whereas the normal lies with 20–30° of plantar flexion.
(c) Simmonds'/Thomson's squeeze test is positive (see *Glossary*).
(d) There may be a palpable gap in the tendon.
(e) The patient cannot rise on tip toe although passive dorsiflexion may be pain-free.
(f) The calcaneo-tibial compression test is negative (see Fig. 13.15) (see *Glossary*).

Cause
Acute overload of the Achilles, possibly with incoordination between the quadriceps and calf muscles, particularly if the calf muscle is actively working whilst the knee is bent. The rupture may occur *de novo* or following existing degeneration or partial tear of the tendon. It is more common in sedentary workers. Note that partial rupture of the Achilles can occur (see Fig. 13.16).

Investigations
None clinically required apart from recognizing the signs. Real-time ultrasound or MRI if in

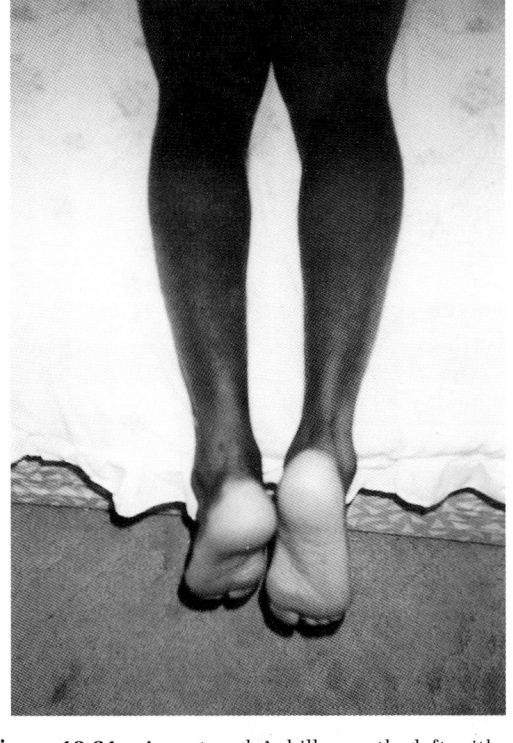

Figure 13.21 A ruptured Achilles on the left with vertical attitude of the foot.

doubt, or if consultation is several weeks after the rupture.

Treatment
(a) Surgery is probably advisable for sports-people.
(b) Cast brace in equinus.
(c) Postoperative rehabilitation via the Achilles ladders (see Chapter 20).
(d) Partial rupture may be treated initially as an Achilles tendinopathy.

Sports
See *Achilles tendinopathy*.

Comment
This diagnosis is still missed too frequently because too much emphasis is put on Simmonds'/Thomson's sign which may produce plantar flexion from squeezing the posterior tibialis muscle. The foot attitude is a very good

indicator. Late surgical repair may be undertaken but best results are obtained when done in the first 2 weeks.

Posterior tibio-fibular ligament

The posterior tibio-fibular ligament is a thickening of the posterior capsule – see below.

Posterior capsule

Findings

A history that fits with the cause given below, such as an inversion sprain of the ankle with plantar flexion, a foot forced into plantar flexion as in kicking a ball or having the kick blocked, a sudden stop which drives the heel into the ground or a sudden drop onto the heel such as missing the kerb or a step. The ankle is swollen with bruising on its lateral, medial and posterior aspects. To stand on tip toe is painful and the calcaneo-tibial compression test is positive (see Fig. 13.15) (see *Glossary*). A soccer player can side foot and chip the football but is not able to drive or volley the ball.

Cause

A compression injury between the calcaneum and posterior aspect of the tibia, bruising the structures that lie at the back of the ankle.

> **Caveat** – Os trigonum (Fig. 13.22)/Stieda process.

Investigations

X-ray to exclude an os trigonum and a Stieda process of the talus which may be fractured. Kager's triangle may be distorted on X-ray (see Fig. 13.14).

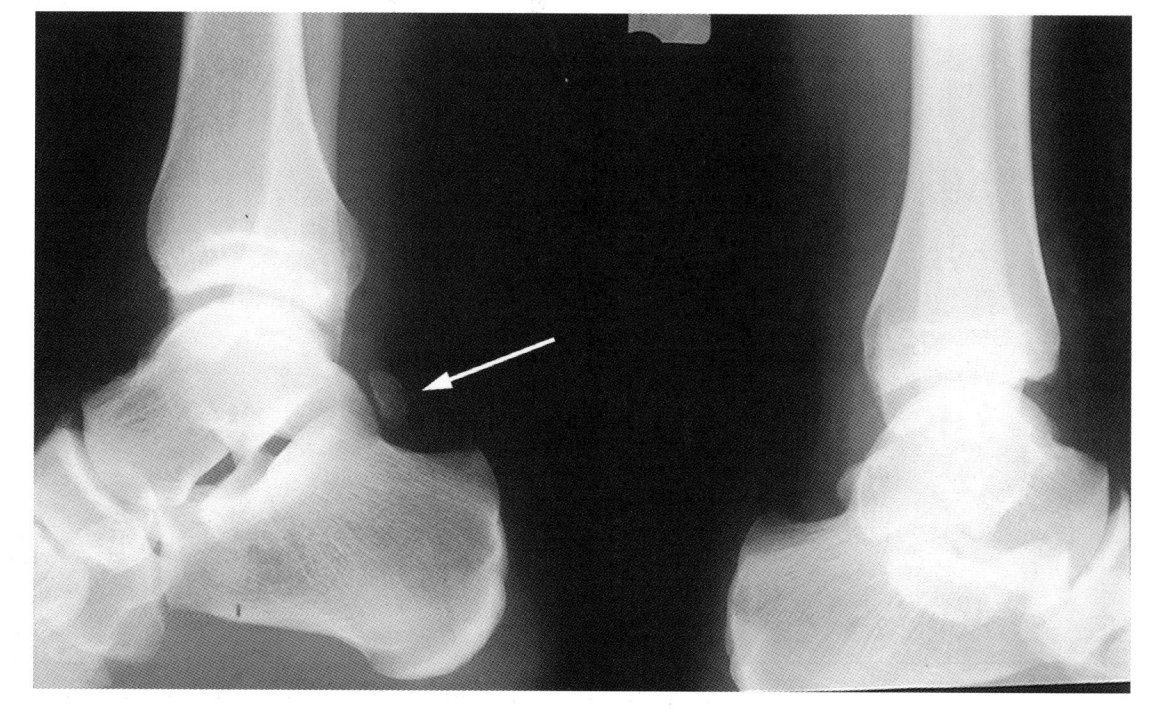

Figure 13.22 An os trigonum (arrow).

Treatment

As for bilateral bruising of lateral ligaments of ankle.

(a) Electrotherapeutic modalities to settle inflammation, such as shortwave diathermy and interferential.
(b) Inject into the posterior capsule and posterior tibio-fibular ligament of the ankle with cortisone.

Sports

(a) Ballet and high jump force this abutment of the calcaneum with the posterior structures of the ankle and must avoid plantar flexion until better.
(b) Footballers can train and use the kicking ladder (see Chapter 20) with side foot and chipping, but can only build into the drive/volley as the injury improves. Strapping to prevent forced plantar flexion may help.
(c) Checking suddenly at field hockey.
(d) Stamping the heel down during a squash shot produces posterior compression.

Comment

This is often the persistent pain, several months after an ankle injury has occurred and is often cured in 2–3 weeks with one or two steroid injections into the posterior structures around the talus and subtalar joint. It is often misdiagnosed as an Achilles problem but achillodynia does not have a positive calcaneo-tibial compression test.

Os trigonum/Stieda process

Findings

Active and passive plantar flexion is painful and the calcaneo-tibial compression test is positive (see Fig. 13.15) (see *Glossary*).

Cause

The os trigonum, a separated ossification centre of the talus, is trapped rather like a nut between the jaws of a nutcracker, the posterior surface of the calcaneum and the posterior tibia, during forced plantar flexion. The Stieda process is the fused os trigonum that leaves an elongated posterior element of the talus.

Investigations

Lateral X-ray of the ankle shows the os trigonum but many radiologists consider this a normal variant and make no mention of its existence, so you may have to request the presence of an os trigonum is to be reported. Both it and the Stieda process may fracture (see Fig. 13.22).

Treatment

(a) Electrotherapeutic modalities to settle inflammation, such as interferential and pulsed shortwave.
(b) Cortisone to the posterior aspect of the talar joint and around the os trigonum.
(c) Surgery to remove the os trigonum [14].

Sports

(a) See *Posterior tibio-fibular ligament*.
(b) Ballet and high jump will require surgery to remove the os trigonum if this is a persistent problem. Other sports only need the acute episode treating conservatively.

Comment

Although not common, it can be very problematical for those requiring large degrees of plantar flexion and surgery is probably the treatment of choice in these cases.

Lateral process of talus fracture

Snow boarders produce some unusual fractures around the ankle of which the lateral process of the talus was the most frequent and, as with all undiagnosed ankle pain, the bone scan is the watershed investigation. CT rather than X-ray or MRI is most suitable [15]. Although most of these fractures are traumatic, a possible stress fracture in this area may occur [16].

Sever's disease

Findings
Pain over the posterior aspect of the calcaneum but also about 2 cm along the medial or lateral side of the calcaneum that is painful to palpation.

Type 1 Is worse on impact but heals faster.
Type 2 Is worse on lift off of the foot and takes longer to heal.

Cause
Not a disease but a calcaneal epiphyseal problem in children.

Type 1 An epiphysitis from impact of the calcaneal epiphysis.
Type 2 An apophysitis from the pull of the Achilles.

Investigations
None clinically required and an X-ray is difficult to interpret as the normal epiphysis is irregular and does show some sclerosis (Fig. 13.23).

Treatment
(a) A heel raise may help type 2.
(b) Reduction in the amount of exercise.
(c) Ensure that the shoes have the best shock absorbability.
(d) If limping during exercise then the child should be removed from exercise.

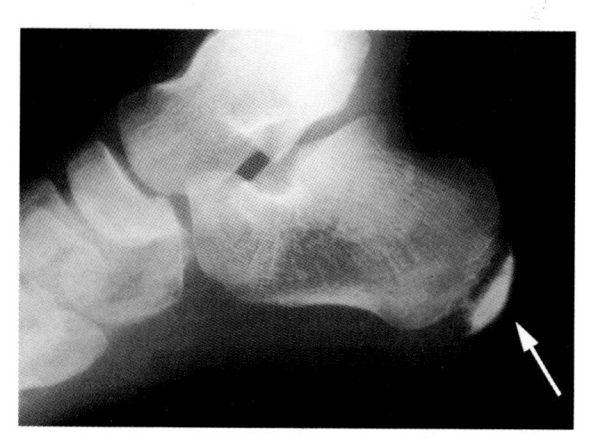

Figure 13.23 An X-ray of a child with Sever's showing the calcaneal apophysis.

(e) If the heel hurts after exercise but is better by morning, maintain the exercise level.
(f) If the heel hurts in the morning when walking then reduce activity by 10–50%.
(g) Occasionally a walking cast brace to rest the heel for 2–3 weeks is required.

Sports
Type 1 is the more general and occurs in those running a lot or playing on hard ground. Type 2 occurs more in gymnasts, jumpers and ballet dancers.

Comment
I have never seen long-term problems with this condition so titrate the amount of exercise against pain and maintain the child in activities with its peers if at all possible. I have seen a very irregular calcaneal epiphysis following a fall and this needed cast bracing and a very long time to settle, suggesting that it was probably a traumatic epiphyseal fracture.

Flexor hallucis tenovaginitis

Pain from the flexor hallucis may be felt immediately behind the medial maleolus and sometimes in its muscle which lies just behind and proximal to the ankle joint. It is particularly associated with ballet dancers and the tendon may rupture (see *Flexor hallucis* – Chapter 13).

Further reading

1. Boytim, M. J., Fischer, D. A. and Neumann, L. (1991) Syndesmotic ankle sprains. *Am. J. Sports Med.* **19**, 294–298.
2. Taylor, D. C., Englehardt, D. L. and Bassett, F. H. (1992) Syndesmal sprains of the ankle. The influence of heterotopic ossification. *Am. J. Sports Med.* **20**, 146–150.
3. Miller, C. D., Shelton, W. R., *et al.* (1995) Deltoid and syndesmosis ligament injury of the ankle without fracture. *Am. J. Sports Med.* **23**, 746–750.
4. Orava, S., Karpakka, J., Hulkko, A. and Takala, T. (1991) Stress avulsion fracture of the tarsal navi-

cular. An uncommon sports-related overuse injury. *Am. J. Sports Med.* **19**, 392–395.

5. Ferkel, R. D., Carzel, R. P., *et al.* (1991) Arthroscopic treatment of antero lateral impingement of the ankle. *Am. J. Sports Med.* **19**, 440–446.

6. Firer, P. (1990) Effectiveness of taping for the prevention of ankle ligament sprains. *Br. J. Sports Med.* **24**, 47–50.

7. Liu, S. H. and Baker, C. L. (1994) Comparison of lateral ankle ligamentous reconstruction procedures. *Am. J. Sports Med.* **22**, 313–317.

8. Kollias, S. L. and Ferkel, R. D. (1997) Fibular grooving for recurrent peroneal tendon subluxation. *Am. J. Sports Med.* **25**, 329–335.

9. Jackson, D. L. and Haglund, B. (1991) Tarsal tunnel syndrome in athletes. Case reports and literature review. *Am. J. Sports Med.* **19**, 61–65.

10. Read, M. T. F. and Motto, S. (1992) Tendo Achillis pain: steroids and outcome. *Br. J. Sports Med.* **26**, 15–21.

11. Read, M. T. F. (1999) Safe relief of rest pain that eases with activity in achillodynia by intrabursal or peritendinous steroid injections: the rupture rate was not increased by these steroid injections. *Br. J. Sports Med.* **33**, 134–135.

12. Hutson, M. A. (ed.) (1996) *Sports Injuries: Recognition and Management*, 2nd edn. Oxford Medical Publications, Oxford.

13. Rossi, F., La Cava, F., Amato, F. and Pincelli, G. (1987) The Haglund syndrome (H.s.): clinical and radiological features and sports medicine aspects. *J. Sports Med.* **27**, 258–263.

14. Marotta, J. J. and Micheli, L. J. (1992) Os trigonum impingement in dancers. *Am. J. Sports Med.* **20**, 533–536.

15. Kilpatrick, D. P., Hunter, R. E., *et al.* (1998) The snowboarder's foot and ankle. *Am. J. Sports Med.* **26**, 271–277.

16. Motto, S. G. (1993) Stress fracture of the lateral process of the talus – a case report. *Br. J. Sports Med.* **27**, 275–276.

Bruckner, P. and Khan, K. (1993) *Clinical Sports Medicine*. McGraw-Hill, New York.

Reid, D. (1992) *Sports Injury Assessment and Rehabilitation*. Churchill Livingstone, Edinburgh.

14

Heel and arch of the foot

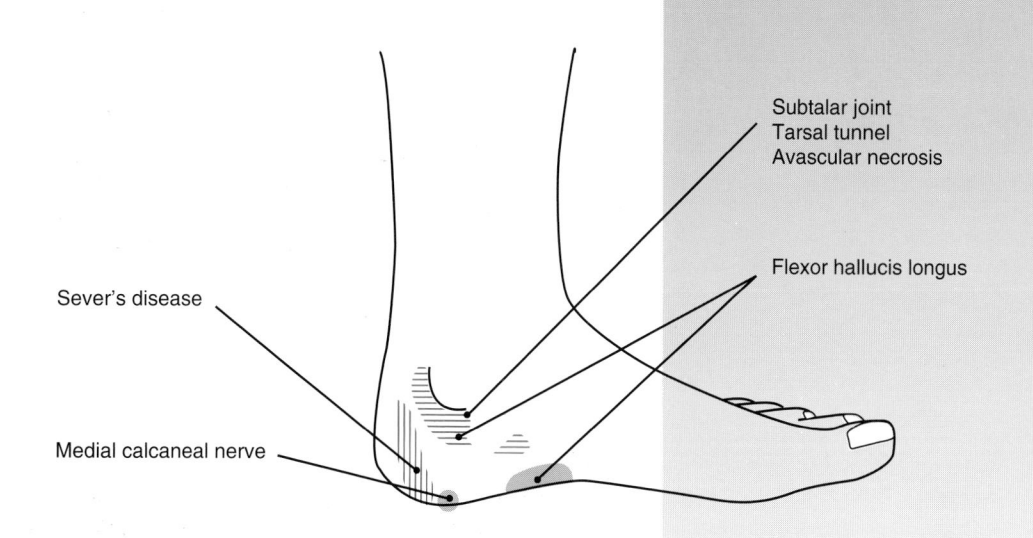

Subtalar joint
Tarsal tunnel
Avascular necrosis

Flexor hallucis longus

Sever's disease

Medial calcaneal nerve

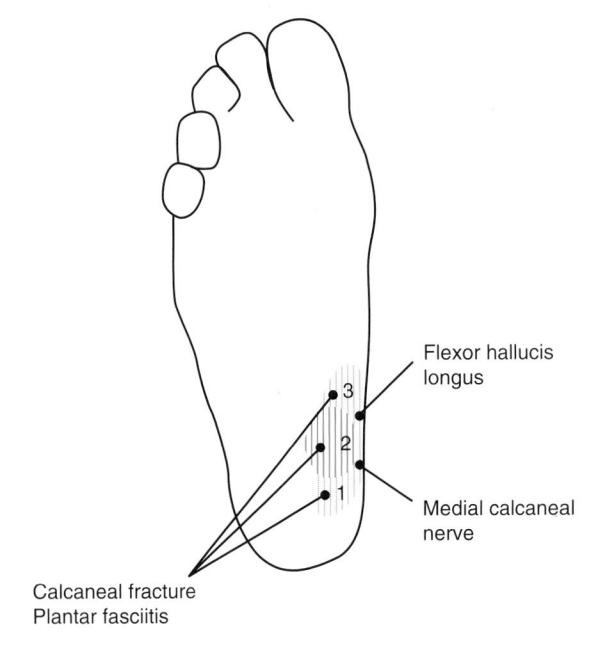

Flexor hallucis longus

Medial calcaneal nerve

Calcaneal fracture
Plantar fasciitis

Plantar fasciitis

Findings

Type 1 Pain over the inferior surface of the calcaneum, worse with direct pressure which is eased by squeezing the margins of the fat pad at the same time.

Type 2 As for type 1, but also the pain can occur with forced dorsiflexion of the foot and toes, and especially rocking up over the balls of the feet and toes at a 45° angle, such as a sprint start position.

Type 3 History of acute or semi-acute pain often under the arch of the foot and the tenderness is not under the calcaneum but over the spring ligament, which may be thickened and tender.

Cause

Possibly plantar fasciitis is a 'catch-all' phrase that may include flexor hallucis and medial calcaneal nerve problems as well.

Type 1 Damage to the fat pad of the heel, often in the more elderly. The fibrous stroma sep-

arates compartments of fat, so that during compression the loculated fat is prevented from spreading and therefore acts as a good shock absorber. When the stroma weakens the fat pad becomes functionally thinner, thus allowing impact to reach the calcaneal periosteum.

Type 2 An enthesitis of the plantar fascia.

Type 3 Plantar fascial tears or a degenerative lesion within the spring ligament.

Caveat – Gout, spondylarthropathies, L5/S1 disc, calcaneal stress fracture, medial calcaneal nerve entrapment and flexor hallucis tendinitis.

Investigations

None clinically required unless failing to respond to treatment, then X-ray. The spur is considered non-causative of plantar fasciitis, but it just might reflect the pull on the enthesis (Fig. 14.1). MRI will help display plantar fasciitis or a tear in the spring ligament. Blood tests (uric acid, AIP, ESR and HLA-B27). Bone scan for damage to the enthesis and to exclude a calcaneal fracture.

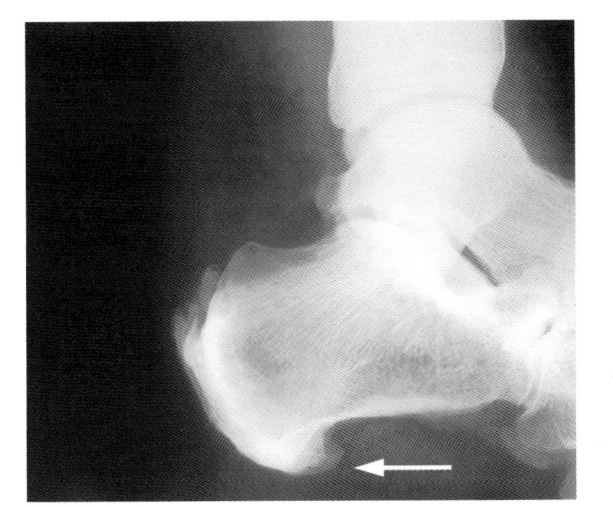

Figure 14.1 A plantar fascial spur. This patient also has an Achilles spur. Some people appear prone to entheseal stress lesions.

Treatment

Type 1:

(a) Orthosis to squeeze the fat pad, diminish impact and correct calcaneo-valgus.
(b) Dye strapping to squeeze the fat pad.
(c) 'Air-soled' shoes which use the same principle as the stroma of the fat pad but will reduce impact.
(d) Non-impact cross-training such as biking, rowing or swimming.
(e) Electrotherapeutic modalities to settle inflammation, such as ultrasound.
(f) Trial of cortisone to settle inflammation in fat and around the periosteum.

Type 2:
(a) Treat as for type 1.
(b) Use a heel raise in the early phase.
(c) Cortisone injection to the enthesis.
(d) Stretch and load the enthesis by rocking over the toes as in a sprint start.
(e) Do heel raises on the edge of a stair so that the heel can be dropped lower to stretch the spring ligament and then load it by standing on tip toe.
(f) Train via the Achilles ladder (see Chapter 20).

Type 3:
(a) Electrotherapeutic modalities to settle inflammation, such as ultrasound.
(b) Rest and shorten the spring ligament with a heel raise, and then gradually reduce the height of the heel raise as the injury repairs.
(c) Gradually introduce stretch and load as in type 2 (d)–(f).

Comment

This is a troublesome condition that takes several months to settle. Defining the lesion will make rehabilitation and treatment easier. A heel raise in types 2 and 3 may be made of sheets of paper reduced by one a day, to gradually stretch out the plantar fascia. I think only type 2 and, occasionally, rather like a peritendinitis, type 3, respond to cortisone. Both need rehabilitation afterwards. My injection rate fell when I used a shock absorbent orthotic with edges that squeeze the heel pad for type 1.

Medial calcaneal nerve

Findings

Linear pain to palpation over the medial inferior calcaneum and a history of heel pain, worse on impact, that may also cause pain at night.

Cause

Compression of the medial calcaneal nerve as it passes over the medial side of the calcaneum into the heel pad. Usually with calcaneo-valgus, though poorly fitting heel wedges or orthotics may cause irritation of the nerve between the shoe and orthotic. The medial calcaneal nerve may be caught in scar tissue of the damaged plantar fascia.

Investigations

As for plantar fasciitis but EMG is not of value.

Treatment

(a) Correct any calcaneo-valgus with a medial heel wedge or orthotic.
(b) Perineural cortisone.
(c) Treat any accompanying plantar fasciitis.

Sports

Avoid impact sports, check the running style and that shoes, especially the heel cups, are not broken down producing a functional calcaneo-valgus. Fit the appropriate orthotics (see *Plantar fasciitis*). Achilles ladder (see Chapter 20).

Comment

This is possibly more common than is usually recognized and is part of the plantar fasciitis complex; however, in spite of the correct treatment, it takes a while to settle.

Sever's disease

Pain over the postero-medial or postero-lateral calcaneum on palpation in a child (see Chapter 13).

Flexor hallucis longus

This muscle is the most distal of the posterior calf muscles, and pain is worse on tip toe and resisted toe flexion (see Chapter 13)

Subtalar joint

See *Sinus tarsi*.

Sinus tarsi

Findings
(a) The sinus tarsi is the route by which an injection may be placed at the ligament at the neck of the talus which when strained may have lateral mid foot and ankle pain.
(b) Subtalar passive movement of inversion and eversion is painful. The range of movement may be reduced and have an obvious calcaneo-valgus.
(c) Sometimes a history of trauma and osteoarthritis of the talar and talo-navicular joints accompanies this problem.
(d) There is frequently pain on impact of the heel but it may be pain-free at rest.

Cause
(a) Osteoarthritis from chronic calcaneo-valgus or secondary to trauma.
(b) Sprain of the ligament to the neck of the talus at the base of the sinus tarsi.
(c) Avascular necrosis (see Fig. 13.8).

Investigations
(a) X-rays for degenerative changes.
(b) Bone scan as a screen, particularly for degenerative osteoarthritis, avascular necrosis or fracture, then MRI or CT scan if the bone scan is hot.

Treatment
(a) Electrotherapeutic modalities to settle inflammation and ease pain, such as shortwave diathermy or interferential.
(b) Cortisone injection of the subtalar joint by a posterior, lateral or sinus tarsi approach.
(c) Orthotic to control subtalar movement.
(d) Avoidance of causes for avascular necrosis, such as alcohol.
(e) Fusion of the joint surgically.

Sports
(a) Sports that impact on the foot prove to be a problem and may have to be abandoned if chronic changes of osteoarthritis have occurred.
(b) Golfers may have to turn their left foot out and open the stance as they cannot roll over this foot during the follow through.

Comment
Not common. Injection via the sinus tarsi is the best initial approach, but they may need manipulation under anaesthetic and injection for the chronic strains that have scarred up the joint. MRI shows up avascular necrosis earlier than CT.

Tarsal coalition

Findings
Usually incidental because a stiff foot does not functionally pronate well and therefore tracking knee problems, recurrent ankle sprain or anterior ankle pain leads to the diagnosis. The mid tarsal joint and subtalar joints are immobile.

Cause
Fibrous cartilage or bony fusion between the calcaneum and the talus, and sometimes cuboid and calcaneum.

Investigations
X-ray (Fig. 14.2) or CT scan.

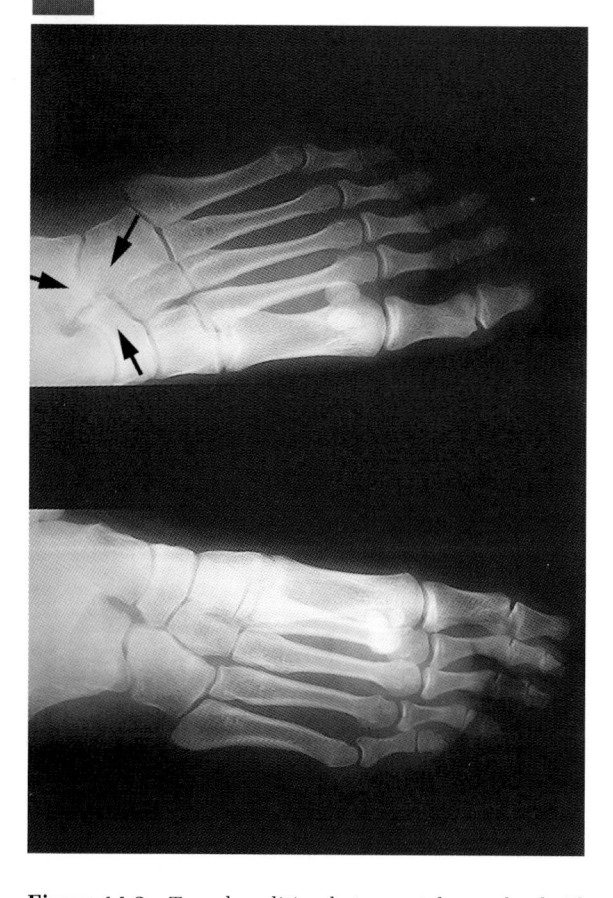

Figure 14.2 Tarsal coalition between talus and cuboid and a bridging of the navicular (arrows).

Treatment
Needs only be directed to the secondary affected areas, although a heel raise may help the patient to move through the foot more easily as this reduces the requirement for pronation.

Sports
Change of direction sports may be influenced by a stiffer foot and running may produce secondary injuries such as knee tracking problems. The ideal is therefore non-impact sports, but slowing down the rate of loading in impact sports will allow secondary areas to adapt.

Comment
Early advice concerning this problem will help the patient to move to a more appropriate sport.

Tarsal tunnel

Heel and arch pain that is accompanied by 'pins and needles', numbness or weakness that is tender over the tarsal tunnel (see Chapter 13).

Avascular necrosis

Subtalar joint pain that is non-diagnostic should have a bone scan. Avascular necrosis often affects the subtalar joint involving the calcaneum and/or talus. Orthotics may help to stabilize the joint and a reduction in causative factors such as alcohol are advised.

Calcaneal fracture

Findings
Pain on impact on the calcaneum from walking and locally tender to pressure.

Cause
From acute impact landing on the heel but it may also present as a stress fracture with insidious onset.

Investigations
X-ray with a history of acute trauma. Bone scan if chronic undiagnosed heel pain and then CT or MRI if the bone scan is positive.

Treatment
A protective cast with a mid foot rocker and later soft absorbent soles rather than hard shoes.

Sports
Jumping into the shallow end of a swimming pool is the most common cause of calcaneal fracture. Continue non-impact sports whilst waiting for bone repair.

Comment

I personally have only seen one stress fracture of the calcaneum in nearly three decades of dealing with sports injuries, though some colleagues feel it is reasonably common.

Further reading

Bruckner, P. and Khan, K. (1993) *Clinical Sports Medicine*. McGraw-Hill, New York.

Reid, D. (1992) *Sports Injury Assessment and Rehabilitation*. Churchill Livingstone, Edinburgh.

15

Mid foot

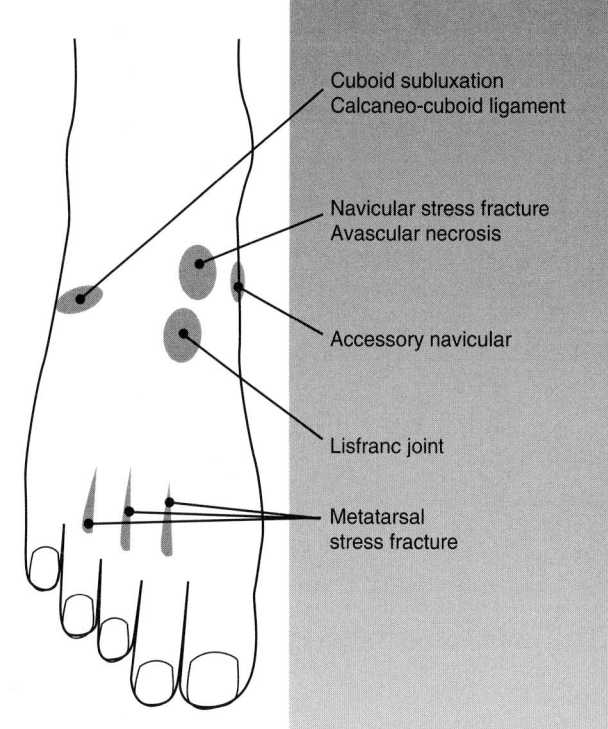

Cuboid subluxation
Calcaneo-cuboid ligament

Navicular stress fracture
Avascular necrosis

Accessory navicular

Lisfranc joint

Metatarsal
stress fracture

Calcaneo-cuboid ligament

Findings
Invariably injured during an ankle sprain when bruising is found also over the mid foot tracking to the toes, but it is often the cause of an ankle injury not getting better. Rough ground is particularly troublesome, and pain is produced on pronating and supinating the mid and forefoot across the mid tarsal joint. There is tenderness to palpation over the calcaneo-cuboid joint.

Cause
Part of the inversion sprain mechanism where more stress has passed through the mid tarsal joint, straining the ligaments between the calcaneum and cuboid.

Investigations
None clinically required.

Treatment
(a) RICE.
(b) Injection of cortisone to the calcaneo-cuboid ligament.
(c) Electrotherapeutic modalities to settle inflammation in the ligament and joint, such as ultrasound, laser and interferential.
(d) Rehabilitation as for a sprained ankle (see Chapter 13).
(e) Soft arch orthotic to rest the joint.

Sports
As for a sprained ankle, but twisting, turning sports may require orthotics and strapping of the mid tarsal joint to reduce movement through this joint for 6–8 weeks after pain-free (see Chapter 13).

Comment
This does not seem to improve with physiotherapy and injection just into the joint capsule works well. It is one of the causes of persistent pain after an ankle sprain.

Cuboid subluxation

Findings
There is no history of an inversion sprain, but there is pain on jumping and landing and rough ground. The mid tarsal joint has pain on passive testing in plantar flexion as well as supination and pronation. It is locally tender to palpation over the calcaneo-cuboid ligament and cuboid.

Cause
Pain in the foot of ballet dancers [1].

Investigations
None clinically required.

Treatment
Plantar flexing manipulations, pivoting over the cuboid.

Sports
Ballet dancers may maintain foot range with self manipulation.

Comment
Well reported and written up in dancers but not other sports. Manipulation seems to be corrective.

Accessory navicular

Findings
May present as rubbing of the skin over the prominent tubercle or as a posterior tibialis tendinitis (see Chapter 13).

Cause
The unfused ossification centre of the tubercle of the navicular or in the adult with fibrous union does not withstand loads as well as the fused tubercle, or it may be rubbed by the shoe and both causes are worse in the over pronator.

Investigations
X-ray but ask for the presence of an accessory navicular to be reported as it is a normal variant

and therefore it is often not commented upon (see Fig. 13.12).

Treatment

As for posterior tibialis tendinitis (see Chapter 13); however, it may require a permanent orthotic to reduce the loads or alter its prominence. It takes longer to heal than expected for the posterior tibialis enthesitis.

Comment

This seems to present mainly in adolescence; adults appear adapted to the problem even when an accessory navicular is visible on X-ray. An explanation to the patient and parents of its longish morbidity is essential (see *Glossary* and Fig. 13.12).

Navicular stress fracture

Findings

Acute or insidious onset of pain over the mid foot, but clinical examination may or may not produce pain on passive mid tarsal joint movements. However, it is usually tender to direct palpation over the navicular.

Cause

Stress fracture of the navicular seems to occur in sprint, jump and interval sprint games, but not in endurance events, perhaps because it gets impacted by the talus in the tip toe position.

> **Caveat** – This fracture is often missed. An index of suspicion or tenderness over the navicular is reason to investigate further.

Investigations

X-ray often misses this sagitally placed fracture and a bone scan is the watershed investigation. If it is hot then investigate further with a CT or MRI scan.

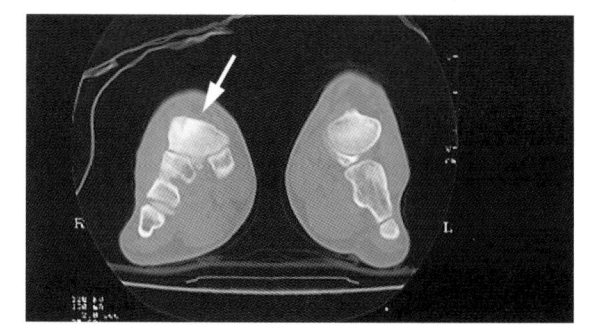

Figure 15.1 CT scan showing non-union of the navicular with sclerosis and separation of fracture.

Treatment

Cast brace and non-weight bearing for 1 month if the scans show no widening of the fracture or sclerosis, then weight bearing for 1 month in cast brace. Later weight-bearing rehabilitation through the Achilles ladders with caution for up to 3–4 months (see Chapter 20) [2].

> **Caveat** – The navicular is prone to non-union (Fig. 15.1) and a compression screw is required.

Sports

(a) Athletics – seems to occur in sprints up to 400 m, jumps and hurdles.
(b) Field hockey – has become more common since the advent of the 'plastic surface'.
(c) Cross-training and local muscle strengthening must be maintained.
(d) Impact should be severely limited until healed but can be introduced on rebound trampettes.

Comment

This is an often missed fracture. Too often this injury presents months after its onset and often when non-union is established. A negative X-ray does not rule out this injury and a bone scan should be ordered if there is any element of doubt whatsoever, because the morbidity of this problem is excessive. If the bone scan is positive do not treat conservatively on this fact alone, do a CT to check on non-union and if in doubt about non-union then it probably should have a compression screw.

Tarsal coalition

Stiffness of the mid tarsal joint may be caused by a coalition (see Chapter 14).

Avascular necrosis of the navicular in young children

Tenderness over the navicular and limping in the young child (*Kohler's disease*; see *Glossary*).

Lisfranc joint – second tarso-metatarsal arthrosis

Findings
A presentation in dancers, especially ballet, of mid foot pain and tenderness over the second tarso-metatarsal joint [3].

Cause
Type 1 A synovitis of this joint.
Type 2 A stress fracture of the proximal second metatarsal.

Investigations
X-ray may show the expected thickening and sclerosis of the second metatarsal, but it does not differentiate the lesion. Bone scan will indicate stress around this joint, but MRI should follow to display an oblique fracture or bony bruising, or a synovitis.

Treatment
Type 1 May be treated with anti-inflammatories, NSAIDs, electrical modalities or cortisone and relative rest. This rest should be in training, avoiding all demi and full point work plus jumps, but performance can be permitted as long as progress is being maintained.
Type 2 Should be removed from dancing and might require a cast brace or even surgery to remove necrotic bone fragments.

Sports
Ballet dancing.

Comment
This is one of those under-diagnosed problems as all dancers expect to have some aches from the Lisfranc joint, but some have a stress fracture.

Further reading

1. Marshall, P. and Hamilton, W. G. (1992) Cuboid subluxation in ballet dancers. *Am. J. Sports Med.* **20**, 169–175.
2. Khan, K. M., Fuller, P. J., *et al.* (1992) Outcome of conservative and surgical management of navicular stress fracture in athletes. *Am. J. Sports. Med.* **20**, 657–666.
3. Harrington, T., Crichton, K. J. and Anderson, I. F. (1993) Overuse ballet injury of the base of the second metatarsal. A diagnostic problem. *Am. J. Sports Med.* **21**, 591–598.

Bruckner, P. and Khan, K. (1993) *Clinical Sports Medicine.* McGraw-Hill, New York.
Reid, D. (1992) *Sports Injury Assessment and Rehabilitation.* Churchill Livingstone, Edinburgh.

16

Forefoot

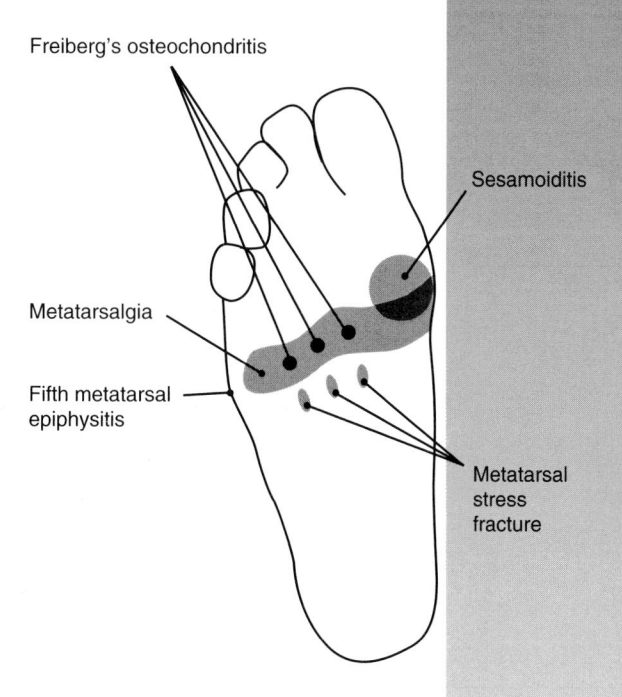

Freiberg's osteochondritis

Sesamoiditis

Metatarsalgia

Fifth metatarsal
epiphysitis

Metatarsal
stress
fracture

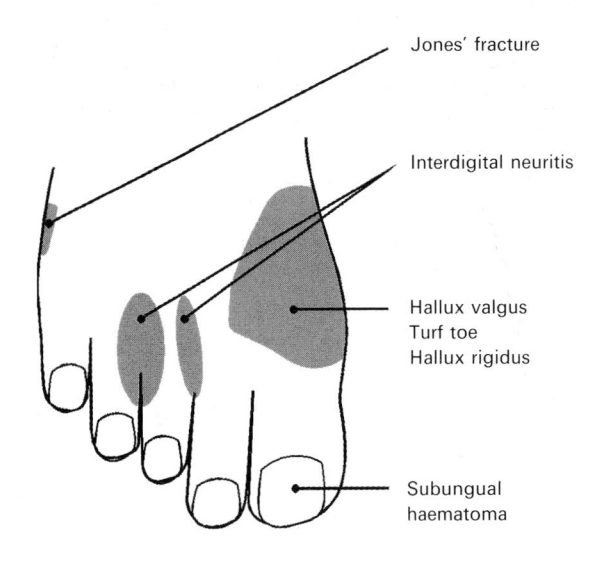

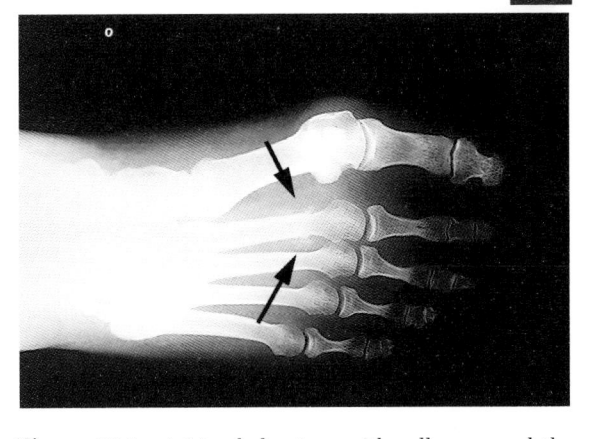

Figure 16.1 A March fracture with callus around the second metatarsal.

Metatarsal stress fracture (march fracture)

Findings
Generally a history of gradual onset of pain with activities, although the onset can be acute. The pain is worse on impact, better with rest. There may be puffy swelling of the forefoot with local tenderness to palpation over the metatarsal shaft on both superior and inferior surfaces. A metatarsalgia and interdigital neuritis may accompany this problem (see *Metatarsalgia* and *Interdigital neuritis*).

Cause
A stress fracture of the shaft of the second, third or fourth metatarsal from too rapid incremental loads. Often seen in army recruits about 3–4 weeks into training.

Investigations
X-ray (Fig. 16.1); however, as the X-ray can be negative for up to 2–3 weeks, bone scan if in doubt.

Treatment
Rest from impact for 6–8 weeks but cross-train, by exercise such as swimming, biking or rowing to maintain fitness. Use firm shoes to act as splint and the Achilles ladder on return to activity (see Chapter 20).

Sports
Usually from running, but can occur with walking and change of direction sports.

Comment
A puffy forefoot with local tenderness is a stress fracture in spite of negative X-rays. Repeat the X-rays 2–3 weeks later or bone scan instead.

Metatarsalgia

Findings
(a) Pain on standing or walking but more particularly on standing on tip toes or running with forefoot impact on the metatarsal heads.
(b) Tender to palpation on the inferior surface and may have pain on passive dorsi- or plantar flexion of the joint.
(c) The foot may have claw toes and be in equinus.
(d) There may be an accompanying interdigital neuritis from the swollen capsule and soft tissue compressing the nerve.

Cause
Impact on the metatarsal heads causing bony bruising, joint and soft tissue swelling. Often

from a clawed or subluxed metatarsal tarsal joint. May be a presentation for systemic joint disease such as rheumatoid.

Investigations
X-ray to exclude Freiberg's infraction in an adolescent and stress fracture in an adult. Blood tests for systemic joint disease. Bone scan may be 'hot' in all three differentials.

Treatment
In a normal foot:

(a) Rest from impact sports, with non-impact cross-training.
(b) Electrotherapeutic modalities to settle inflammation, such as interferential, ultrasound and laser.
(c) NSAIDs.
(d) Metatarsal transverse arch orthotic proximal to the metatarsal heads to raise the metatarsal head from impact.
(e) Reintroduce impact with an orthotic and increment into sprints via the Achilles ladder (see Chapter 20).

In the equinus foot:

(a) A cast made orthotic to spread the loads and silicone pads under the tips of the toes to help them exert pressure on the ground.
(b) Chiropody for calluses.
(c) Avoid impact sports.
(d) Surgery.

Caveat – The diabetic foot and rheumatoid.

Sports
(a) This develops in a normal foot with sprint drills, especially in a runner who has a low knee carry and in a shuffle runner unused to impacting and driving through the forefoot for speed as sprinting requires forefoot propulsion. These drills need to be introduced more slowly to allow adaptation.
(b) Stop/start games, especially netball, where the sudden stop is mandatory, will impact on the metatarsals.

Comment
The equinus foot should be introduced to non-impact sports, but many have adapted over the years producing large calluses, and they too often have tried something new or incremented their activity too fast and only require treatment of the immediate problem.

Freiberg's osteochondritis/infraction

Findings
Local tenderness over the metatarso-phalangeal joint in adolescents with a history of pain on impact of foot on the ground.

Cause
Osteochondritis, possibly avascular, of the distal head of the metatarsus, usually second or third in adolescents. Sometimes known as Kohler's second disease.

Investigations
X-ray shows squaring of metatarsal head (Fig. 16.2).

Treatment
This takes several years to settle with a transverse arch or metatarsal pad to help. Avoid impact sports and high heels; well-padded shoes are required. NSAIDs can help as required. Surgery can have a place [1].

Sports
Avoid impact sports. May try impact games on soft surfaces to tolerance until the problem settles.

Comment
This is a real nuisance as it requires a quantum shift from impact to non-impact sport until the problem settles, although the patient may play goalkeeper in team games, for instance.

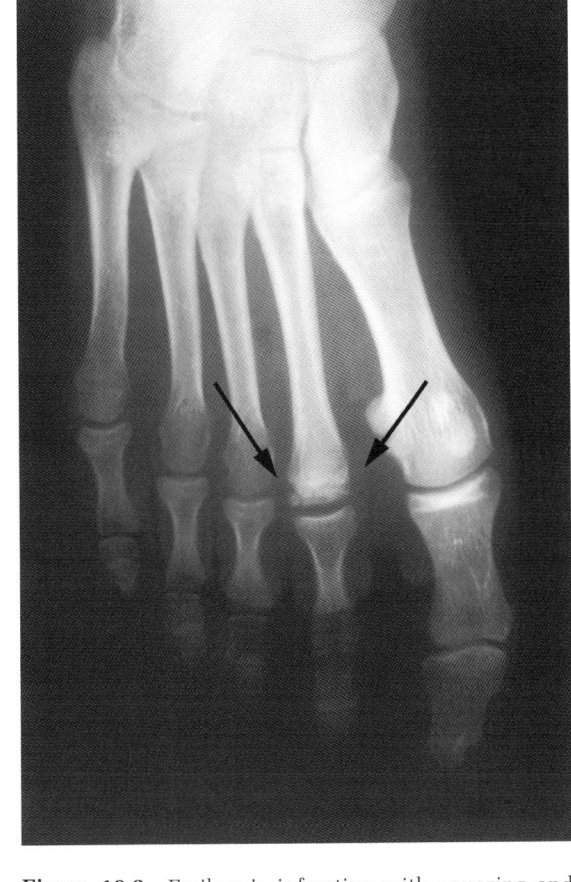

Figure 16.2 Freiburg's infraction with squaring and fragmentation of the second metatarsal.

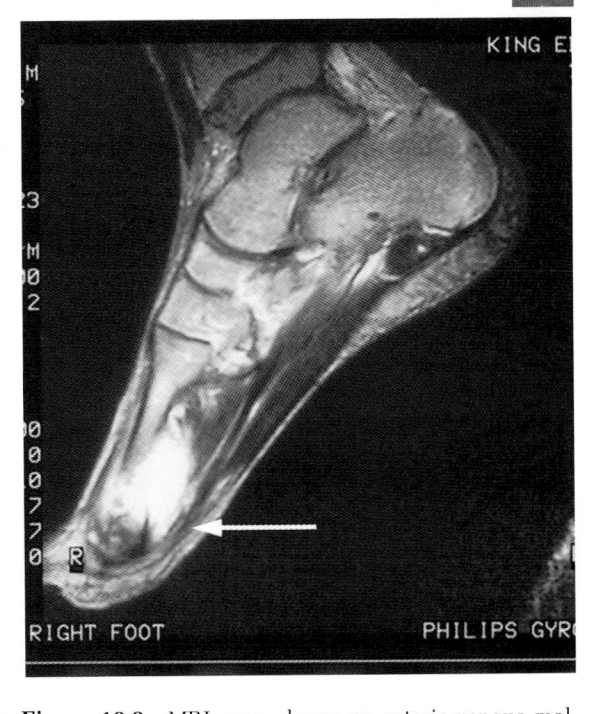

Figure 16.3 MRI scan shows an arterio-venous malformation that mimicked interdigital neuritis.

Cause

Irritation of the interdigital nerve between the head of the metatarsal or a neuroma in this area, known as Morton's neuroma. Most often caused by compression from shoes that are too narrow.

Investigations

X-ray or bone scan for possible provoking causes such as a fracture (see Fig. 16.1). MRI may be required for rare soft tissue lesions involving the nerve (Fig. 16.3).

Treatment

(a) Widen the shoes.
(b) Metatarsal transverse arch orthotic just proximal to the metatarsal heads.
(c) Treat other causes.
(d) Perineural steroid.
(e) Surgery for interdigital neuroma (Morton's neuroma).

Interdigital neuritis

Findings

Pain around the metatarsal heads that may refer down adjacent sides of the relevant two toes, usually 2/3 and 3/4. There may be pain on non-weight bearing as well as weight bearing which can wake the patient at night. Squeezing the metatarsal heads together provokes pain, and this can be worse in tight shoes and better with bare feet. Look also for factors that provoke the problem such as increased pronation, metatarsalgia and march fracture (see *Glossary*, *Metatarsalgia* and *Metatarsal stress fracture*).

Sports

Avoid impact sports and cross-train, non-impact, such as cycling, rowing or swimming, but may have to pedal cycle by using the arch of the foot and not the ball, and may not be able to use a rowing machine, again because of pressure over the ball of the foot. When walking has become pain-free, may try running.

Comment

Wider shoes and corrective orthotics often are curative and probably if seen early enough prevent a neuroma from forming. Locally placed orthopaedic felt as a transverse arch elevator can prove sufficient to widen the interdigital space in the early stages as long as the narrow shoes which caused the nerve irritation are changed.

Hallux valgus

Findings

Painless, occasionally painful, valgus of the great toe and accompanying findings that fit with the causes. When painful, all movements of the great toe hurt, but usually it is superficial over the medial aspect, where the bursa is inflamed and may be red and swollen (the bunion).

Cause

As part of the first ray adductus valgus or secondary effect to overpronation, especially with forefoot varus. The shoe may be too pointed, thus constricting the toes, and it may occur with Morton's toe (second toe longer than the first toe).

Investigations

None clinically required, but X-ray to assess metatarso-phalangeal joint for osteoarthritis.

Treatment

(a) Correction of overpronation. However, in the mobile foot with forefoot varus the first ray should be allowed to drop towards the ground by only correcting the hind foot and supporting the longitudinal arch, but with a fixed first ray, correction of the varus defor-

mity with forefoot wedges in the orthotics is required.

(b) Press out an area in the shoes to create room for bunions and use softer, wider shoes.

(c) Gel preparations over the bursa to reduce friction.

(d) NSAIDs.

(e) Electrotherapeutic modalities to settle inflammation, such as ultrasound and laser.

(f) Inject the bursa with cortisone.

(g) Surgery to correct the valgus.

Sports

(a) Overpronation problems (see Glossary).

(b) Although ballet shoe blocks should hold onto the forefoot rather than the toes themselves, stress often produces osteoarthritic and valgus deformity at the metatarso-phalangeal joint.

Comment

It is cheaper and less invasive to alter the shoes than the foot so that early correction of overpronation is very successful and may even be so in established problems. This should be tried before surgery.

Subungual haematoma

Findings

Acute trauma leaves a throbbing purplish nail; when it becomes chronic, a dark brown coloured nail that grows out leaving normal nail near the base is found. The nail becomes thickened, ridged and detaches later with the new nail growing underneath.

Cause

Driving the foot into the front of the shoe in stopping games or long-distance running when perhaps downhill running may cause the problem, or direct trauma that causes bleeding under the toe nail.

Investigations

None clinically required.

Treatment

Trepination of the nail in the acute case when a red hot needle or paper clip can be used to burn through the nail and immediately releases the haematoma which is under pressure. This produces instant relief of pain. Observation of the chronic staining is required just to confirm it is moving with the growing nail and is not a discoloration on the nail bed from a melanoma.

Sports

Using padding over the dorsum of the mid foot allows the laces to be tied tight, thus holding the foot firm but leaving room for the toes to be moved and not impact on the front of the shoe. Make certain shoes do not cramp the toes.

Comment

Immediate relief is obtained from trepination, thus I always have a needle holder, paper clip and cigarette lighter in my sports medical bag.

Turf toe

Findings

Red, swollen great toe, often with a subungual haematoma, but also there is pain on all movements of the great toe, including lateral stretching.

Cause

Traumatic arthritis or even fracture of the great toe from driving the foot into the front of the shoe. Particularly occurs on artificial surfaces when the increased friction between the studs and surface permits no slide and therefore drives the toe into the front of the shoe.

Investigations

X-ray to exclude a fracture.

Treatment

(a) Preventative – 1 cm space between toes and inside of the shoe is preferable, but padding over the arch and forefoot so that the laces may be tightened to hold the foot firmly will help if the shoe needs to be snug.
(b) Inject the great toe joint with cortisone.
(c) Electrotherapeutic modalities to settle inflammation, such as ultrasound and laser.
(d) Splinting if fractured – the shoe itself may act as a sufficient splint.

Sports

All those played on artificial plastic surfaces are at risk, although water and sand filling have decreased the deceleration friction, allowing some slide and thus reducing the incidence of the injury.

Comment

Although often mentioned in American literature, I have not often seen this problem, probably because the pitches are nowadays permitting some slide of the foot.

Hallux limitus/rigidus

Findings

May be asymptomatic but the symptomatic have pain, especially on tip toe, and with running and change of direction sports. The pain, which is worse on dorsi- or plantar flexion of the big toe, is localized to the joint area which is swollen and may be tender to palpation. Dorsiflexion may be limited. See *Hallux valgus*.

Cause

Osteoarthritis of the first metatarso-phalangeal joint. There may be a congenital tendency. An overpronated foot may prevent full dorsiflexion of the toe.

Investigations

None required as usually some osteophytic lipping and early osteoarthritis is present anyway, but may X-ray to assess the bony state. Uric acid if gout suspected.

Treatment
(a) Avoid high heels which produce extension of the toe.
(b) Try simple correction of overpronation.
(c) Widen the shoes and use a metatarsal bar or a kinetic wedge orthotic.
(d) If painful, use electrotherapeutic modalities, such as ultrasound and shortwave diathermy.
(e) Cortisone injection of the joint if it is inflamed.
(f) Surgery may be required.

Sports
(a) Runners and joggers will have to shorten the stride length and lift off from the ball of the foot rather than the toe, as running around this problem may produce an everted foot with accompanying overpronation, genu valgus and hallux valgus.
(b) Serve at tennis may require a 'jump' to avoid rolling through this joint.
(c) Dancers, at the start of their career, should be filtered out as this will certainly cause problems requiring surgery which then probably will not take dancing loads.

Comment
Steroids are very successful to relieve pain, but alteration of movement patterns orthotics and adjustment of shoes are as vital before surgery is considered.

Sesamoiditis – fractured sesamoids of the great toe

Findings
Pain and tenderness over the sesamoids of the great toe. Not worse on passive adduction and abduction of the great toe, but may be worse on passive dorsiflexion and resisted plantar flexion of the toe. The forefoot may have increased varus with functional pronation and an abducted hallux.

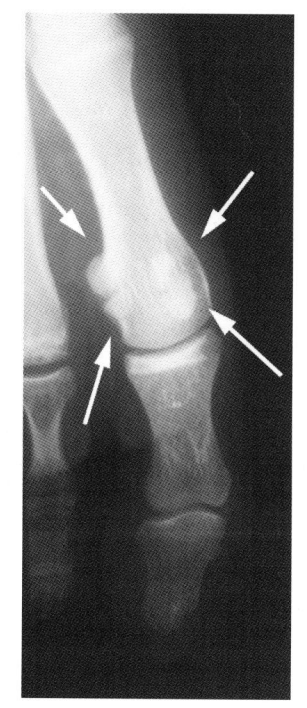

Figure 16.4   The sesamoids have not fractured but are quadripartite.

Cause
From impact over the great toe joint, which may be severe enough to fracture a sesamoid.

Investigations
X-ray with specific views for the sesamoids and bone scan if there is a doubt about the sesamoid integrity.

Caveat – Halluceal sesamoids may normally be uni-, bi-, tri- or quadripartite (Fig. 16.4).

Treatment
(a) Cross-train using non-impact sports returning via the Achilles ladder (see Chapter 20).
(b) Electrotherapeutic modalities to settle inflammation, such as ultrasound and laser. Steroids if the bone scan is not hot.
(c) Correct pronation with orthotics.

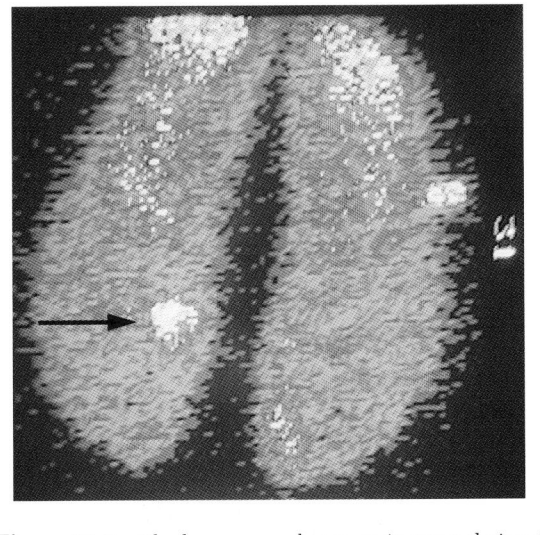

Figure 16.5 The bone scan shows an increased signal from the sesamoid fracture or bone bruising.

Sports

High-impact sports such as repetition starts in track and field sprinters and lunge drills at badminton.

Comment

Not common and I personally have only seen this condition in sprinters and badminton players (Fig. 16.5).

Fifth metatarsal enthesitis

Findings

Acute traumatic or insidious onset of pain localized to the proximal end of the fifth metatarsal that is worse on walking, rough ground and resisted peroneals. It is locally tender over the proximal fifth metatarsal head.

Cause

Apophysitis or enthesopathy or an avulsion fracture of the proximal end of the fifth metatarsal from overuse of the peroneals.

Investigations

X-ray of the foot for avulsion and to exclude Jones' fracture if traumatic (see *Fracture of the proximal shaft of the fifth metatarsal*).

Treatment

(a) Rest from activities.
(b) Wear shoes at all times except in bed to act as a splint.
(c) Perhaps cast brace.
(d) Electrotherapeutic modalities to settle inflammation, such as ultrasound, laser and interferential, and cortisone for the enthesopathy when no avulsion is present.
(e) Check for peroneal weakness and rehabilitate when the pain permits.

Sports

Rest from impact and cross-train non-impact, such as cycling, rowing and swimming; when walking without pain gradually reintroduce running via the Achilles ladder (see Chapter 20).

Comment

This usually heals without resorting to cast bracing and the apophysitis in the young is rare.

Fracture of the proximal shaft of the fifth metatarsal (Jones' fracture)

(a) May present with a history of a sudden pop or trauma to the fifth metatarsal and be tender over the proximal metaphysis. These lesions are seen on X-ray and may represent an unfused apophysis, symptomatic sesamoid or non-union and surgical management may involve shelling out or a compression screw. Take a surgical opinion [2].
(b) May involve a fracture across the proximal shaft and is prone to non-union, the Jones' fracture.
(c) Spiral fractures of the distal shaft occur in dancers and may be displaced. They may be treated non-operatively or operatively [3].

Oddities

(a) *Logo pain.* Plastic logos may not stretch as much as leather and cause compression of the foot under this area.

(b) *Big toe nail.* Some athletes run with dorsi-flexed toes, rubbing a hole in the shoe. They are often mid foot strikers who are trying to firm up the foot for impact. Encourage heel strike.

(c) *Plantar fascial pain near the arch.* Several insoles are manufactured with the arch support of the shoes rising up too near the heel and thus do not match the shape of the foot arch, causing rub of the foot.

(d) *Shoe heel tags.* May rub the Achilles causing peritendinitis. Tags should be soft and easily pulled backwards. If not, cut the tags off or slit down to the heel cups either side of tags but not so close together that the sides can close in again (see Glossary).

(e) *High sides of the shoe.* These can rub under the maleolus irritating the tendons of the peronei or posterior tibialis.

(f) *High arch of the foot.* May be rubbed by shoe lacing on the dorsum of the foot.

(g) *Tibialis anterior.* Tendons may be rubbed by too tight a shoe lacing.

(h) *Extensor hallucis.* May pull up into the shoe causing rubbing. Pad either side of the tendon to direct pressure onto this area and away from the tendon.

(i) *Shoe nail or stud.* May rub through onto the foot. Note any unequal wear of studs that alters the action of the shoe, usually encouraging overpronation.

Caveat – Gout, spondylarthropathies, Reiter's, rheumatoid and DISH (disseminated idiopathic skeletal hypertrophy).

Further reading

1. Sproul, J., Klaaren, H. and Mannarino, F. (1993) Surgical treatment of Freiberg's infraction in athletes. *Am. J. Sports Med.* **21**, 381–384.
2. Rettig, A. C., Shelbourne, K. D. and Wilckens, J. (1992) The surgical treatment of symptomatic non-unions of the proximal (metaphyseal) fifth metatarsal in athletes. *Am. J. Sports Med.* **20**, 50–54.
3. O'Malley, M. J., Hamilton, W. G. and Munyak, J. (1996) Fractures of the distal shaft of the fifth metatarsal. Dancer's fracture. *Am. J. Sports Med.* **24**, 240–243.

Bruckner, P. and Khan, K. (1993) *Clinical Sports Medicine.* McGraw-Hill, New York.

Reid, D. (1992) *Sports Injury Assessment and Rehabilitation.* Churchill Livingstone, Edinburgh.

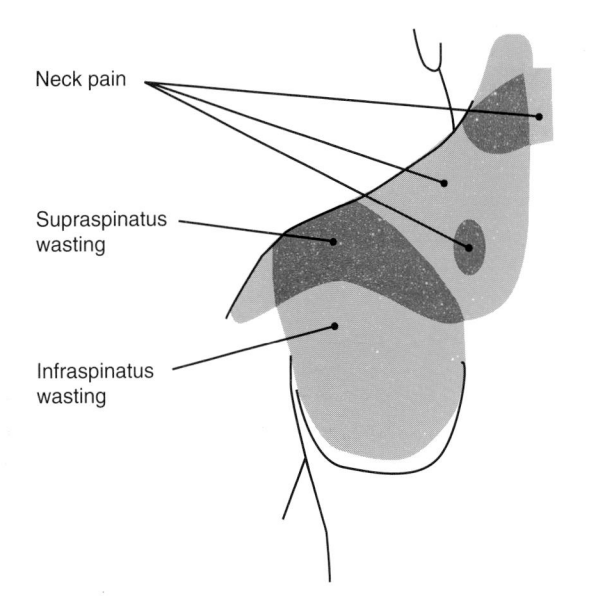

Neck pain

Supraspinatus wasting

Infraspinatus wasting

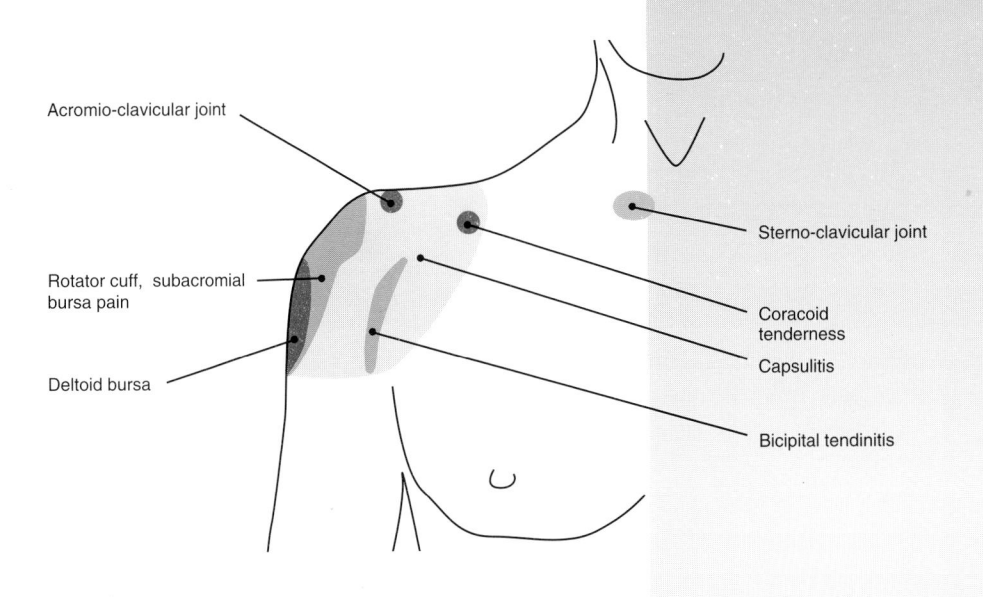

Acromio-clavicular joint

Rotator cuff, subacromial bursa pain

Deltoid bursa

Sterno-clavicular joint

Coracoid tenderness

Capsulitis

Bicipital tendinitis

Introduction

The shoulder movement requires gleno-humeral movement plus scapulo-thoracic movement. During this combined movement the humeral head rises up in the glenoid to impinge on the inferior surface of the acromion. The elevation of the humeral head is prevented and controlled by the rotator cuff. Damage to the rotator cuff allows the humeral head to rise, compressing the rotator cuff and the subacromial bursa, and this produces a cycle of rotator cuff injuries from compression, malfunction of the cuff, elevation of the humeral head, compression of the subacromial bursa and bruising of the rotator cuff. Treatment is required to break this vicious cycle.

Scapulo-thoracic movement rotates the acromion away from the humeral head to avoid impingement and keeps the humeral head applied to the glenoid rather like a seal balancing a ball on its nose. The plane of movement is along the posterior thoracic wall, i.e. about 20° anterior to the coronal plane between both shoulders. Thus movements posterior to this scapulo-thoracic plane (scaption) will inhibit scapular rotation and thus encourage impingement. Many weight training exercises will therefore produce impingement such as:

(a) Wide placed hands on a bench press or lateral pull-downs.
(b) Too high an elbow position on pectoralis decks will cause impingement, and no posterior stop to prevent excess external rotation will stress the anterior capsule and produce subluxation of the joint as in an anterior dislocation.

Throwing and serving at tennis require scapulo-thoracic rotation first before humeral acceleration. This can be seen in the 'set' position adopted by the tennis professionals just before they hit the serve. The movement is exaggerated by knee bends and lumbar extension (Figs 17.1 and 17.2).

Equally muscle/tendon damage can occur from concentric overload, too much too soon, or from eccentric overload, decelerating the shoulder

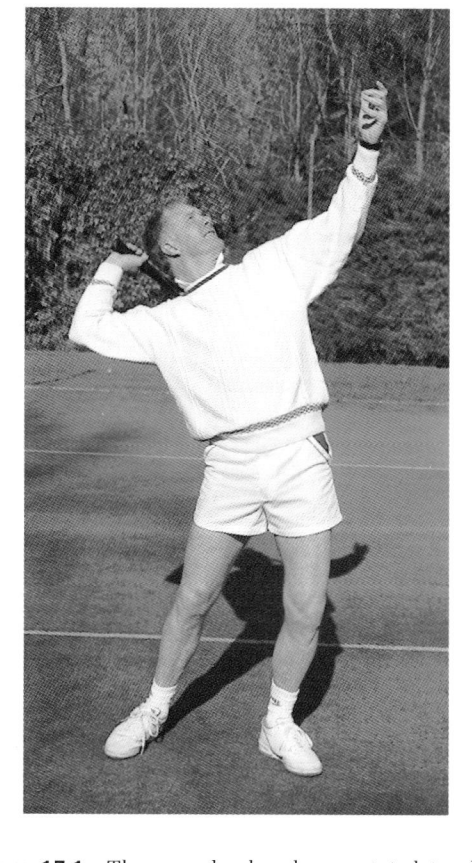

Figure 17.1 The scapular has been rotated to allow the shoulder to drop into the set position.

after the shot. A sudden block or loss of resistance to these movements may produce an acute tear.

Trauma to the shoulder may damage the capsule and supporting ligaments, and when more severe the glenoid labrum, rotator cuff and bone, plus the other 'shoulder' joints, the acromio- and sterno-clavicular may be involved. This pectoral instability may be caused by 'front-on' techniques with racket and throwing sports (Figs 17.3 and 17.4) as the failure to rotate the upper body forces retraction of the whole pectoral girdle. Thus, closely interlinked movement patterns can easily develop secondary injuries following damage to one element and treatment should be directed at the primary damage, but relief of pain is insufficient without restoration of normal function and correction of the secondary 'trick' moves.

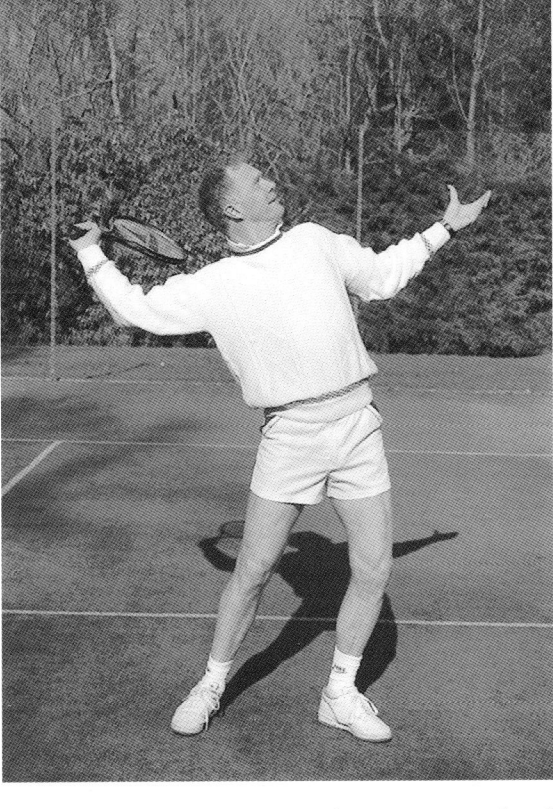

Figure 17.2 Scapular rotation has not occurred and this hitting position will cause subacromial impingement.

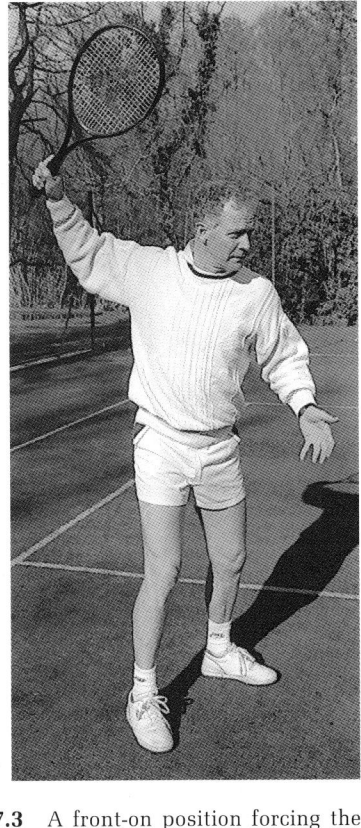

Figure 17.3 A front-on position forcing the shoulder backward by retraction rather than rotation of the dorsal spine. Attempts to hit harder from this position may destabilize the whole pectoral girdle.

<table>
<tr><td></td></tr>
</table>

Referred pain from the neck

All examinations of the shoulder must rule out referred pain from the neck, particularly from C5/6 (see Chapter 3).

Acromio-clavicular joint (shoulder separation)

Findings

(a) May occur acutely with a fall, but can appear gradually.
(b) Classically pain occurs with overhead work, but carrying heavy weights and lying on the shoulder produce pain over the acromio-clavicular joint in the shoulder.
(c) Often accompanied by the 'point sign', when the patient points at the acromio-clavicular joint as the site of pain (see Fig. 22.20).
(d) Referral of pain often goes up towards the neck as well as down into the arm and elbow.
(e) It may hurt to lie on the elbows such as whilst reading a book.
(f) The acromio-clavicular joint is the great mimic of the shoulder, so that if signs are confusing inject the acromio-clavicular joint and review in 7–10 days.
(g) Classically sore at the end of circumduction, worse on internal rotation and forced adduction across the body, with the shoulder at 90° of abduction.

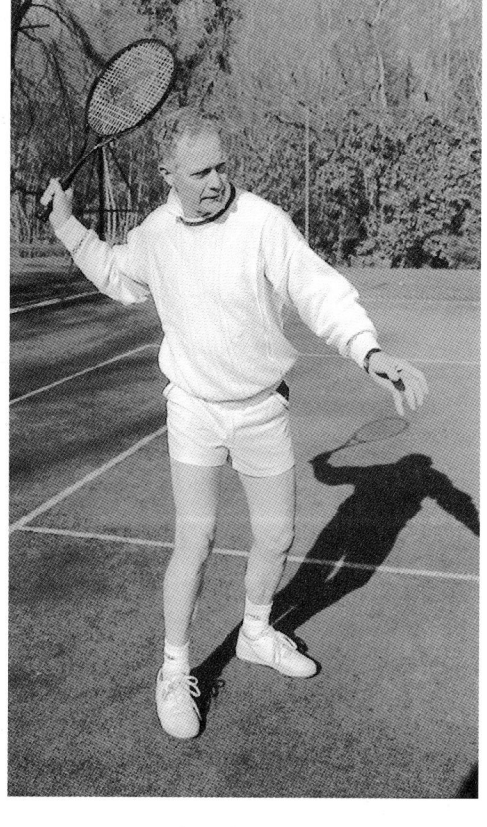

Figure 17.4 Even though the stance is front-on, the shoulder girdle has been rotated rather than retracted.

(h) Palpable tenderness over the acromio-clavicular joint which may appear swollen and displaced with an obvious step.

Cause

Most commonly seen following a fall onto the tip of the shoulder, but it can occur whilst sleeping with the arm pulled across the body and also carrying heavy weights and during overhead work.

Grade 1   Swelling and bruising. No deformity. A tear of the superior ligament but with a stable joint.

Grade 2   A more extensive tear of the superior ligament with increased mobility and some subluxation of the joint but not more than half shaft thickness.

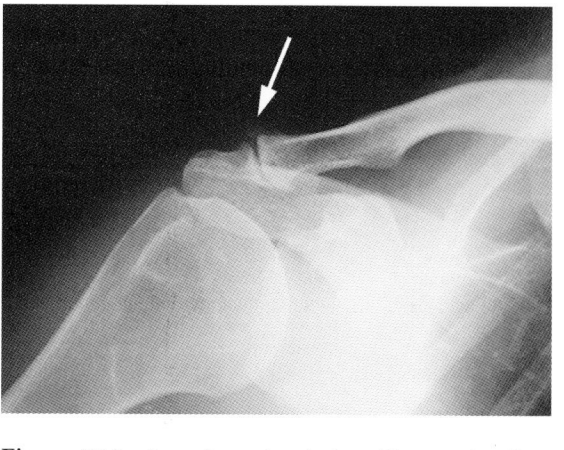

Figure 17.5 Superior osteophyte with superior ligament calcification in the acromio-clavicular joint.

Grade 3   A tear of the conoid and trapezoid ligaments with considerable deformity (more than half the shaft distance) and increased mobility plus some tearing of the deltoid from the clavicle.

Grades 4–6 display more severe disruption with displacement and are graded by the surgeons.

Investigations

X-ray of acromio-clavicular joint and X-ray of acromio-clavicular joint weight bearing for comparison. X-rays may show subluxation of the acromio-clavicular joint, inferior osteophytes or sclerosis and lysis from osteoarthritis (Fig. 17.5).

Treatment

(a) Grades 1 and 2. Electrotherapeutic modalities to settle inflammation, such as ultrasound and laser to the ligament. An injection of the acromio-clavicular joint with cortisone, especially for grade 2.

(b) Grade 3. The much larger deformed step in grade 3 in fact causes less problems and often requires an injection of hydrocortisone, but rarely requires stabilization [1]. Ultrasound and laser may help. Some authorities believe these should be repaired in sportspeople [2]. Failure to improve from grades 1 and 2 may require burring of osteophytes or excision of the distal end of the clavicle.

(c) Treatment may vary between the dominant and non-dominant shoulder, a more active approach being taken for the dominant. Rarely wiring or screwing of the clavicle to the corocoid may be required in high level contact sports.

(d) Grades 4–6 require surgery.

(e) If in doubt about the diagnosis, inject the acromio-clavicular joint and review 7–10 days later.

> **Caveat** – Entrapment of the supraspinatus by an inferior osteophyte of the acromio-clavicular joint. Conoid and trapezoid ligament strain. Impingement of the short head of biceps by the clavicle and coraco-brachialis origin strain.

Sports

(a) Usually no problem with below shoulder sports, although carrying heavy weights may flare the acromio-clavicular joint.

(b) Flared by press-ups, overhead weights, overhead badminton shots, volleyball and serving at tennis. As the overhead shot is uncommon in squash, it is the racket game of preference for rehabilitation.

(c) A high take away technique into adduction of the shoulder in the backhand at tennis and squash may hurt.

(d) There can be a problem with contact sports, although many play without problems after the injury has settled [3]. Padding anterior and posterior to the clavicle to bring the point of contact away from the acromio-clavicular joint may help.

Comment

Most acromio-clavicular joints will be pain-free rapidly following a cortisone injection and really only grade 1 can be treated by physiotherapy. Many patients live within the tolerance of the shoulder, avoiding causative factors.

Subacromial bursitis

Subacromial bursitis can exist alone but is often accompanied by rotator cuff injury and scapulo-humeral disassociation.

Findings

(a) It invariably follows overarm activity such as throwing, hedge cutting or painting the ceiling.

(b) There is pain lying on the shoulder, doing hair, putting on a coat, driving (hand over top of the wheel) and reaching into the back seat.

(c) The patient indicates the deltoid area and below as painful, and sometimes the presentation of pain will be over the lateral epicondyle, being confused as a tennis elbow. Local anaesthetic into the bursa should resolve the diagnostic dilemma.

(d) There may be a painful arc between 80° and 120° but often only at 180° with active and passive circumduction depending whether the patient shrugs their shoulder or not during the test.

(e) Passive and active circumduction may be pain-free but resisted circumduction at 90° will hurt as the deltoid lifts the humerus into the bursa.

(f) Resisted rotator cuff isometrics are pain-free.

(g) The impingement signs are positive (see *Glossary*).

(h) There may only be a history of not being able to throw with no positive clinical signs.

Cause

Compression of the subacromial bursa between the humeral head and acromion. Usually because arm elevation is produced at the gleno-humeral joint without any accompanying scapulo-thoracic rotation (see Chapter 17), but the shape of the acromion may make impingement more likely.

Investigations

None clinically required unless failing to respond to treatment; use X-ray to assess the shape of the

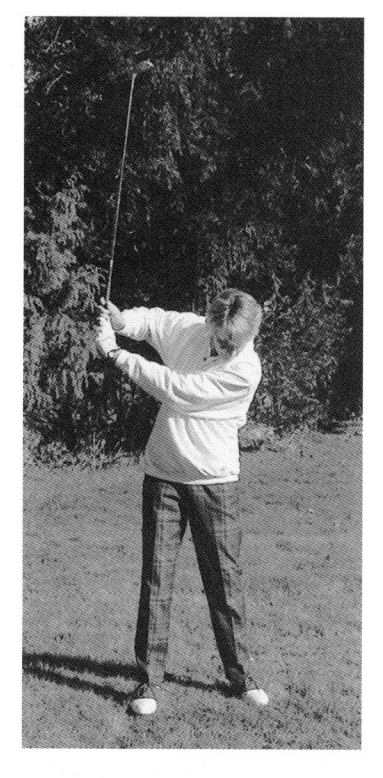

Figure 17.6 The 'flying' right elbow at golf.

acromion and MRI to look for accompanying problems.

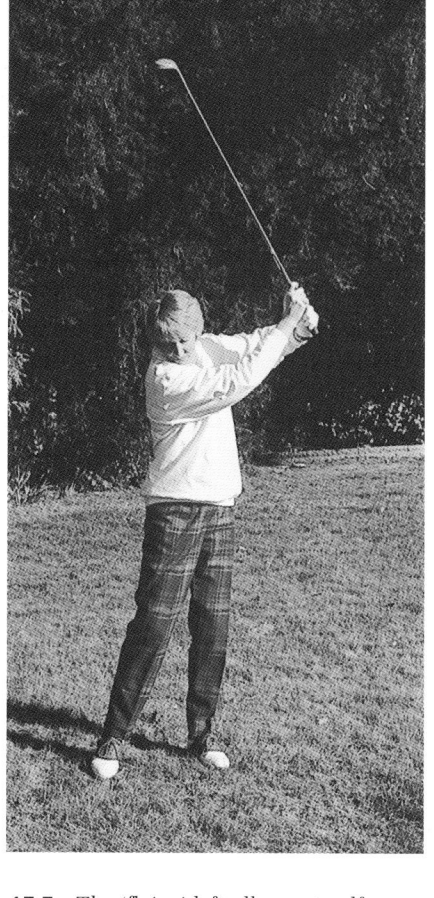

Figure 17.7 The 'flying' left elbow at golf.

Treatment

Inject the subacromial bursa with cortisone and local anaesthetic, and at the same time correct any faulty technique to improve scapulo-humeral disassociation and strengthen the rotator cuff.

Sports

(a) Golf. Right shoulder. Correct the flying elbow and too flat a plane of swing (Figs 17.6 and 17.7).

(b) Racket sports. Correct the flying elbow (Figs 17.8 and 17.9).

(c) Squash. Correct the chest front-on position for the forehand high volley without upper body rotation (see a coach).

(d) Throwing. Not enough scapulo-thoracic rotation and upper body turn, throw side to side underarm whilst troublesome. Can often bowl at cricket but not throw overarm.

(e) Swim. Freestyle. Not pulling far enough back to allow scapulo-thoracic rotation. Too low a recovery position of the elbow.

(f) Tennis serve. Hitting before the 'set' position is obtained so that scapulo-thoracic rotation has not been achieved (see Fig. 17.2). Try taking the racket directly back to the 'set' position (see Fig. 17.1) with extended but not externally rotated upper arm.

(g) Archery. The draw elbow is taken too high with the final movement being external rotation of the humerus, rather than scapular retraction.

(h) Running. Tight shoulders, arms held across the body whilst running with high elbows.

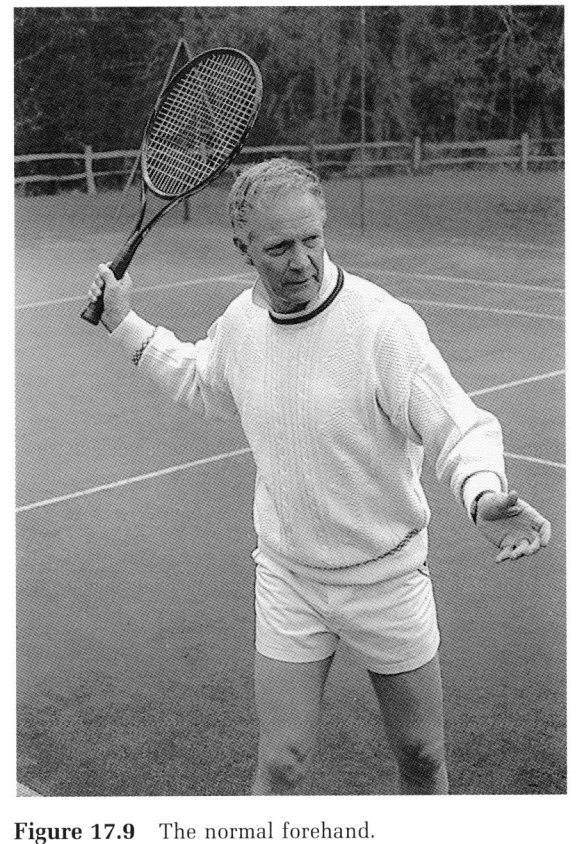

Figure 17.9   The normal forehand.

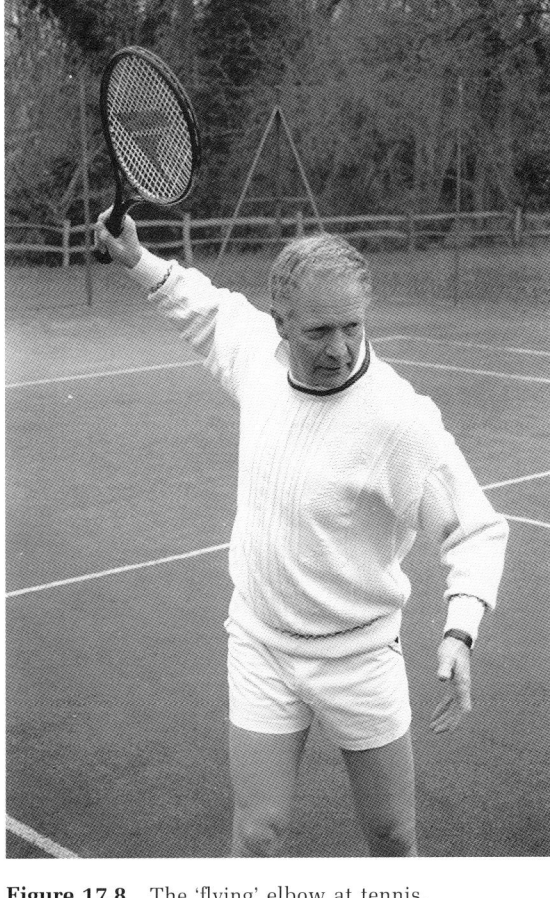

Figure 17.8   The 'flying' elbow at tennis.

(i)   Weights. Too wide a grip and working the lifts behind the scapulo-thoracic plane (see *Introduction*). Especially with deltoid exercises. Narrow the grip on the bench press to correct. 'Flies' and pectoralis machines are worked too close to or above the horizontal plane and cause impingement. Work these exercises below the horizontal plane.

Comment

Although physiotherapists treat this injury, I feel the bursa is best treated with cortisone as an anti-inflammatory because physiotherapy modalities do not reach the bursa in its protected position between the bones. Physiotherapy to the rotator cuff and/or correction of the scapulo-humeral dis-

association can then follow immediately the vicious cycle is broken (see *Introduction*).

Subdeltoid bursitis

Findings

Gradual development of pain over the inferior deltoid area with pain on active circumduction, but resisted rotator cuff is pain-free and the impingement signs are negative. Resisted deltoid is painful but at 90° this may stress the subacromial bursa.

Cause

Inflammation of the subdeltoid bursa which may well be an extension of the subacromial bursa under the deltoid. Uncommon.

Treatment

Treat the subacromial bursa first and if this fails then try electrotherapeutic modalities to settle inflammation, such as ultrasound, interferential and laser. Massage techniques such as frictions to prevent intrabursal adhesions can help as can a locally placed injection of hydrocortisone to the subdeltoid bursa.

> **Caveat** – Beware of attrition to the circumflex humeral nerve.

Sports

(a) Usually internal and external rotation of the shoulder in the circumducted position such as a 'front-on' tennis service hit wide out from the shoulder.

(b) Dancing and skating – carrying or supporting the partner with the elbow at 45–90° circumduction.

Comment

Pain on resisted deltoid release may be a subacromial bursa as this test allows the humeral head to elevate and cause impingement. Generally treat the subacromial bursa first.

Rotator cuff injuries

Findings

(a) An acute episode of pain, followed by weakness suggests a rupture.

(b) Gradual onset of pain referred to the deltoid may refer to the elbow or the forearm and may be diagnosed as a tennis elbow.

(c) Pain particularly with the elbow elevated above the shoulder, such as drying hair or reaching forwards or backwards.

(d) Reaching behind the back towards the dorsal spine.

(e) Acute shoulder pain, getting worse over 4–5 days, suggests the possibility of calcific tendinitis (see *Calcific tendinitis*).

(f) The patient indicates the top of arm and deltoid as being the localization of pain.

(g) There is a painful arc on active movements and especially on eccentric movement, although passive movement is pain-free (technically).

(h) Pain on resisted internal rotation suggests subscapularis, pain with resisted external rotation suggests infraspinatus and abduction supraspinatus, and these may be either weak and/or painful. However, note that the eccentric stabilizing effects of the other muscles of the shoulder may produce pain so that the infraspinatus, acting to stabilize the shoulder, may produce some discomfort on resisted internal rotation.

(i) Localized tenderness. Subscapularis anteriorly, supraspinatus over the greater tuberosity, the palpation being made easier with the arm in internal rotation. Infraspinatus – lying prone leaning on the elbows, as in reading a book, when the posterior humeral head is tender.

(j) The impingement signs are invariably positive (see *Glossary*).

Cause

Damage to subscapularis, supraspinatus or infraspinatus. Clinically teres major and minor which are part of the rotator cuff have not had their injuries well defined. The rotator cuff stabilizes the shoulder and decelerates the shoulder movements to prevent the arm following the ball in a throw. The injury may be a tear often during eccentric movements or tendon degeneration from compression of the rotator cuff between the humeral head and acromion causing localized avascularization. The other action of the rotator cuff is to depress and stabilize the humeral head away from the acromion. Rotator cuff damage allows elevation of the humerus which impinges on the acromion which inflames the rotator cuff and so a vicious cycle is introduced.

> **Caveat** – C5/6 neck injury and acromio-clavicular joint with an inferior osteophyte pressing on the supraspinatus muscle.

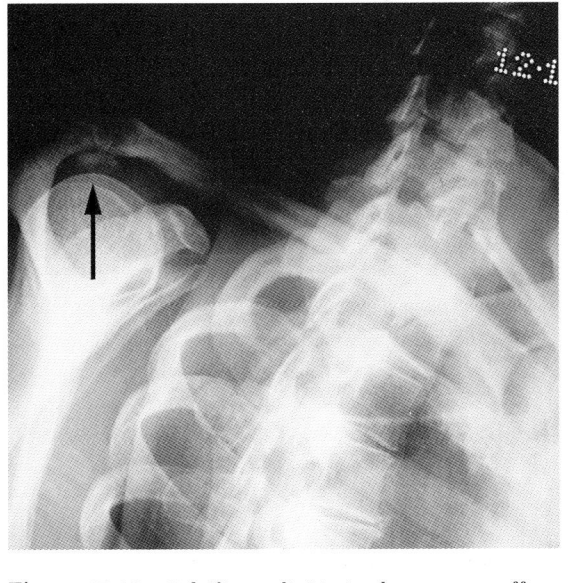

Figure 17.10 Calcific tendinitis in the rotator cuff.

Investigations

(a) Not clinically required unless failure to progress.

(b) X-ray – looking for calcific tendonitis (Fig. 17.10) and to assess acromial angulation if impingement is a major problem and surgery is considered.

(c) MRI scan may show supraspinatus degeneration or localized tear. These are less easy to see in the infraspinatus and subscapularis which may only show on dynamic views.

Treatment

(a) Treatment is designed to break the vicious cycle where an injection of the subacromial bursa calms the inflammation, decreases pain and allows the rotator cuff to work, and thus prevents humeral elevation and subsequent impingement which irritates and inflames the rotator cuff.

(b) Electrotherapeutic modalities to settle inflammation, such as ultrasound, laser and interferential.

(c) Massage techniques to control and organize scar tissue.

(d) Local injection of the rotator cuff if inflammation is present, but this is usually placed in the subacromial bursa over the rotator cuff. Injection of cortisone into the tendon area, especially if acute calcific tendonitis is present.

(e) Proprioceptive strapping to encourage scapular rotation and prevent shoulder elevation during circumduction, i.e. improving scapulo-humeral disassociation.

(f) Isometrics for the rotator cuff.

(g) Isotonics or isokinetics for the rotator cuff.

(h) Throwing, hitting rehabilitation.

(i) Arthroscopy to repair any rotator cuff tear, debridement of adhesions, and debridement of the inferior surface of the acromion, the coraco-acromial ligament and the acromio-clavicular joint to create more space for the rotator cuff, especially with mal-shaped acromia.

Sports

(a) Golf. An arm take away with no shoulder rotation injures the left shoulder, particularly the infraspinatus and supraspinatus. The right arm taken flat but with a flying elbow compresses the infraspinatus at the posterior aspect of the shoulder.

(b) Tennis. Hitting too soon on the serve before the scapulo-thoracic 'set' position is obtained; this problem is often accompanied by a subacromial bursitis (see Fig. 17.2).

(c) All throwing events – when too much power, too soon is used. Many people train their legs to run or kick but few train their shoulders with graduated exercises, in the off season, to build sufficient strength in the decelerators, the rotator cuff.

Comment

Although there may be a local tender area, my first treatment is an injection of the subacromial bursa, and then physiotherapy and rehabilitation to the rotator cuff muscles. Persistent discomfort may require local infiltration and resistant problems often resolve when the infraspinatus is injected. Some authors suggest three injections and then surgery, but many patients do not want surgery. If only resisted rotator cuff testing is sore then rehabilitation is required. If the impingement signs become positive again, then repeat the cortisone injection as the still weak rotator cuff has allowed impingement and subacromial bursitis to recur and the vicious cycle to restart. Proprioceptive strapping to display to the patient when they are shrugging is beneficial.

Calcific tendinitis

Findings
Chronically, contributing to a rotator cuff injury that is not settling, whereas acute calcific tendinitis has excruciating pain which may develop over 4–5 days. There may be localized swelling and always tenderness on palpation over the damaged area. The patient does not want to move the arm and all movements hurt, as do resisted movements (see *Rotator cuff injuries*).

Cause
Calcium hydroxyapatite deposition in the rotator cuff tendon. This may be found incidentally and be pain-free or form acutely when it produces excruciating pain.

Investigations
X-ray at once for the acute presentation and when a shoulder is not progressing (see Fig. 17.10).

Treatment
(a) Acute. Sling. Analgesia. Intralesional injection of cortisone and local anaesthetic, then treat as for chronic calcific tendonitis. However, one injection may be curative.
(b) Chronic. If incidental, leave alone. Local friction makes this worse and, when painful, intralesional injections of cortisone and local anaesthetic may be curative. If recurrent may try needling the tendon and injecting with local anaesthetic to work out the calcium; however, lithotripsy may be the best answer rather than surgical debridement of the calcific area.

Sports
Particularly from implemental games requiring shoulder power or throwing which must be rested in the acute phase. Check scapulohumeral disassociation and re-educate this movement, perhaps with a proprioceptive taping to prevent shrugging.

Comment
The finding of calcium does not warrant treatment, only the painful phase. The acute calcific tendinitis reveals itself by the acute presentation and the intensity of pain description and immobility. This responds well to cortisone injection but does need resting in a sling and strong analgesia for 48 hours.

Bicipital tendinitis

Findings
(a) Acute pain with resisted or overloaded biceps or with a gradual onset of pain either referred to the shoulder or down the belly of the biceps muscles.
(b) Passive shoulder internal and external rotation is pain-free.
(c) Circumduction may have a painful arc but the rotator cuff isometrics are pain-free.
(d) The impingement signs may be positive (see *Glossary*).
(e) It is differentiated from subacromial bursitis by a positive resisted biceps test and Yergason's and Speed's tests (see *Glossary*).

Cause
Attritional degeneration or a partial tear of the tendon due to acute resistance of biceps contraction or eccentric overload. Damage is probably created in the bicipital groove where some impingement on the acromion may contribute to the injury. Probably not as common as is often diagnosed. Maybe a partial degenerative tear with subsequent synovial inflammation and adhesions binding down the tendon and causing pain (see *Ruptured biceps*).

Investigations
None clinically required unless failing to progress, when a diagnostic ultrasound or MRI scan will show synovitis and perhaps a partial tear.

Treatment

(a) Electrotherapeutic modalities to settle inflammation in the sheath, such as ultrasound and laser.
(b) Massage techniques to control adhesions, such as frictional massage to the tendon sheath.
(c) Injection with cortisone of the sheath within the bicipital groove.
(d) Isometrics progressing to dynamic exercises and heavier weights.
(e) Extension and external rotation shoulder stretches plus extension of the shoulder with pronation of the forearm.

> **Caveat** – The lesion may well be a partial tear whose integrity is maintained by the adhesion but these cause the pain. Local cortisone frees the adhesion and relieves the pain but exposes the tendon to pain-free loads thus causing a rupture. Some surgeons in the past have severed the tendon to treat the lesion, relieving the pain and then treating it in the same way as a ruptured biceps. Patients should be warned of the possible consequence of injection, which may cure the pain but permit a rupture, this having the same effect as surgery (see *Ruptured long head of biceps*).

Sports

Those requiring bicipital strength, often weightlifting. Check for anabolic steroid abuse.

Comment

This diagnosis is often quoted but any tendon lesion should have pain on resisted biceps testing; in practice this rarely occurs with shoulder pain, and it therefore seems to be an overdiagnosed lesion and is rarer than quoted. The treatment of the subacromial bursa is preferable to local bicipital groove or tender point injection unless there is positive resisted pain with the biceps. Sometimes bicipital tendinitis will not heal until the rupture occurs and then it heals to a functional norm, hence the surgical division of the long head.

Ruptured long head of biceps

Findings

Bruising over the biceps muscle with a 'Popeye' shape to the long head of biceps muscle. Bicipital function is intact but in the early stages may be weaker and painful, but rapidly becoming pain-free. Resisted biceps testing and Speed's and Yergason's tests are painful (see *Glossary*).

Cause

Acute blocking resistance of bicipital contraction or the end-point of chronic bicipital tenosynovitis. Indeed chronic bicipital tenosynovitis may not settle until a rupture has occurred, traumatically or surgically (see *Bicipital tendinitis*).

Investigations

None clinically required.

Treatment

(a) RICE.
(b) Electrotherapeutic modalities to settle inflammation and remove tissue debris, such as ultrasound, laser and interferential.
(c) Massage techniques to remove tissue debris and organize scar tissue.
(d) Allow the long head of biceps to reattach itself by adhesions lower down the humerus but maintain normal elbow movements and add controlled isometric resistance exercises to the biceps.
(e) Full extension of the elbow must also be maintained and later full extension of the shoulder with a pronated forearm.
(f) Add isotonic and isokinetic exercises to pain onset (general muscle ladder; see Chapter 20).

Sports

Weight training – check for anabolic steroid abuse. Biceps curls, preacher curls, upright rowing, rowing machine, etc., may all have to be introduced only to pain onset.

Comment

Normal function can return without treatment as I have seen a Commonwealth weightlifting gold won by an athlete with a conservatively managed reattached long head of biceps.

Supraspinatus impingement

Findings

Similar to the acromio-clavicular joint but resisted or active movement of the supraspinatus produces pain so the symptoms may reflect acromio-clavicular and/or supraspinatus injury. Tenderness can be just posterior rather than on the acromio-clavicular joint, and it may produce actual disuse wasting of the supraspinatus as well as pain-induced weakness. An X-ray may show an inferior osteophyte from the acromio-clavicular joint (see *Acromio-clavicular joint* and *Supraspinatus weakness*).

Cause

Impingement of the supraspinatus muscle beneath the acromio-clavicular joint.

Treatment

An injection of cortisone is placed behind and beneath the acromio-clavicular joint onto the muscle fascia as it passes beneath the acromio-clavicular joint. The inferior osteophytes may require surgical debridement.

Sports

As for acromio-clavicular joint, supraspinatus weakness and rotator cuff.

Comment

Not common. The patient often indicates that the pain is just behind the acromio-clavicular joint and it can do well conservatively, but recurrence is best treated surgically.

Supraspinatus weakness

Findings

Weakness and incoordination on active circumduction and weakness on resisted abduction of the shoulder:

Type 1 As for rotator cuff with a supraspinatus tear.

Type 2 An amyotrophy.

Type 3 Gradual onset of muscle weakness and incoordination commonly in racket players with some diffuse shoulder, neck and arm pain. Weak and wasted supraspinatus and infraspinatus. Normal glenohumeral movements, but there may be some discomfort on side flexion of the neck to the opposite side.

Cause

Type 1 Rotator cuff damage (see *Rotator cuff injuries* and *Supraspinatus impingement*).

Type 2 Amyotrophy (see *Infraspinatus weakness*).

Type 3 Damage to the suprascapular nerve as it passes through the suprascapular notch.

Investigations

See *Infraspinatus weakness*.

Treatment

Type 1 See *Rotator cuff injuries* and *Supraspinatus impingement*.

Type 2 Treat with analgesia in painful initial stages. Attempt rehabilitation of muscle as far as possible when the inflammatory stage has settled down.

Type 3 Release of nerve at the suprascapular notch, followed by appropriate rehabilitation of the shoulder muscles, but see in conjunction with *Infraspinatus weakness*.

Sports

Racket sports and volleyball. Usually after surgery, type 3 may be rehabilitated back to racket sports and volleyball, but see *Infraspinatus weakness*. If there has been nerve damage then this will take time to regenerate. Do not introduce shot making with a racket too soon, before the rotator cuff strength has returned, otherwise subacromial problems will occur.

Comment

Damage at the suprascapular notch will affect both the nerve supply to the supraspinatus and the infraspinatus, whereas damage at the spino-glenoid notch only affects the infraspinatus. Not a common lesion but release of the nerve may help.

Infraspinatus weakness

Findings
Type 1 Residual weakness following a rotator cuff tear.
Type 2 Amyotrophy with localized pain and tenderness in the muscle and weakness which gets better with time.
Type 3 Suprascapular nerve damage, often presenting as gradual weakness and incoordination in racket or ball control rather than the poorly localized shoulder and arm pain. There is invariably a wasted, weak infraspinatus muscle at presentation.

There are no accompanying gleno-humeral signs and surprisingly little functional deficit. There are no abnormal neck signs, although side flexion to the opposite side may provoke some discomfort.

Cause
Type 1 Rotator cuff damage (see *Rotator cuff injuries*).
Type 2 Amyotrophy – probably a localized viral neuromyositis.
Type 3 Damage to the suprascapular nerve as it passes round the scapular spine at the spinoglenoid notch, usually in a racket or volleyball player, sometimes weight with training either because of a traction neuropathy or a cyst compressing the nerve. If the supraspinatus is weak as well the damage is at the suprascapular notch (see *Supraspinatus weakness*).

Investigations
(a) MRI may show a cyst at the spinoglenoid notch that is compressing the infraspinatus branch of the supraspinatus nerve.
(b) EMG may show localized denervation or evidence of amyotrophy.

Treatment
Type 1 See *Rotator cuff injuries*.
Type 2 Analgesia for amyotrophy. Maintain normal activities as far as possible.
Type 3 Surgical release of the nerve if there is a cyst. Increasing the notch size to reduce tension on the nerve seems to help any pain but does not regenerate muscle bulk [4]. Followed by appropriate rehabilitation.

Sports
Outside a ruptured rotator cuff, the gradual onset infraspinatus weakness is almost entirely a racket or volleyball sport injury. The serve in volleyball may be part of the problem [4]. Release of the nerve entrapment allows rehabilitation and return to sports, but increasing the notch size to reduce traction on the nerve does not seem to alter muscle bulk and function.

Comment
Neither amyotrophy nor localized nerve damage are common; however, as one gets better and the other is treatable, if there is a cyst present then the clinical diagnosis of the cause should be established and appropriate investigations instituted.

Anterior dislocation

Findings
A history of trauma, especially forced external rotation and abduction. There is pain and an inability to move the arm away from the side. The shoulder appears squared off with a hollow below the acromion.

Cause
Trauma to the shoulder where the humeral head dislocates anteriorly and inferiorly.

Investigations
X-ray to exclude fracture and Bankart lesion (Fig. 17.11) (see *Glossary*).

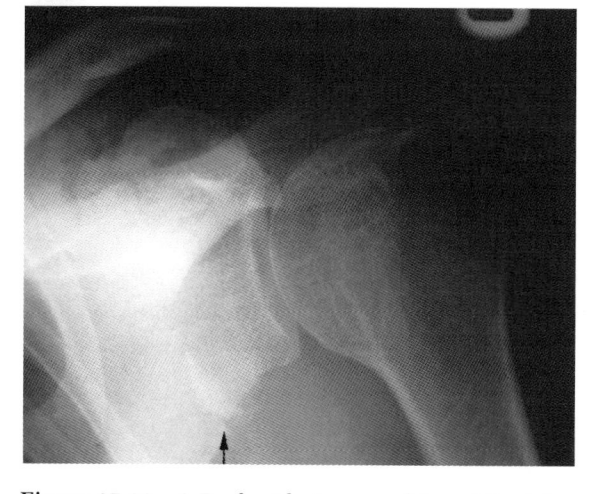

Figure 17.11 A Bankart lesion – avulsion of the inferior glenoid margin. (Mr. Basil Helal.)

Treatment

(a) Relocation preferably after an X-ray to exclude any humeral fracture.

(b) Support for 3–4 weeks in internal rotation held by a sling and start isometrics to the rotator cuff.

(c) Maintain hand movements to prevent swelling from a shoulder–hand syndrome and dependent oedema.

(d) After 3–4 weeks regain the range of movement, continue isometrics, and add isotonics and then gradually introduce throwing over a short distance to encourage concentric and eccentric muscle activity.

(e) Avoid external rotation in abduction until all subluxation tests are negative (see *Glossary*).

(f) Surgery if a Bankart lesion is present.

Sports

See *Subluxing shoulder.*

> **Caveat** – A patch of numbness over the deltoid equals damage to the axillary nerve. Swelling in the hand and fingers, and loss of pulse equals damage to artery and axillary plexus, and is likely to have a fractured humerus.

Comment

Although many surgeons await further dislocation, the young seem to be destined for recurrence and an arthroscopy may reveal a labral Bankart lesion that can be repaired. Hence the dominant shoulder in the young should be considered for repair; the non-dominant may be treated conservatively. One must remember that the young do change their sporting activities as they get older, often giving up the causative sport, and this must influence decision making for or against surgery.

Recurrent dislocation

Findings

A previous history of dislocation. The arm jumps out and may be relocated by the patient with a trick move. The arm may be relocated easily or have relocated itself. Apprehension and relocation tests are positive (see *Glossary*).

Cause

As for anterior dislocation, but when externally rotated and abducted the arm is forced beyond the range of the anterior capsule and the arm may dislocate anteriorly and inferiorly, often without pain. There is usually labral or bony glenoid deficiency.

Investigations

X-ray to look for a Bankart lesion and/or Hill–Sach's lesion (Hatchet lesion) (see *Glossary*) (Figs 17.11 and 17.12)

Treatment.

(a) Dominant arm. Withdraw from precipitating events until stabilized surgically, such as Bankart, Putti Platt or Bristow operations.

(b) Non-dominant arm. Avoid the dislocate position and try a restraining strap to racket sports until stable (Fig. 17.13). However, if on X-ray a Bankart's or Hill–Sach's lesion is present it will require surgery.

Sports

See *Subluxing shoulder.*

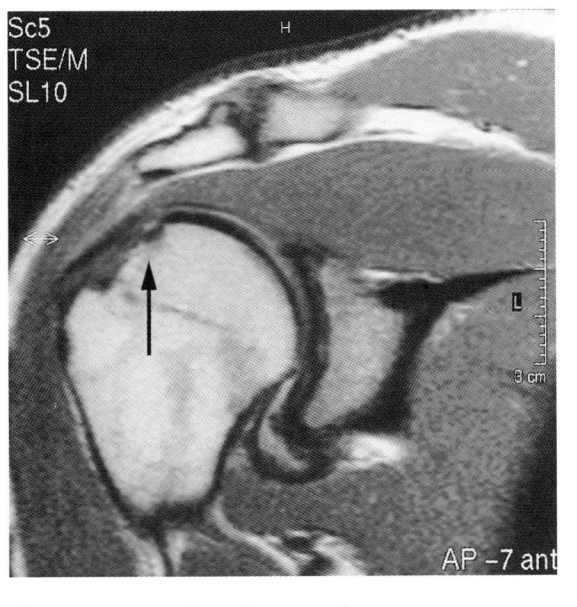

Sc5
TSE/M
SL10

H

L

3 cm

AP –7 ant

Figure 17.12   Hill–Sach's lesion from recurrent trauma between the head of the humerus and the acromion.

Comment

Surgical stabilization is invariably required in throwing and hitting sports with the dominant arm, and rugby with either, unless the athlete gives up these sports. Before deciding on a treatment policy for your patient, one must remember that many athletes change or give up their sport as they grow older and time without a recurrence will tighten and stabilize the capsule.

Subluxing shoulder

Findings

(a) The shoulder may jump and catch with some movements.
(b) The patient may talk of a 'dead arm' after throwing or hitting which may have 'pins and needles'.
(c) There can be capsular or rotator cuff signs because of the recurrent stresses, but often a full range of shoulder movements is present. The rotator cuff may be weak, or weak and painful.

(d) Anterior apprehension test is positive (see *Glossary*).
(e) Relocation test is positive (see *Glossary*).
(f) In multidirectional instability, with a high Beighton–Horan score, the sulcus sign is positive for inferior instability and anterior and posterior draw is increased (see *Glossary*).

Cause

(a) Previous dislocation.
(b) Hypermobility with congenital ligamentous laxity.
(c) Atraumatic repetitive stretching of the anterior capsule, as in throwing, bowling or serving at tennis.
(d) Weak rotator cuff muscles.

Investigations

X-ray to exclude Bankart's and Hill–Sach's lesions (see Figs 17.11 and 17.12). Possible MRI scan.

Treatment

(a) Non-dominant unidirectional – rehabilitation of rotator cuff muscles and a shoulder strap restraint (see Fig. 17.13).
(b) Dominant unidirectional – surgery and avoidance of causative mechanisms.
(c) Multidirectional (dominant and non-dominant) – muscle rehabilitation of the rotator cuff and large shoulder muscles, plus reinforce scapulo-humeral associative movements.
(d) Restriction of activity to avoid subluxing.

Sports

(a) All overarm throwing or hitting are at risk but the patient may get away with side arm throwing.
(b) The non-dominant arm can be at risk when it abducts and rotates to check or stop a spin as in skating or when being turned suddenly at squash to chase a ball.
(c) Rugby. Diving with the arms outstretched to touch down, the fall backwards tackle with the tackle arm externally rotated and abducted, propping and hooking in the scrum, are all at risk.
(d) Swimming. Diving in, butterfly, backstroke, particularly and freestyle are at risk.

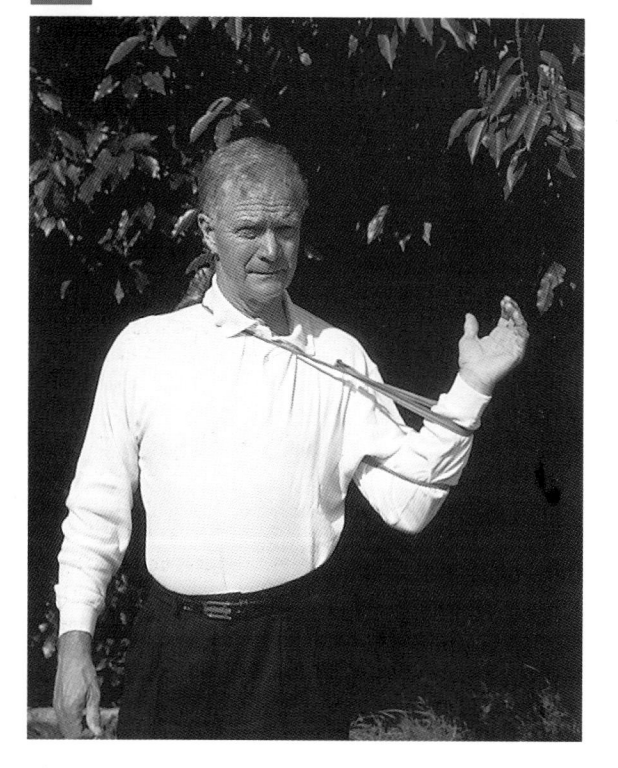

Figure 17.13   The non-dominant arm may be strapped to prevent subluxation. The strap circles the forearm, and travels behind the shoulder and around the neck to the wrist. If the wrist flies wide, the elbow is pulled downwards; if the elbow flies wide the wrist is pulled in towards the body. Both mechanisms prevent the dislocation position being reached.

    Encourage high elbow clearance and reduce length of pull backwards until the shoulder is more stable.

(e) Weightlifting. The pectoralis deck may cause a problem when it is used so that the elbows are at the level of or above the shoulders and if there is no stop to prevent the shoulder being forced backward too far into external rotation, when fatigue sets in. Always have a limiting stop level with the coronal plane of the shoulders and work the elbows below shoulder tip level.

Comment
Athletes who present with a strange feeling or popping in the shoulder often have subluxing

shoulders. Proper rest and avoidance of activity, plus shoulder rehabilitation is essential. It may mean 2–3 years away from the causative activity. Hypermobility and a high Beighton–Horan score will always cause trouble and the patient should find another sport!

Posterior dislocation

Findings
Loss of the normal rounded appearance with a limitation in external rotation. The shoulder should be viewed superiorly and when palpated the humeral head will be noted to lie posteriorly to the acromion. Atraumatic subluxation/dislocation may have a recurrent popping and sliding of the shoulder without pain, and the patient may be able to perform the dislocate as a trick movement. Posterior subluxation test is positive and the Beighton–Horan score may be high and may be part of multidirectional instability (see *Glossary*).

Cause
Uncommon dislocation of the humerus posteriorly from the glenoid cavity. Traumatically with the shoulder being taken into extension but more commonly atraumatic in those with multidirectional instability during functional overstretching.

Investigations
X-ray with true lateral and axillary views should be requested if there is any doubt, as standard views of a shoulder may not display this lesion.

> **Caveat** – Missed diagnosis is common.

Treatment
(a) Relocation under general anaesthetic if acute trauma and if posterior lateral disruption which may require surgery.
(b) Atraumatic require training with biofeedback of deltoid posterior fibres as the posterior deltoid fibres hold and relocate the humeral head. Multidirectional instability does not do well with surgery.

Sports

Butterfly swimming stroke may produce posterior dislocation.

Comment

Not nearly as common as anterior dislocation. Multidirectional instability tends to present as clicking and can do quite well with biofeedback but the patient probably should be moved out of racket games and rugby.

Intracapsular ligament tear

Findings

Generalized shoulder pain which disturbs many activities, e.g. doing the hair, putting on a coat, driving, etc. There may be a click or catch and it disturbs sporting activities. On examination there may be a discomfort and limited movement in external, internal and gleno-humeral abduction and possibly a subacromial bursitis. A click or jump on the Crank test may suggest a capsular tear and the active compression test may be positive (see *Glossary*) [5].

Cause

Acute traumatic or chronic overuse damage to the capsular ligaments, particularly the superior labral, anterior and posterior, the so-called SLAP lesion.

Investigations

May be seen on MRI or not discovered until arthroscopy.

Treatment

(a) Electrotherapy to settle inflammation, such as shortwave diathermy and interferential.
(b) Functional training and strengthening of the rotator cuff in the non-dominant shoulder.
(c) Earlier arthroscopic repair in the dominant shoulder.

Comment

This lesion often presents as a subacromial bursitis or capsulitis. There may be signs from the rotator cuff. Attempts to calm the inflammation with cortisone and rehabilitate the rotator cuff are valid; however, failure to progress warrants an MRI. A positive Crank test or active compression test may be sufficient and cost-effective enough to ignore the MRI, which is often negative, and proceed to arthroscopy.

Traumatic capsulitis of the shoulder

Findings

Rapid increase in pain around the shoulder and down the arm following a traumatic incident. The arm is stiff and painful at night, hurts to lie on, or whilst doing the hair, putting on a coat or a bra. It is eased by resting in a sling. External rotation, internal rotation and gleno-humeral abduction are limited and painful on active and passive movements. Resisted rotator cuff testing is pain-free, though it may be damaged as well by trauma, when it produces its own signs (see *Rotator cuff injuries*).

Cause

A wrench of the shoulder or trauma to the shoulder, or a gradual wrench of the shoulder from forced external rotation.

Investigations

If major trauma, X-ray to exclude fracture or dislocation – otherwise not clinically required.

Caveat – Acute calcific tendonitis and signs of shoulder subluxation.

Treatment

(a) NSAIDs.
(b) Intra-articular injection of cortisone.
(c) Electrotherapeutic modalities to settle inflammation, such as interferential and shortwave diathermy until pain-free.
(d) Isometrics to the rotator cuff.
(e) After 48 hours rest and NSAIDs, capsular stretching and rotator cuff isometrics should start.

Sports

(a) Usually traumatic in any sport.

(b) Cricket. A wide open, chest-on, style of delivery with an exaggerated external rotation of the shoulder may produce an anterior capsulitis. This usually occurs in adolescents trying to bowl too fast – slow down, learn to swing the ball and build up pace when matured. Perhaps bowling a fast ball should be limited to a certain number per week in growing children (see *Spondylolisis*; Chapter 5).

Comment

Not that common in its pure form when it responds rapidly to cortisone, but even when pain-free one must recheck the shoulder for signs of subluxation. Early intra-articular injection is very effective. Follow this with shortwave diathermy and interferential whilst the range of shoulder movements is re-established.

Atraumatic capsulitis of the shoulder (frozen shoulder)

Findings

Stage 1 Diffuse pain in the shoulder, worse when doing one's hair, putting on coat or bra and it may wake the patient at night, especially when lying on the shoulder and may have stabs of pain, caused by movement that suddenly pulls on the capsule. There is a pain-free inner range, but pain at the outer range of external rotation, internal rotation and glenohumeral abduction in the so-called capsular pattern [6], and monitored over time this range of movements becomes reduced. Resisted rotator cuff testing is pain-free.

Stage 2 Limited range of movement, with external rotation limited to 0–5°, internal rotation to the hip pocket and gleno-humeral abduction 30–40°. End of range is pain-free unless forced.

Stage 3 A gradual increase in gleno-humeral

movements which are essentially pain-free.

Separated into thirds:

- Stage 1 of gradually increasing pain and decreasing range of movements.
- Stage 2 of very limited range of movement, but effectively pain-free.
- Stage 3 of increasing range of movement back to normality, almost pain-free.

In total lasting 9 months to 3 years.

Cause

(a) Synovial inflammation and contraction of the shoulder capsule, especially the lax inferior portion, and this may follow trauma, dislocation or subluxation of the shoulder.

(b) More common in the over 40s age group.

(c) This could be a reflex sympathetic dystrophy as it may often follow a cervical lesion.

> **Caveat** – Sometimes the patient develops a greater use of the scapulo-thoracic range of movement that gives the appearance of improvement in the condition, whereas the gleno-humeral range has actually remained the same.

Treatment

Stage 1 Intra-articular injection of cortisone but if there is no improvement after four injections, the cortisone is unlikely to help. Concomitant analgesia and NSAIDs should be given.

Stage 2 Encourage scapulo-thoracic range of movements, wait for stage 3 or manipulation under anaesthetic.

Stage 3 Therapeutic mobilization and stretching exercises. Manipulation under anaesthetic.

Sports

Not associated with any particular sport but very limiting to any arm-related sports. Maintain general fitness.

Comment

Physiotherapy in the first stage is useless but effective in stage 3. Intra-articular cortisone can be successful enough to warrant its use but can also prove ineffective so that analgesia and advice about the natural history of healing become the treatment of choice. Guanethidine, oral or intra-articular, may have a place if there is a reflex sympathetic element. Manipulation under anaesthetic in stage 2 can be very effective but may produce a flare and many patients are happy to leave well alone.

Subscapular crepitus

Findings

Diffuse shoulder pain, sometimes over the posterior thorax but pain-free gleno-humeral movements and pain-free resisted shoulder movements. Rotation and compression of the scapula on the thorax produces grating and pain.

> **Caveat** – The grating may be pain-free and in that case probably is not the cause of the symptoms. Check then for dorsal, costal and vertebral problems (see Chapter 4).

Cause

Roughened underside of the scapula, sometimes with an osteophyte pressing against the thorax which is made worse by a hunched back and shoulders.

Investigations

None clinically required, but if failing to improve, or a suggestion of trauma, then X-ray to exclude scapula fracture or exostosis and consider a bone scan to exclude a stress fracture of the rib.

Treatment

(a) Relax the shoulder position and retrain the rhomboids to release scapulo-thoracic pressure.

(b) Electrotherapeutic modalities to settle inflammation, such as shortwave diathermy and interferential.
(c) Occasionally subscapular injection of cortisone.
(d) Occasionally surgery to remove any obvious osteophyte.

Sports

(a) Golf. At the address position, forced straight arms, hunched shoulders and a forced scapula thoracic compression cause pain. Encourage the sit back position and more relaxed arm tension at the address.
(b) Running. Tight shoulders and a high arm position can cause pain.

Comment

I once cured a golfer's pain and reduced his handicap by four strokes just by altering the 'hunched' shoulder position. A common finding but not a common cause of problems.

Stress fracture of the humerus

Cause

Rare. Sometimes occurs in throwing events and can occur at the epiphysis in children [7].

Coracoid tenderness

Findings

May have pain on full shoulder internal and external rotation and circumduction and the site of the pain is over the coracoid process. Resisted rotator cuff testing is usually pain-free, whereas resisted adduction from the fully externally rotated and circumducted arm is painful. There is local point tenderness on the coracoid and conoid and trapezoid ligaments.

Cause

The causes may be variable, possibly impingement of the clavicle onto the coracoid process, strain of the conoid or trapezoid ligaments, strain of the short head of biceps and coraco-brachialis insertion. Produced by forced or excessive external rotation in abduction or muscle power being produced from this externally rotated and abducted position without upper body rotation (see *Traumatic capsulitis*).

Investigations
None clinically required.

Treatment
Avoid excessive externally rotated shoulder position. The tenderness may respond to local ultrasound or laser and is responsive to local corticosteroid and controlled isometrics of adduction in external rotation and 90° circumduction.

Sports
(a) Uncontrolled pectoralis deck machine exercises when the elbow height is worked too high and no block is put onto the machine to prevent excess external rotation when the muscles fatigue.
(b) Throwing and bowling with a wide open chest and front-on position.
(c) Swimming freestyle when the catch phase is applied with power and followed by an immediate pull phase with no intervening glide phase. Excessive shoulder mobilizing exercises in swimming.

Comment
This element always responds well to local injection of cortisone over the coracoid and then appropriate rehabilitation of the adductors plus correction of the technical fault, but it is often part of a pectoral girdle instability, where all the elements, anterior capsule, acromio-clavicular joint and sterno-clavicular joint, are involved and all must be treated. I have not seen shoulder mobilizing exercises produce this problem in gymnasts, possibly because they are naturally more supple than the swimmers.

Triceps origin strain or tear

Findings
Pain and tenderness on the posterior aspect of the humerus at the triceps origin. Resisted triceps in the triceps curl position are painful.

Cause
An uncommon injury produced by supine lying triceps curls with too big a weight or whilst lying at the end of a bench so that the eccentric phase of contraction leaves the weight unsupported at the end of the movement.

Investigations
None clinically required, although diagnostic ultrasound can aid monitoring the injury.

Treatment
(a) RICE.
(b) Electrotherapeutic modalities to settle inflammation, such as ultrasound and laser.
(c) Controlled triceps rehabilitation following the general muscle ladder principles (see Chapter 20).

Sports
Weight training – beware anabolic steroid abuse.

Comment
Very rare. I have only seen one.

Sterno-clavicular joint strain

Pain and tenderness over the sterno-clavicular joint that may have a swelling (see Chapter 6).

Further reading

1. Tibone, J., Sellers R. and Tonino, P. (1992) Strength testing after third degree acromio clavicular dislocations. *Am. J. Sports Med.* **20**, 328–331.
2. Krueger-Frank, M., Siebert, C. H. and Rosemeyer, B. (1993) Surgical treatment of dislocations of the

acromio clavicular joint in the athlete. *Br. J. Sports Med.* **27**, 121–124.

3. Webb, J. and Bannister, G. (1992) Acromio clavicular disruption in first class rugby players. *Br. J. Sports Med.* **26**, 245–247.

4. Ferretti, A., De Carli, A. and Fontana, M. (1998) Injury of the suprascapular nerve at the spinoglenoid notch. The natural history of infraspinatus atrophy in volleyball players. *Am. J. Sports Med.* **26**, 759–763.

5. O'Brien, S. J., Pagnani, M. J., *et al.* (1998) The active compression test: a new and effective test for diagnosing labral tears and acromio-clavicular joint abnormality. *Am. J. Sports Med.* **26**, 610–613.

6. Cyriax, J. H and Cyriax, P. J. (eds) (1993) *Cyriax's Illustrated Manual of Orthopaedic Medicine*, 2nd edn. Butterworth-Heinemann, Oxford.

7. Boyd, K. T. and Batt, M. E. (1997) Stress fracture of the proximal humeral epiphysis in an elite badminton player. *Br. J. Sports Med.* **31**, 252–253.

Bruckner, P. and Khan, K. (1993) *Clinical Sports Medicine*. McGraw-Hill, New York.

Hutson M. A. (ed.) (1996) *Sports Injuries: Recognition and Management*, 2nd edn. Oxford Medical Publications, Oxford.

Reid, D. (1992) *Sports Injury Assessment and Rehabilitation*. Churchill Livingstone, Edinburgh.

18

Elbow

ANTERIOR

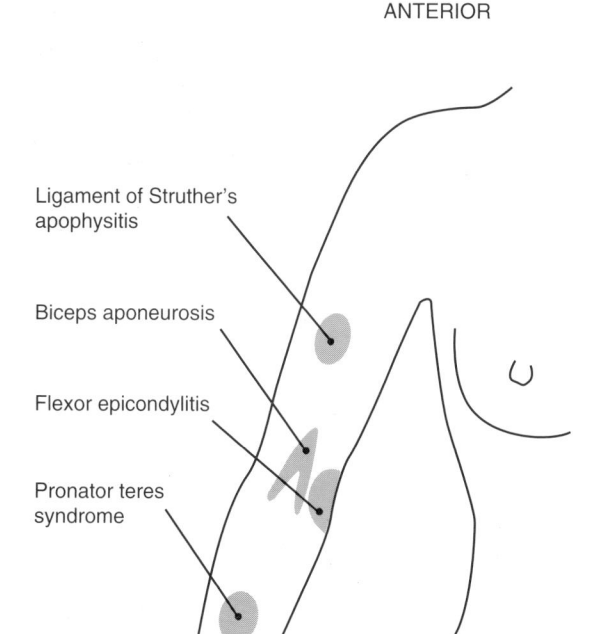

Ligament of Struther's apophysitis

Biceps aponeurosis

Flexor epicondylitis

Pronator teres syndrome

LATERAL

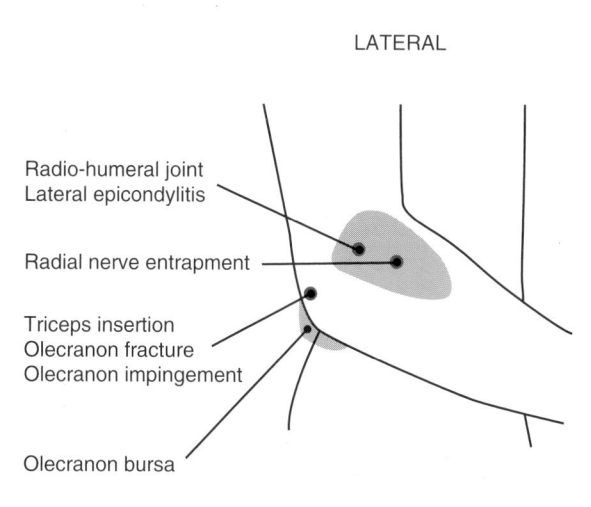

Radio-humeral joint
Lateral epicondylitis

Radial nerve entrapment

Triceps insertion
Olecranon fracture
Olecranon impingement

Olecranon bursa

POSTERIOR

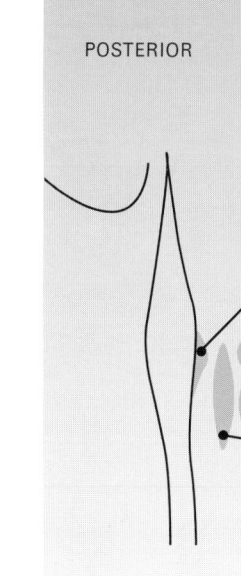

Flexor epicondylitis

Triceps insertion
Olecranon fracture

Olecranon impingement

Ulnar nerve

Referred pain from the neck

Referred pain from the C5/6 roots must be excluded (see Chapter 3).

Referred pain from the shoulder

Particularly the subacromial bursa and occasionally the rotator cuff may be the only presenting symptoms. Always check the shoulder first; if in doubt, inject the subacromial bursa with local anaesthetic and review the signs afterwards (see Chapter 17).

Lateral epicondylitis (tennis elbow/pitcher's elbow)

Findings

Gradual or acute onset of pain over the lateral epicondyle or wrist extensor muscles, which is worse when gripping, hitting, digging, hammering, using a screwdriver and carrying a heavy brief case with palms down. It is worse on making a fist, lifting a cup or kettle, or sometimes writing. Resisted wrist and finger extension are painful. Classically the third and fourth finger, but if the index (second) and thumb are painful then the sports technique is possibly wrong. Tenderness to palpation will differentiate:

Type 1 Tenoperiosteal.
Type 2 Musculo-tendinous.
Type 3 Muscular.
Type 4 Posterior annular.

Cause

Tear or sprain of the extensor origin, particularly the extensor carpi radialis, and this may include impingement of the synovium from the radio-humeral joint.

Investigations

None clinically required, but if getting worse over the first 5 days of an acute injury then X-ray for myositis ossificans (Fig. 18.1); otherwise to

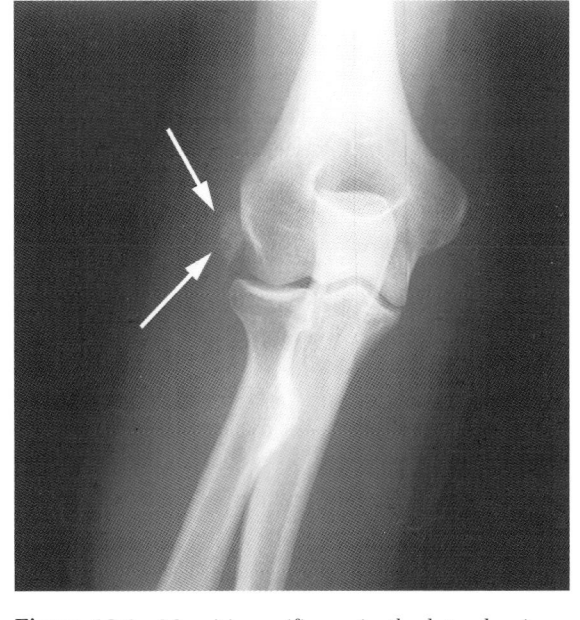

Figure 18.1 Myositis ossificans in the lateral epicondyle of a skier who had been performing rapid turns.

exclude calcified ligament or radio-humeral arthrosis. Possibly diagnostic ultrasound.

> **Caveat** – Pain referred from cervical root C6, subacromial bursa or rotator cuff, radial nerve entrapment and forearm compartment syndrome.

Treatment

(a) RICE.
(b) NSAID gel or ointment or iontophoresis during the acute phase.
(c) Electrotherapy to settle inflammation, such as ultrasound, laser and interferential.
(d) Massage techniques to control scar tissue, such as frictions.
(e) Stretching of the muscle to stimulate the enthesis and prevent scar contraction.
(f) Isometrics of the extensors to organize scar tissue and strengthen the muscles.
(g) Dynamic exercises to increase muscle strength.
(h) Type 1 (tenoperiosteal) responds to physiotherapy and cortisone injections; type 2

(musculo-tendinous) responds to physiotherapy and cortisone injections; type 3 (muscular) responds to physiotherapy; type 4 (posterior annular) usually involves the extracapsular synovium of the radio-humeral joint and does not respond well to physiotherapy, requiring cortisone injection.

(i) Tennis elbow ladder (see Chapter 20).

(j) Chronic adhesions with fixed flexion but no radio-humeral arthrosis – Mills' manipulation after injection of cortisone and local anaesthetic into enthesis (see *Glossary*).

(k) Epicondylitis clasps help some people, but are often applied too tightly and some compress the radial nerve/anterior interosseous nerve.

(l) Failure to progress – rest for 1 year, work through the pain, or surgery.

> **Caveat** – If the radio-humeral joint is involved, this must be treated before the epicondylitis. Myositis ossificans gives a history of getting much worse after about 5 days from the acute injury. Rest, sling, NSAIDs, but may try cortisone, plus analgesia.

Sports
Golf (left)
(a) Left wrist is forced high, so that the extensors are over-stretched.

(b) Left wrist at the address is in front of the hands and take away is with flexion of the left wrist, not with shoulder rotation, so that when hitting, the ground will acutely resist and block the extensors' movement into the shot (Fig. 18.2).

Golf (Right)
Closed grip with the right hand (Fig. 18.3).

Tennis and squash
Pain, usually with backhands, serve or overhead shots.

(a) A grip that is too tight with the thumb and index finger prevents the full wrist flexion that the shot requires and stresses the restraining extensors. Treat by releasing the

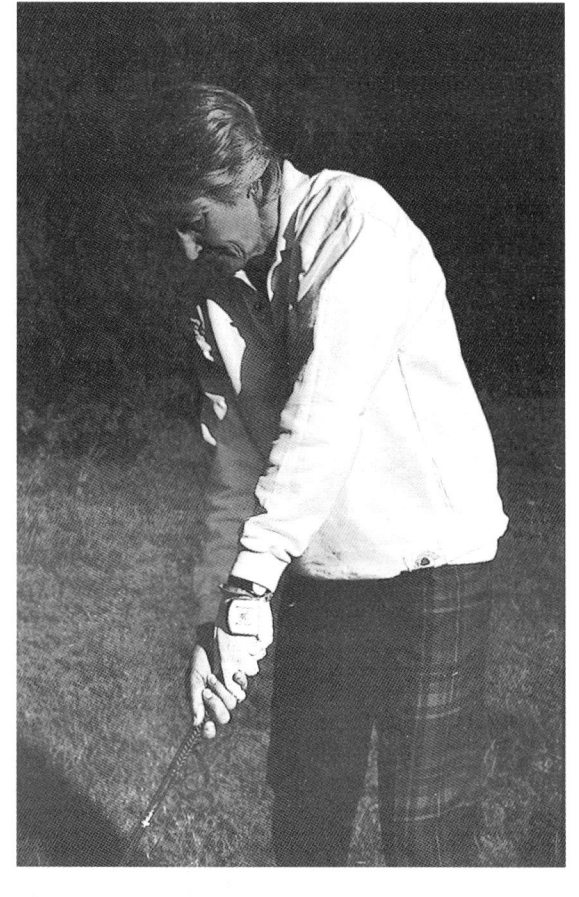

Figure 18.2   The left wrist is forced forwards, increasing the tension on the wrist extensors and the shoulder is shut, preventing proper release through the ball.

tension of the thumb and finger grip (Fig. 18.4), and grip with the third, fourth and fifth fingers.

(b) Check other causes for gripping being too tight, such as a slippery handle, too thin a handle, too thick a handle, tension of the racket strings, tension of the player, etc. (Figs 18.5 and 18.6).

(c) Backhand problems, such as leading with the elbow and wrist into the shot (Fig. 18.7) and dropping the racket head below the wrist (Figs 18.8 and 18.9).

(d) The top spun single handed backhand may overload the extensors if over-practised without developing appropriate strength.

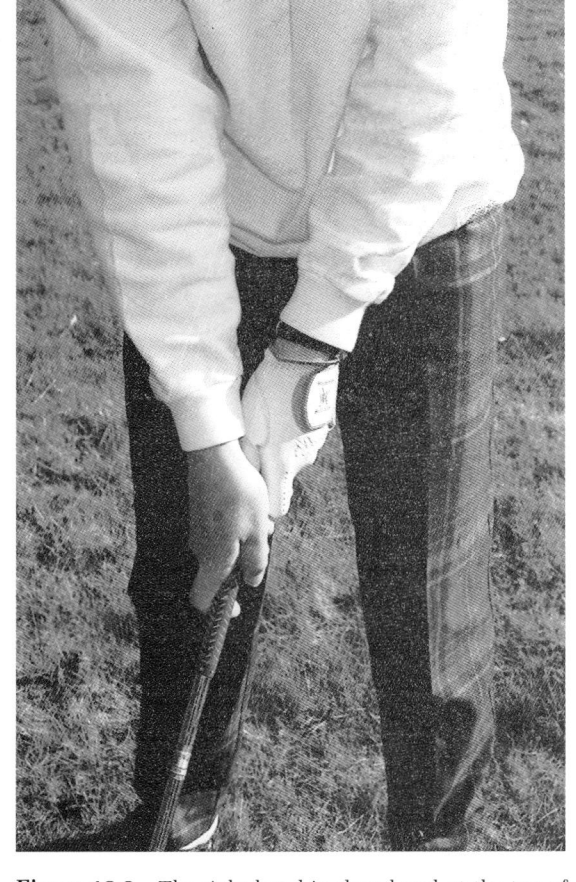

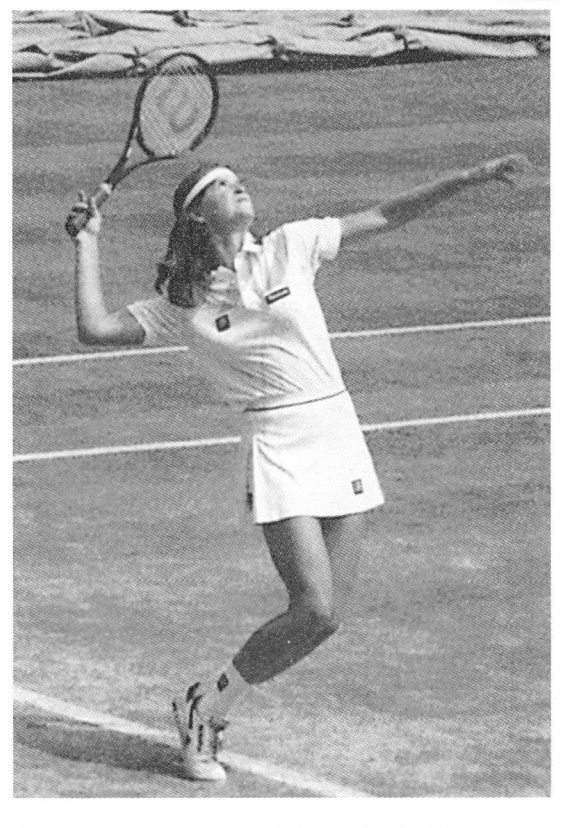

Figure 18.4 Hanna Mandlikova clearly demonstrates release of the thumb and index finger.

Figure 18.3 The right hand is closed and at the top of the back swing will not lie under the club but be forced into ulnar deviation. Unless the thumb and index finger are released, tension will develop in the extensor mechanism. Correction of technique is required.

Badminton

(a) See tennis and squash.
(b) The net player tends to intercept the shuttle and hit the shuttle acutely towards the floor when a tight grip, with thumb and second finger, transfers the forces to the elbow, especially the radio-humeral joint, as well as the extensor complex, causing tennis elbow.

Water skiing

Usually beginners with the tow bar held horizontal can be helped by using a vertical hold as this uses the flexors and rests the extensors.

Snow skiing

Can occur in good skiers, but as an acute overload as the poles are used at speed on repeated rapid turns. Hold on to the tow bar of a drag lift with palms up.

Fly fishing

Too much wrist and not enough elbow and shoulder in the casting technique.

Office

(a) Writing. Thicken the grip and hold the pen between the second and third fingers.
(b) Files. Lift out from a shelf with palm up grip or use both hands.
(c) Computer mouse. Work with a bent elbow and relax the grip to move the mouse but especially select a size of mouse that allows

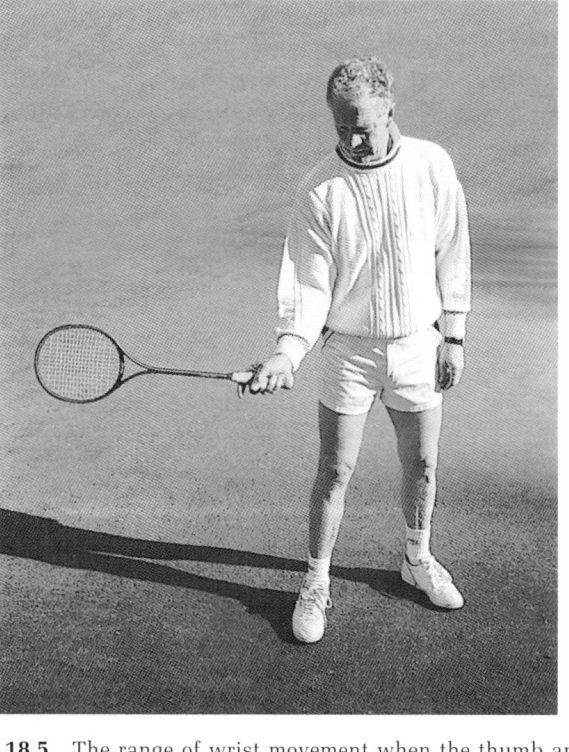 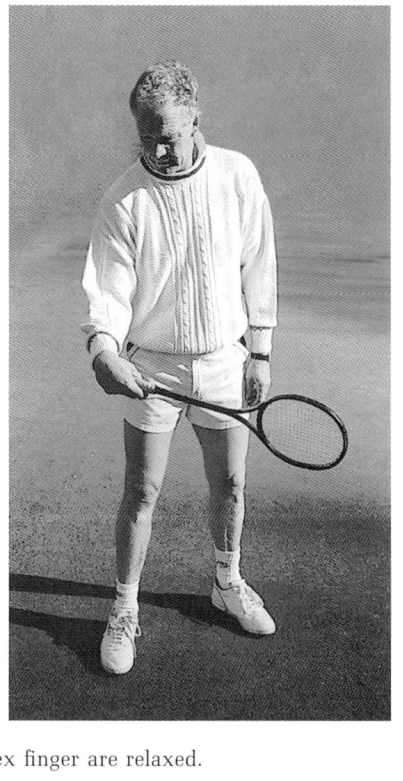

Figure 18.5   The range of wrist movement when the thumb and index finger are relaxed.

a relaxed grip. Change the click 'pressing finger'.

(d) Brief case. Carry with palm up grip and carry two light rather than one heavy case or use a rucksack style case. Do not throw the case into the car.

DIY and garden

Carry, weed and dig palm up. Use a long handle or powered screw driver to reduce the force onto the epicondyles at the elbows. Avoid hammering or use a thicker grip and release the second finger and thumb. Use hand-, not finger-held, secateurs.

Comment

Most cases that have failed physiotherapy are posterior annular. These have often been treated for months before being referred on. One posterior annular injection including the radio-humeral joint often relieves the pain and then rehabilitation of the extensors can be started as soon as the pain level permits. There seem to be three groups:

those that settle after one episode, those that settle but return whilst the technique or the strength is improved and those who seem to improve but are never entirely cured with the problem constantly returning. This is the group who often end in surgery to the extensor origin. I cannot emphasize enough how many presentations of elbows are referred pain from the neck or shoulder. All examinations of the elbow must include the neck and shoulder, and, if in doubt, inject the shoulder, usually the subacromial bursa, with 2% local anaesthetic to see if this relieves the elbow pain.

Radio-humeral joint

Findings

Similar to a tennis elbow, with which it is often associated, so it is painful making a fist and gripping with the palm down, as described in tennis

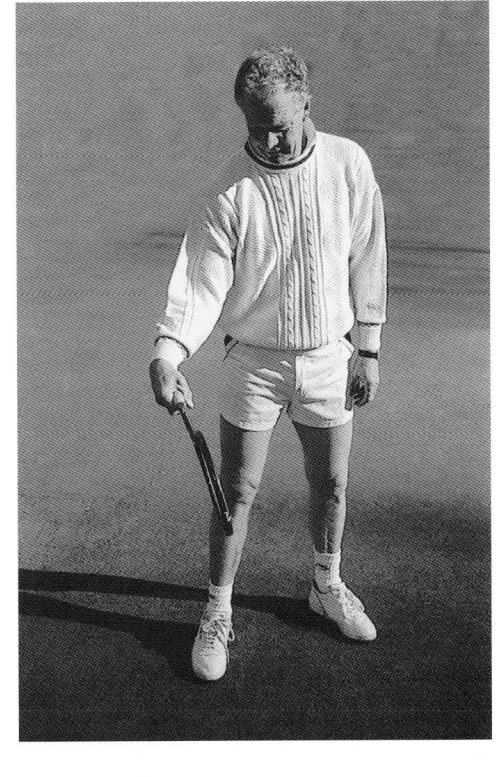

Figure 18.6   The reduced range when the thumb and index finger grip is tight.

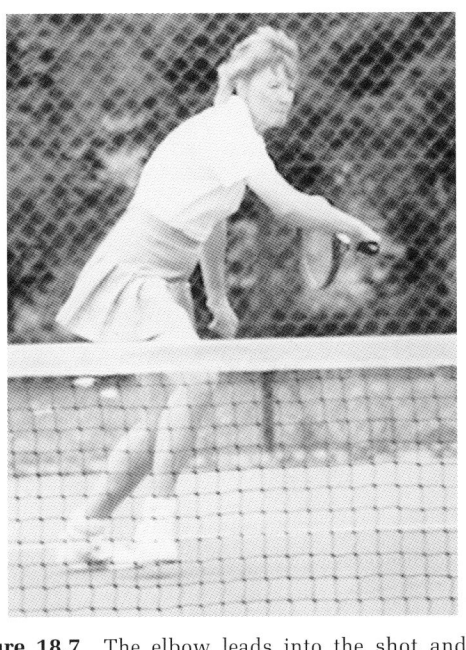

Figure 18.7   The elbow leads into the shot and the wrist is excessively cocked.

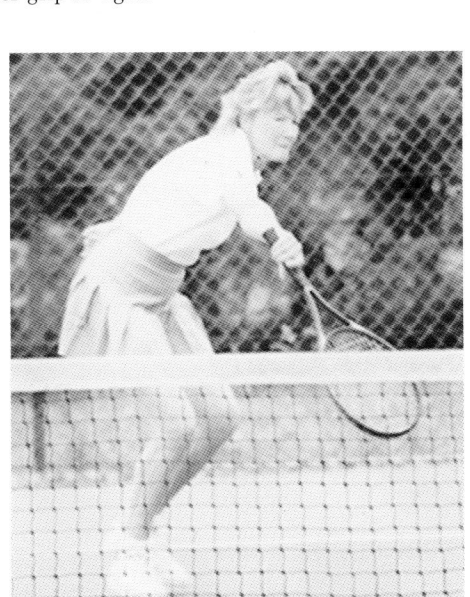

Figure 18.8   The racket head has now dropped below the wrist increasing tension on the wrist extensors.

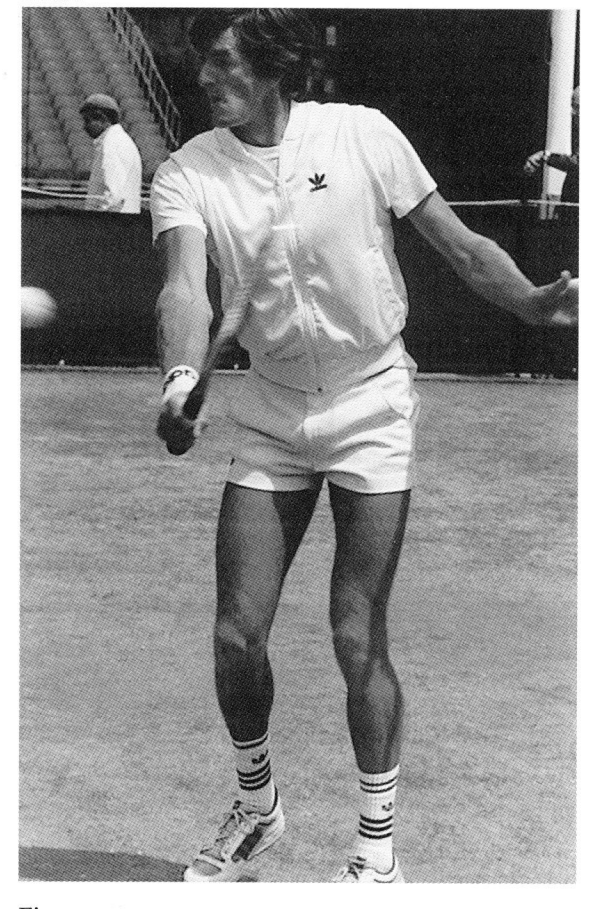

Figure 18.9 Kevin Curran shows a racket head above the wrist and the elbow not leading into the shot.

elbow (see *Lateral epicondylitis*), but it may also cause night pain and straightening of the elbow hurts, as sometimes does full flexion. Passive flexion, extension, and sometimes pronation and supination are painful at the end of the range.

Cause
Traumatic arthrosis of the joint plus the extracapsular synovium may be impinged, and sometimes becomes atrophied and necrotic.

> **Caveat** – Gout, degenerative or inflammatory arthritis, fracture of the radial head if a history of trauma.

Investigations
None clinically required, but X-ray for degenerative changes if failing to settle.

Treatment
(a) Treat the radio-humeral joint before any accompanying lateral epicondylitis.
(b) NSAIDs.
(c) Electrotherapeutic modalities to settle inflammation, such as interferential, pulsed short-wave diathermy and ultrasound.
(d) Injection of cortisone into the joint.

Sports
Tennis
(a) Backhand grip for serve and hitting the top spin serve with pronation. In the early stages of learning to use this technique, the service shot snaps the radio-humeral joint into pronation and extension.
(b) Snatching the wrist movements to get on top of the serve when trying to induce top spin.

Badminton
Usually the net player gets tense and has too tight a grip between the thumb and second finger, so that the wrist will not release as easily into flexion whilst intercepting at the net and this restricted wrist range snaps the force into the radio-humeral joint. The correct shot should be a 'karate chop' with an angled racket, not a forced flexion of the wrist to drive the shuttlecock to the floor, but most net players want to kill the shot!

Golf
Gripping tightly and forcing extension of the elbows at the address, particularly the left. Try a thicker grip on the clubs as this releases the grip pressure and relaxes the elbows, which may prove less easy to do when tense.

Comment
Tennis elbow does not hurt on passive flexion and pronation/supination, a soft block to extension is suggestive of joint involvement. If the techniques are not corrected the injury will return. Treating the epicondylitis before the radio-humeral joint

does not seem to work. Treat the radio-humeral joint first.

Radial nerve entrapment

Findings

(a) An impression of a persistent tennis elbow but with a description of intense pain that often wakes the patient at night, and the pain is worse stretching out for something and is easier in the foetal flexed arm position. The pain can radiate to the back of the hand or up the arm.

(b) The signs at the elbow may be confusing with no definite tennis elbow pattern (see *Lateral epicondylitis*) with the extensor muscle group tender locally to palpation over the radial nerve.

(c) Nerve tensioning tests may be positive, but neck movements do not seem to make it worse (see *Glossary*).

Cause

Radial nerve, the posterior interosseus branch is caught under the ligament of Frohse (the band between the two heads of the supinator).

> **Caveat** – C6/7 referral, referred shoulder pain.

Investigations

An EMG may or may not show nerve conduction deficit.

Treatment

Surgical release.

Sports

Probably not causative but implemental sports may make this worse.

Comment

The clues seem to be night pain with an intensity of pain description that seems too strong for a 'tennis elbow'. A preference for the foetal arm pos-

ition and unclear epicondylar signs. The surgical scar is much bigger than the patient expects.

Flexor epicondylitis (golfer's elbow)

Findings

(a) Pain on pulling (weeds up), carrying boxes palms up or scratching one's back with finger tip pressure as in cleaning or polishing a small object. No history of 'pins and needles' or night pain.

(b) Classically the right elbow of golfer and dominant arm of the tennis player with a Western grip, or a baseball pitcher.

(c) The joint has a pain-free range.

(d) The ulnar nerve is not pathologically tender to palpation.

(e) It is always worse on resisted pronation though, finger tip curl (flexor digitorum profundus), mid phalanx (flexor digitorum superficialis), especially the third (mid) and fourth (ring) fingers are usually, but not invariably, painful.

Cause

Enthesopathy at the flexor origin from overload of pronator and flexors of the wrist and fingers.

> **Caveat** – Neck C8, T1, ulnar nerve entrapment at elbow and avulsion of the medial humeral epicondyle (Little League elbow – apophysitis in children).

Treatment

(a) RICE, but beware of ice irritating the ulnar nerve.

(b) Electrotherapeutic modalities to settle inflammation, such as laser and ultrasound.

(c) Cortisone to the locally tender area.

(d) Massage techniques to control scar tissue orientation.

(e) Stretch fingers and wrist into extension to prevent scar contraction and orientate scar tissue.

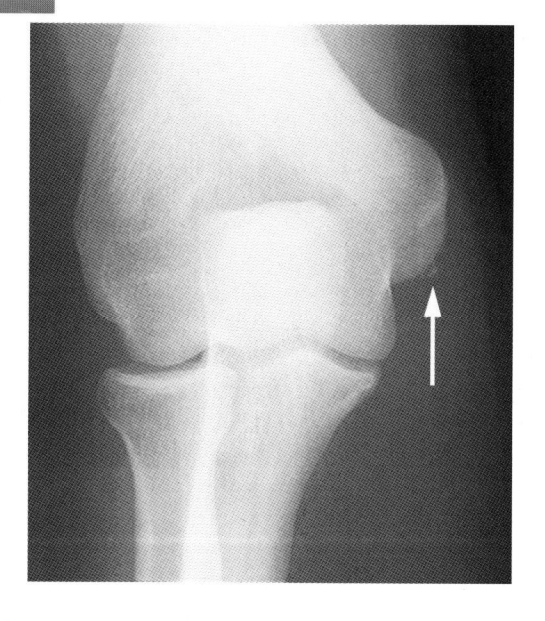

Figure 18.10 A small avulsion fragment from the medial epicondyle (arrow).

(f) Isometric resisted exercises against pronation, scratch the back over the top of the shoulder with finger pulp pressure and squeeze objects with finger tip grip, to put a controlled load on the enthesis and scar tissue and to maintain muscle strength.

(g) Gradually introduce larger loads (see Chapter 20).

(h) This injury takes time to heal, usually because rehabilitation is taken too fast and thus it has episodes when it reflares.

(i) Failed conservative treatment requires a surgical release of the enthesis.

Investigations

None clinically required unless failing to improve or following an acute, severe episode, then X-ray to exclude avulsion and apophysitis (Fig. 18.10).

Sports

(a) Throwing or hitting with strong finger and wrist flexion to increase acceleration, such as javelin, and in baseball, the fast ball and curve ball.

(b) Rotational shot putt – if the shot slides off the tip of fingers and thumb.

(c) Golf. Strong right arm pull through the swing, especially with the right-hand grip being too open.

(d) Tennis. Semi-Western forehand – top spun shots.

(e) Winching out sails.

(f) Pulling, weeding and polishing with a tight finger grip.

Comment

This is not as common as tennis elbow but it is fairly resistant to treatment. Cortisone removes the pain, but rehabilitation which then follows will take several months. Do not take the patient up the rehabilitation ladder too fast. Proportionally, more of my patients with flexor epicondylitis have come to surgery than my patients with extensor epicondylitis.

Ulnar neuritis

Findings

(a) Pain at the elbow which may refer upwards or down to the wrist and may wake at night.

(b) 'Pins and needles' and possibly numbness at the fourth and fifth fingers and ulnar half of the third finger.

(c) Tenderness to palpation of the ulnar nerve in the condylar groove or just distal to the groove which refers pain and 'pins and needles' to fingers.

(d) Adverse neural tensioning tests, if positive, are not worse with neck movements.

(e) Muscle weakness of interossei and hypothenar eminence wasting. May have clawing of the third and fourth finger; the Pope's sign and Froment's sign can be positive (see *Glossary*).

Cause

Irritation of the ulnar nerve in the condylar groove, often from local pressure, such as the edge of the desk and window of the car when driving.

Occasionally post-trauma to the elbow when it is bound into the scar tissue.

Investigation
Electromyogram.

Treatment
Avoid local pressure but with night pain can try perineural cortisone ×1 at the elbow. Surgical release and transposition if not settling with conservative means.

Sports
No sport is particularly relevant (see Chapter 19).

Comment
Referral to the ulnar two fingers can be from the carpal tunnel as the ulnar and median nerves may link in the forearm. Damage to the superficial branch of the ulnar at the pisiform (Guyon's canal) has no muscle weakness as this superficial branch is sensory. Avoidance of local pressure settles most of the problems and perineural steroids can reduce a flare, but chronic problems require transposition.

Triceps insertion

Findings
Acute or chronic onset of pain at the insertion which is worse with extending the elbow actively or on resisted extension. Passive elbow extension is pain-free and there is local tenderness to palpation on the enthesis.

Cause
Strain of the triceps insertion into the olecranon, usually in sports that accelerate extension at the elbow (see Chapter 19).

> **Caveat** – Cervical spine C6/7 and ruptures at the triceps insertion have been reported [1].

Investigations
X-ray as there is a well-recorded incidence of stress fractures and avulsion of the apophysis; a bone scan may be required if healing appears slow.

Treatment
(a) RICE and NSAIDs.
(b) Electrotherapeutic modalities to settle inflammation, such as ultrasound and laser.
(c) Massage techniques to control scar tissue such as frictions.
(d) Injection of cortisone to the enthesis.
(e) Stretching with passive flexion of elbow on flexed shoulder to prevent scar tissue contraction and to load the enthesis.
(f) Graded resisted isometrics to stress the enthesis and prevent scar tissue contraction.
(g) Incrementation of loads (see Chapter 20) but particularly through triceps curls, shoulder presses, dips and throwing.

Sports
(a) Weightlifting. Driving the arm into extension when pressing weights and triceps dips.
(b) Tennis, where there is a tendency to an arm-only serve that tries to hit the top spin serve but does not transfer the body weight to the back foot and then forwards through the service on to the front foot and net.
(c) Pitchers – particularly throwing the 'change up' which snaps the elbow into extension.
(d) Martial arts when the elbow is snapped into extension.

Comment
Like all entheses the inflammation responds well to anti-inflammatories such as cortisone but rehabilitation of the teno-osseous junction is also required.

Olecranon impingement

Findings
Acute or chronic onset of pain at the posterior aspect of the elbow which is worse on passive or active elbow extension but not with resisted isometrics testing of the triceps. It is locally tender along the lateral olecranon, humeral condylar

groove and is usually not swollen. Check Beighton–Horan score for hypermobility (see *Glossary*) as patients often have increased elbow extension.

Cause

Synovial or fat pad entrapment between the olecranon and olecranon fossa of the humerus, usually because the elbow is whipped into extension or because the elbow hyper extends as a result of increased ligamentous laxity.

> **Caveat** – C6/7 referral from neck, triceps strain, stress fracture of olecranon, avulsion of olecranon and gout.

Treatment

(a) Avoid the causative mechanisms. See a coach.
(b) Electrotherapeutic modalities to settle inflammation, such as interferential and ultrasound.
(c) Inject cortisone to the tender area within the olecranon fossa by a lateral approach as the medial risks the ulnar nerve. You need to get into the olecranon condylar groove and occasionally inject the fossa behind the triceps tendon.

Sports

(a) Weightlifting. Locking out 'presses' may cause impingement in hypermobile elbows and too heavy a weight in biceps curls can snap out extension in the eccentric phase.
(b) Pitchers – particularly throwing the 'change up' which snaps the elbow into extension.
(c) Martial arts – snapping the elbow into extension.
(d) Gymnastics – sway back elbows. These gymnasts are most unlikely to survive four-piece gymnastics if they possess a high Beighton–Horan score. Rhythmic gymnastics may be preferable (see *Glossary*).
(e) Squash. The backhand shot is played too close to body with a straight elbow and especially a little angled shot from the backhand corner to the forehand front wall can lock out the elbow into extension (Fig. 18.11).

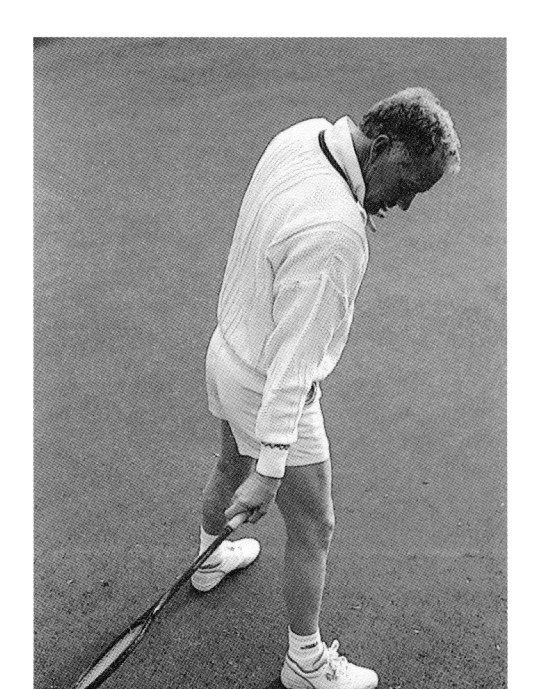

Figure 18.11 A backhand shot at squash played with an extended elbow, racket below the wrist that jams the olecranon into its fossa.

Comment

Does not do well with physiotherapy. Cortisone and altered technique is the treatment of choice.

Olecranon bursa

Findings

Pain-free palpable fluctuant swelling or swelling that occurs post local trauma. There is stiffness of the elbow but the joint movement is pain-free, although flexion may be stiff or if inflamed painful at the bursa. Inflammatory disease, infective or systemic produces a red, warm and painful swelling as may a haembursitis.

Cause

(a) Frictional from leaning on the elbow or repetitive full flexion at elbow as reported by darts throwers.

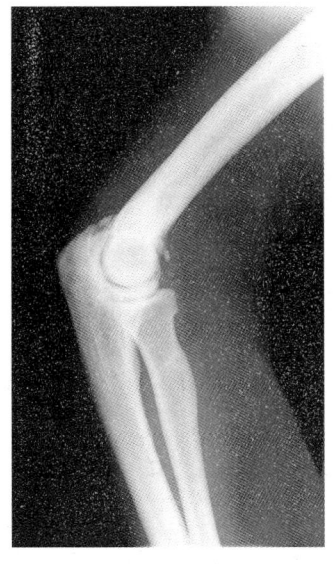

Figure 18.12   Degenerative changes in the elbow.

(b) Traumatic – haembursitis of the olecranon bursa.
(c) Systemic – such as gout and the inflammatory arthritides.

Treatment

(a) Avoid causative factors.
(b) Aspirate and check for crystals or culture.
(c) Hydrocortisone if required for comfort.
(d) Rarely surgical ablation.

Investigations

X-ray for osteoarthritis osteophytes or synovial chondromatosis (see Figs 11.3 and 18.12) and aspirate for polarized light microscopy (gout or pseudogout). Culture if infection suspected.

Sports

Said to occur in darts throwers during early training.

Comment

Unless painful, most patients will accept the bursa. Try aspiration and cortisone, but if this does not settle after two then leave well alone. Surgery may be required if synovial chondromatosis or osteophytes are troublesome.

Olecranon fracture

Apart from local trauma to the elbow the olecranon can suffer a stress fracture or in children avulsion of the apophysis. The problems are those of a triceps insertion but the bony damage requires longer to heal and a loose fragment may require surgical screwing (see *Triceps insertion*).

Osteoarthritis of the elbow

Findings

(a) Possibly a history of previous trauma followed much later by a gradual increase in pain and decrease in range, first noted by limitation of extension.
(b) Swelling, plus or minus limitation in passive flexion and extension with pain at the limit of movement.
(c) Pronation and supination are not limited unless the radio-humeral joint has been involved.
(d) Occasionally osteophytes may cause ulnar nerve pressure and symptoms in the hand.

Cause

Degenerative changes which are mainly post-traumatic.

Investigations

X-ray for osteophytic lipping (see Fig. 18.12).

Treatment

(a) NSAIDs.
(b) Electrotherapeutic modalities to settle inflammation, such as shortwave diathermy and interferential.
(c) Allow movement in the pain-free range.
(d) Surgery.

Caveat – Systemic arthritis, gout or synovial chondromatosis.

Sports

Most problems occur with hitting sports as in golf or racket shots when the elbow straightens rapidly, extending the joint into the painful range, and this is a difficult problem to get round. Forcing weight lifts into an extended arm or the weight being too heavy and forcing extension of the elbow can also be causative.

Comment

Fortunately not that common but really quite limiting when it does occur.

Loose bodies

Findings

A history of intermittent or persistent restriction or locking of the elbow with swelling of the elbow joint which may have followed trauma. There is a restricted range of flexion and extension with pain, and with a radio-humeral loose body, pronation and supination are restricted and painful.

Cause

Osteochondral fragment or a traumatic fragment in the ulnar humeral or radio-humeral joint.

Investigations

X-ray is usually sufficient and the best investigation to show a loose body or osteochondral defect on the humeral condyle, but a cartilaginous loose body may not show (Fig. 18.13). CT or MRI may be required, but these are also not good for visualizing a cartilaginous loose body.

Treatment

Surgical removal.

Sports

(a) Gymnastics. The injury may be the end for four-piece gymnastics for the gymnast, as this has been produced by an osteochondral defect, but gymnasts may be able to try the asymmetric bars, balance beam and build into walkovers, and only later add flicks and

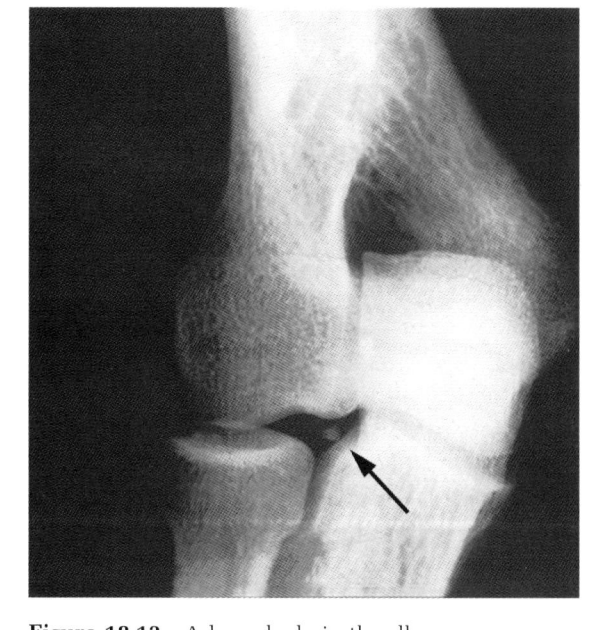

Figure 18.13 A loose body in the elbow.

somersaults and vaults with careful monitoring.
(b) It is usually post-traumatic in other sports.

Comment

The osteochondral defect may be a compression stress fracture. The elbow does seem to suffer a reduction in range after the injury and whether this elbow is truly capable of further attrition from gymnastics is highly debatable, fortunately it is not a common injury.

Osteochondral defect

A history of a loose body or of pain and swelling in an adolescent elbow should have an X-ray and possibly MRI to look for osteochondral damage (see *Loose bodies*).

Biceps aponeurosis

Findings

(a) Usually gradual onset associated with elbow flexion under loads.

(b) There is pain on resisted supination and flexion, and Yergason's and Speed's tests may be positive (see *Glossary*).

(c) There is tenderness to palpation along the aponeurosis to the radial insertion.

(d) Very rarely, may rupture at the distal end of the biceps [2].

Cause

Uncommon consequence of strong biceps loading, usually with flexion and supination. Consider anabolic steroid abuse.

> **Caveat** – C5/6 referral from neck, referral from the shoulder or radial neck fracture.

Investigations

None clinically required apart from the rupture when ultrasound or MRI will help.

Treatment

(a) The rupture requires surgery [2].

(b) The tendinopathy is poor to respond and may take months, so it is best to reduce load and use controlled biceps exercises while the lesion heals over time.

(c) Can try local cortisone along the aponeurosis but this has variable results.

Sports

(a) Any requiring strong elbow flexion and supination.

(b) Archery. Can be caused by beginners drawing the bow with elbow flexion rather than scapula retraction. Correct the fault and use a lighter draw weight until the injury has settled.

(c) Weightlifting and body building – avoid biceps curls and 'hand under' pull-ups. Check for anabolic steroid abuse.

(d) Cricket – a violent square cut from one of my patients produced this injury as the right hand is whipped into supination during this shot.

Comment

Fortunately rare, as this heals so slowly. I now inform patients that treatment is time and controlled activities as anything else does little to help.

Pronator teres syndrome

Findings

(a) A history of acute pain locally over the mid anterior forearm and some anterior elbow pain that is locally tender to palpation.

(b) Gripping with the finger tips or middle phalanges, especially the third and fourth, give pain.

(c) Resisted flexor superficialis (middle phalanges) of the third and fourth fingers give pain in the forearm. Other authors have found that the profundus hurts (distal phalanges).

(d) Pain on forehand shots.

Cause

Restriction of the median nerve through the pronator teres.

(a) Acute – a one-off retrieving shot (tennis) when the ball is behind the player and the shot is played forehand with a straight arm and extreme flexion of wrist to achieve the correct direction of return.

(b) Chronic – the acute mechanism as above employed regularly, usually in squash.

(c) Perhaps these mechanisms in fact pull on the flexor muscle belly and this is a muscle injury, but the findings are similar to that of the nerve entrapment reported as pronator teres syndrome.

Investigations

None clinically required.

Treatment

For the acute type, local cortisone to the tender area and alter technique, especially so for the chronic problems. Rest from gripping as in shot making in tennis and squash for 12–18 months may be required. Surgery to release the tight pronator restriction band.

Sports

(a) Tennis – a one-off shot (see *Cause*).
(b) Squash – instead of facing the back wall to hit the boast or drive out of the forehand back corner, the player faces the front wall to the side wall and tries to direct the shot straight to the front wall with a straight arm and extreme wrist flexion.

Comment

A rare condition. Although it is reported to do well with surgery to release the median nerve, my patients seem to have had an extreme resisted flexion injury which should be a tear of superficialis with scar tissue. The symptoms of the two descriptions seem to be similar but they may be different conditions. Two did very well with steroid injections, two settled with altered technique but one took a long time to rehabilitate. The technical fault was consistent with all four.

Supinator strain

Findings

Pain over the upper forearm that is worse with resisted supination. However, the passive elbow range is pain-free, passive supination is pain-free, resisted wrist and finger flexion is pain-free, and pure resisted elbow flexion is pain-free, and the biceps aponeurosis is not tender to palpation.

Cause

Rare. Biceps curls with hyper extended elbow and over-supinated hand position. Sometimes called 'preacher curls' when the weight is too heavy and produces pain of supinator origin. There is acute pain during exercise, which appears then to come with a number of different weight exercises, but careful analysis shows often that the supinated position has been achieved.

Investigations

None clinically required.

Treatment

Difficult, but electrotherapeutic modalities, such as ultrasound, laser and interferential, plus reduced loading of the supinator might help.

Sports

Weight training 'preacher curls'.

Comment

I have only seen two cases which took a long while to settle, but one player continued to play hockey during the problem – both had been performing preacher curls.

Ligament of Struther's apophysitis

The ligament of Struther attaches to the humerus and may pull out a bony spur at its attachment. This can become vulnerable to direct trauma as in boxing (Fig. 18.14).

Compartment syndrome of the forearm

Findings

A history of forearm flexor pain, worse with increasing length of exercise. No evidence of referral from the neck or shoulder is found and resisted flexors do not hurt unless seen acutely.

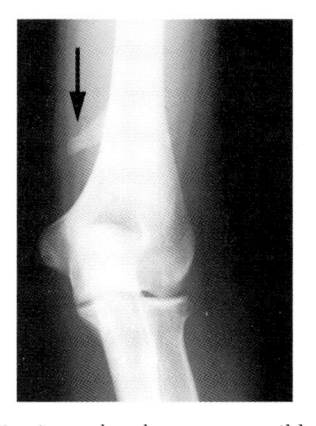

Figure 18.14   An ecchondroma or possibly the attachment of the ligament of Struther's has been hit and fractured in this boxer.

Cause

Possibly swelling of the flexor muscles within a fascial sheath that does not allow for this expansion which then reduces oxygen supply to the muscle.

> **Caveat** – Carpal tunnel syndrome.

Investigation

Flexor compartment pressure studies.

Treatment

(a) RICE.
(b) NSAIDs.
(c) Electrotherapeutic modalities to settle inflammation, such as ultrasound, laser and interferential.
(d) Surgical release of the tight fascia.

Sports [3]

(a) Water ski racing. Caused by the pure endurance of holding the tow bar, even though elbow and shoulder holds are used to relieve the problem.
(b) Motor-cross. As the rider stands most of the time the clutch and brakes must be set at an angle about 45° to the horizontal. Sometimes they are set nearly horizontal for the sitting position but when the rider stands the forearm flexors become continually stretched and work from this position.
(c) Rowing. Occurs infrequently from the flexed grip.

Comment

These are not common, but in these sports an index of suspicion should be aroused.

Further reading

1. Stannard, J. P. and Bucknell, A. L. (1993) Rupture of the triceps tendon associated with steroid injections. *Am. J. Sports Med.* **21**, 482–485.
2. D'Alessandro, D. F., Shields, C. L., *et al.* (1993) Repair of distal biceps tendon ruptures in athletes. *Am. J. Sports Med.* **21**, 114–119.
3. Wasilewski, S. A. and Asdourian, P. L. (1991) Bilateral chronic exertional compartment syndromes of forearm in an adolescent athlete. Case report and review of literature. *Am. J. Sports Med.* **19**, 665–667.

Bruckner, P. and Khan, K. (1993) *Clinical Sports Medicine*. McGraw-Hill, New York.

Hutson M. A. (ed.) (1990) *Sports Injuries: Recognition and Management*. Oxford Medical Publications, Oxford.

Reid, D. (1992) *Sports Injury Assessment and Rehabilitation*. Churchill Livingstone, Edinburgh.

19

Wrist and hand

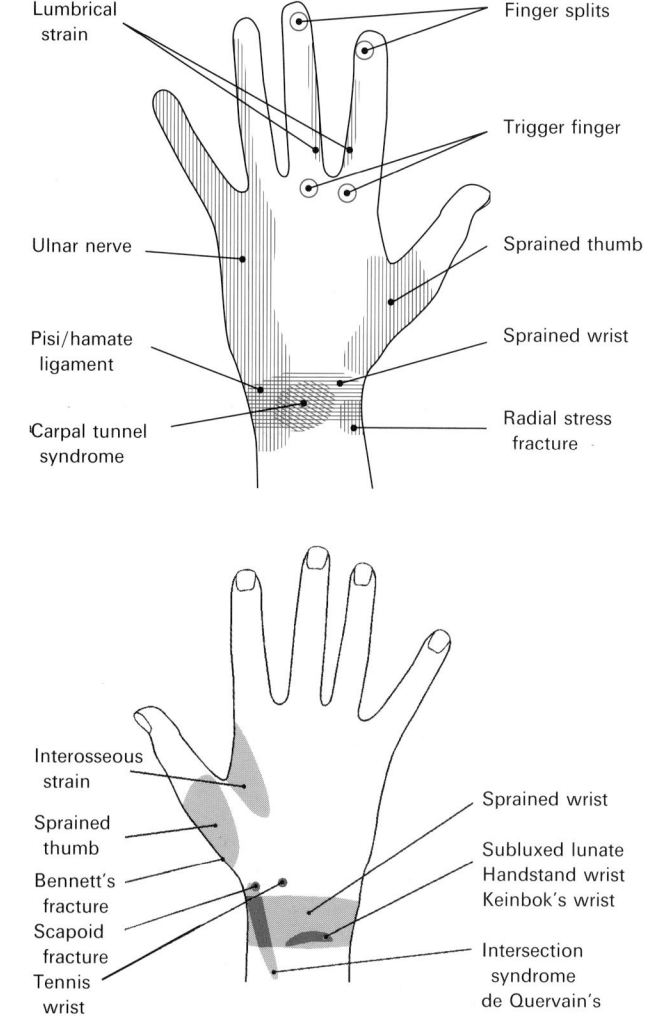

Lumbrical strain

Finger splits

Trigger finger

Ulnar nerve

Sprained thumb

Pisi/hamate ligament

Sprained wrist

Carpal tunnel syndrome

Radial stress fracture

Interosseous strain

Sprained wrist

Sprained thumb

Subluxed lunate
Handstand wrist
Keinbok's wrist

Bennett's fracture

Scapoid fracture

Tennis wrist

Intersection syndrome
de Quervain's tenosynovitis

Acute traumatic injuries

Falls, implemental trauma or karate blows may produce fractures and internal ligament derangement. X-rays should be taken when the Terry Thomas sign and Watson test suggest scapholunate disassociation which can cause on-going problems (see *Glossary*). A bone scan will often show chronic bony stress, and will display the scaphoid and hamate fracture, but generally management is for experts in hand and wrist problems because internal ligamentous damage is difficult to diagnose and often requires arthrograms. Finger fractures, avulsions and ligament sprains are common, and although the adjacent fingers may act as splints, mallet and boutonnière deformities and spiral fractures do require specific management by a hand specialist. The attitude of the open hand and clenched fist will give clues to metacarpal and phalangeal stress fractures, where a spiral fracture will distort the alignment. The distal end of the fourth and fifth metacarpals are classically broken with a punch, but a subluxation of the second metacarpal also occurs in boxers at the proximal end. Triangular fibro-cartilage tears can be caused by impingement with excessive ulnar deviation but is usually traumatic and MRI may show the damage, but arthrogram may also be required.

Impingement injuries

The wrist has a rotatory movement between the radius and the ulnar. The major movements are ulnar and radial deviation between the radius and ulnar, on one side, and the proximal carpal bones, scaphoid, hamate and triquetral, on the other. A hinge joint is formed between this proximal row and the distal row of hamate, capitate, trapezoid and trapezium. The hinge movement is especially prone to impingement in extension and distraction of intracarpal ligaments in flexion.

(a) Tennis wrist is caused by impingement at the base of the second and third metacarpals with a full Western grip (Figs 19.1–19.3), where the very open hand grip takes all the impact of the forehand tennis shots over this area. The grip must be weakened to a semi-Western style.

(b) Handstand wrist is an impingement in extension whilst doing a handstand or press-up. Turning the hand out into ulna deviation will relieve this. A half glove filled with padding over the butt of the hand or performing press-ups on a pile of books or a bench so that the wrist is held in a neutral position aids training.

Subluxed lunate

The lunate may sublux with wrist flexion. Manipulation and splinting in a cock-up splint may help.

Keinbok's avascular necrosis of lunate

Rest in cast brace or cock-up splint may help. Surgery may be required in chronic cases (Fig. 19.4).

Sprained thumb: metacarpo-phalangeal joint

Findings
A history of an acute injury with swelling and bruising of the thenar eminence. Pain is centred around the metacarpo-phalangeal joint. Passive abduction of the first metacarpo-phalangeal joint is painful and the range of movement may be increased. However, this range must be checked against the contralateral thumb for the normal range of movements which may be extreme. The patient may not be able to lift a bottle or a glass in a one-hand grip.

Cause
Forced abduction of the thumb or thumb caught in clothing during a tackle or forced abduction from

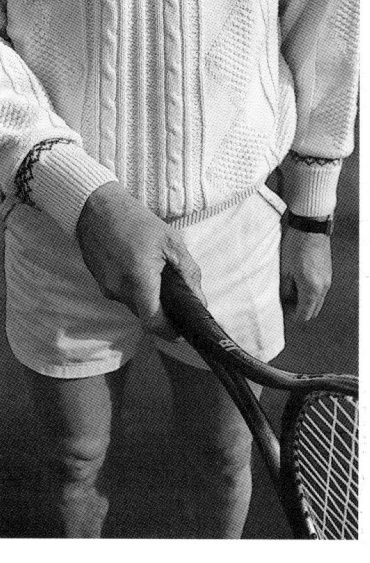

Figure 19.1   Standard grip.

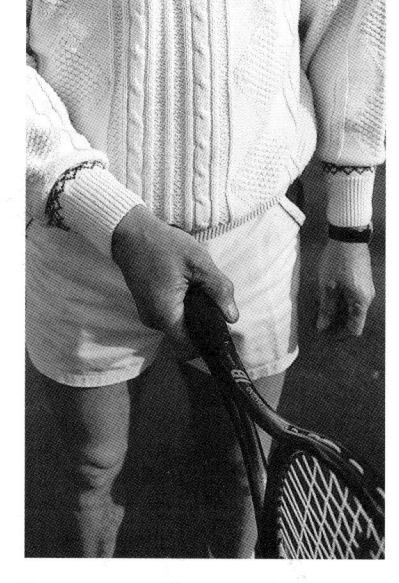

Figure 19.2   Semi-Western grip.

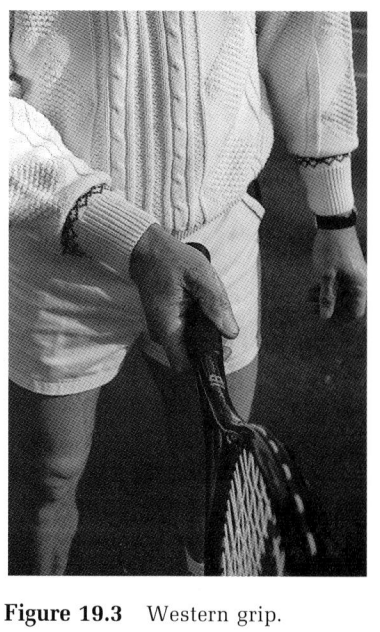

Figure 19.3   Western grip.

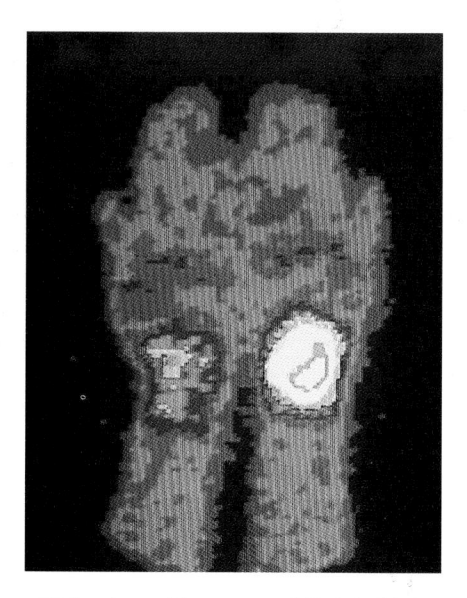

Figure 19.4   A positive scan of Keinbok's avascular necrosis of the lunate.

a ball or implement where the ulnar collateral ligament and capsule and occasionally radial collateral ligament are damaged.

Investigations
X-ray for flake fracture of the ulnar collateral ligament.

Treatment
(a) RICE.
(b) NSAIDs.
(c) Strapping of the joint but encourage flexion and extension.
(d) Electrotherapeutic modalities to settle inflammation, such as ultrasound and laser.
(e) If the range is increased, it will probably require surgery to the ulnar collateral ligament.

Sports
(a) Strap for activities; in sports that permit this form of strapping, strap between the thumb and base of the index finger, like a web between the fingers.
(b) Skiing. Caused by the thumb catching in the diamond of a dry ski slope. A pair of socks over the gloves or taping the first metacarpophalangeal joint may help prevent this problem. Safety straps for ski poles pull on the thumb when the skier falls. Use release handles on ski poles or allow the strap to hang over the wrist so they are not held down by the hand grip. Thermoplastic ski splints may be appropriate.

Comment

A very common lesion. The major problem is strapping the thumb in sports that need to hold an implement. Probably best to tape during activities and use an elasticated bandage for normal use. Unfortunately the unstable ulnar collateral ligament is often overlooked.

Sprained thumb: metacarpo-trapezial joint

Findings

Either acute but more usually gradual onset with pain at rest in the metacarpo-trapezial joint which is worse with writing, gripping, polishing or picking up a glass. There is pain on extension and circumduction and opponation of this carpo-phalangeal joint. It is tender to palpation over both the dorsal and volar aspect of the joint.

Cause

Strain of the joint capsule usually from hyper extension (see *Osteoarthritis of the metacarpo-trapezial joint* and *Bennett's avulsion fracture*).

Investigations

X-ray and CT scan for degenerative changes if failure to progress, and also blood tests for rheumatoid factors and autoimmune profile if systemic disease suspected.

Caveat – Rheumatoid arthritis.

Treatment

(a) NSAIDs.
(b) Injection of cortisone to first carpo-phalangeal joint.
(c) Electrotherapeutic modalities that settle inflammation, such as shortwave diathermy and interferential.
(d) Strapping or thermoplastic splint for sport.
(e) Surgical replacement of trapezium.

Sports

(a) Fishing. May have to relax thumb pressure on the grip or slide the thumb around the side of the rod as opposed to holding on the top when casting.
(b) Golf. Similarly, may have to relax thumb pressure on the golf club or thicken the grip. This problem can occur with a split grip in either the take away when the top of the back swing extends the thumb further or in the follow through with a drawn shot. A power fade seems to relieve the pressure on the thumb.

Comment

An acute flare is a capsulitis that responds very well in 48 hours to an intra-articular injection of cortisone but the chronic stresses seem to return with minor loads.

Osteoarthritis of the metacarpo-trapezial joint

Degenerative change is very common in this joint and responds to conservative measures (see *Sprained thumb: metacarpo-trapezial joint*) but a splint or support during activities is essential and surgical replacement of the trapezium may be required.

Bennett's avulsion fracture

Findings

A history of an acute injury with swelling and bruising around the thenar metacarpal eminence. There is a painful or painless increased range at the first metacarpo-trapezial joint in abduction and the patient cannot hold a wide grip such as holding a bottle or glass. Although the range of movement is increased, the painful side must be checked against the normal side as a great variation in the normal range can exist.

A Practical Guide to Sports Injuries

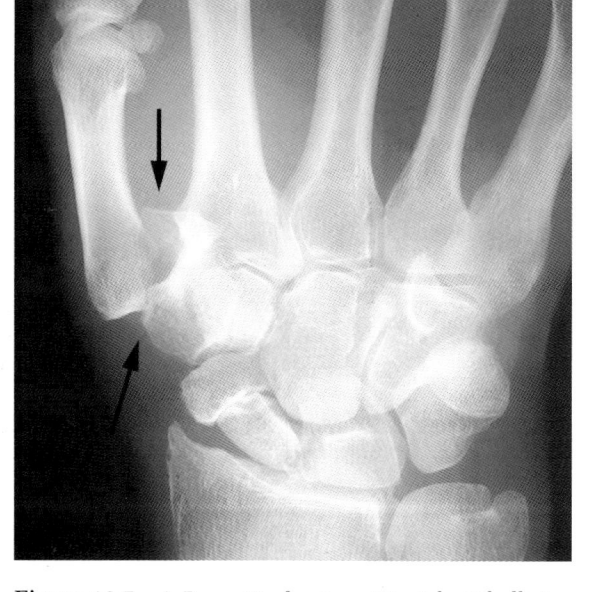

Figure 19.5   A Bennett's fracture (Mr. John Challis).

Cause

Abduction injury with a trans-articular fracture dislocation of the first metacarpal at the meta-carpo-trapezial joint, in which a small fragment remains held *in situ* by the strong volar ligament. In sport, particularly whilst skiing, when the wrist straps or 'diamond' of the dry ski slope forces the thumb into abduction. This fracture may be further graded by the surgeons.

Investigations

X-ray thumb (Fig. 19.5).

Treatment

Immediate cast bracing for comfort but surgical repair is usually required for stability.

Sports

Certainly after injury of this joint and perhaps prophylactically, strongly advise a thermoplastic splint, particularly for skiing, and if permitted in any other relevant sport, even after surgery. Wearing socks over gloves may help infill the first interdigital space and prevent abduction when falling on a dry ski slope, whilst clip re-

tainers for ski poles will spring out to prevent the thumb from catching.

> **Caveat** – A permanent unstable or weak grip will occur if the thumb is not repaired successfully.

Comment

This injury is much more likely to end in Accident and Emergency where the history of the mechanism of injury should alert to the need for X-raying and surgical referral.

de Quervain's tenosynovitis

Findings

Pain over the radial aspect of the wrist that may radiate up over the distal radial half of the forearm that is worse with resisted or active movement of the abductor policis. Finklestein's test is positive (see *Glossary*).

Type 1   The radial styloid is tender and may be swollen.

Type 2   The junction is tender where the abductor policis tendon is crossed by the extensor communis and there may be crepitus in the early stages.

Type 3   Resisted abduction of the thumb is painful over the muscle due to a tight fascial band.

Cause

Tenosynovitis of the abductor policis longus and extensor policis brevis from overuse, usually with a wide spread grip. The thumb is spread into abduction, such as the feathering hand in rowing, opening jam jars and polishing.

> **Caveat** – Referral from neck C6/7, arthrosis of the trapezium first metacarpal joint, scaphoid fracture, tenosynovitis of extensor policis longus and extensor carpi radialis strain.

Investigations

None clinically required.

Treatment

Type 1 Injection of cortisone around the tendon at the radial styloid. If this does not settle after two injections then surgery over the radial styloid to free the tendon sheath.

Type 2 NSAIDs, laser, ultrasound, frictions, injection of cortisone, surgery to free the sheath. It can recur.

Type 3 As for type 2.

Sports

(a) Rowing. Usually in the feathering wrist, when a smaller oar grip may be tried, and the 'gate' for the oar must not be too tight and resist rotation of the oar. Rough water does not always let the oar clear and can produce a resistance to feathering.

(b) Ten pin bowling. When the thumb hole is too far away from the finger holes.

(c) Golf. Over forcing the, mainly right, thumb down the handle with a high wrist – relax the wrist and thumb or thicken the grip or pad under the thumb.

(d) Kayaking. Several adaptations of paddle shape are available that may help the grip and reduce the functional spread of the thumb.

(e) General. Avoid wide abduction of the thumb.

Comment

Rowers often get the 'intersection' de Quervain's and some surgeons release the sheath on the first occasion. The radial styloid de Quervain's almost never responds to physiotherapy, and early cortisone and correction of the technical problem is the treatment of choice.

Intersection syndrome

Pain and swelling over the distal radial forearm that may have crepitus and be tender to palpation, and is worse with resisted abduction or extension of the thumb (see de Quervain's tenosynovitis type 2).

Carpal tunnel syndrome

Findings

Pain in the wrist and forearm which may even spread more proximally, and often wakes the patient at night and may be eased with elevation of the hand. There is classically numbness and 'pins and needles' of the thumb and index finger and radial side of the middle finger. Because of an anatomical higher anastomosis between the ulnar and median nerve, up to 30% may have referral in the ulnar two fingers. Phalen's test and Tinel's sign may be positive (see *Glossary*). Wasting of the thenar eminence will be apparent when chronic or severe.

Cause

Compression of the median nerve as it passes through the carpal tunnel.

Caveat – Referral from the neck.

Investigations

Clinically not required, but when the diagnosis is in doubt:

(a) A trial of local carpal tunnel injection therapy.

(b) EMG if doubt about the forearm pain, but if thenar wasting is present it is probably not required.

(c) Thyroid function for hypothyroidism and systemic or local fluid retention.

Treatment

(a) Treat the systemic causes and also with diuretics as this may be used acutely to ease the pain.

(b) Injection of cortisone into the carpal tunnel.

(c) Surgical release, especially if muscle wasting is present.

Sports

Occurs in cycling and motor cycling if the break or gear levers force the wrist into extension. Tribars may also produce the same problem [1]. Treat by moving the gears downwards out of the horizontal plane to lessen wrist extension and also reduce the angle of extension at the wrist when holding tribars.

Comment

Does well with cortisone injection but muscle wasting and failure to respond long-term should be treated by surgical release.

Ulnar neuritis

Findings

Pain, 'pins and needles' and numbness in the hypothenar eminence and ulnar two fingers (fourth and fifth) but this is not accompanied by weakness, as the motor and sensory nerves divide at the wrist, and only damage more proximal will cause motor weakness as well. There may be a definable sensory disturbance. Pope's and Froment's signs are negative (see *Glossary* and Chapter 18, *Ulnar nerve*).

Cause

Pressure on the ulnar nerve around the pisiform at Guyon's canal.

Caveat – Pisi-hamate ligament strain, ulnar nerve damage proximal to Guyon's canal, C8 T1 lesion, carpal tunnel and ulnar artery occlusion [2].

Investigations

Electromyogram is probably unhelpful but X-ray for Hook of Hamate views if trauma is suspected.

Treatment

Remove the cause of pressure and surgery if a

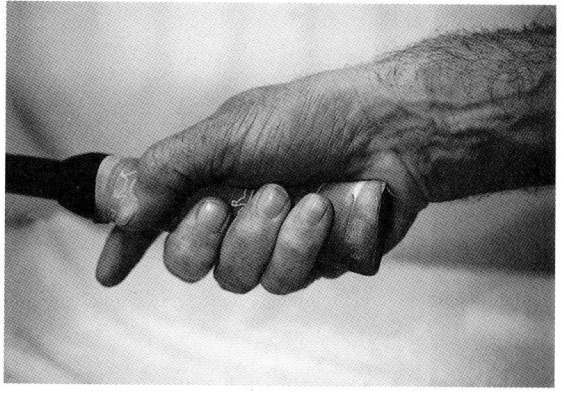

Figure 19.6   The racket handle is held too long so that the handle end levers across the Pisi–hamate ligament and Guyon's canal.

hamate fracture or gross pisiform instability is present.

Sports

(a) Reported in cyclists holding the curve of handle bars with the ulnar border compressed. Pad the handle bars and avoid this grip and use tribars if permitted, but note tribars can produce a carpal tunnel syndrome (see *Carpal tunnel syndrome*).

(b) Tennis players or golfers may hold the handle at the end of the grip which digs into the ulnar nerve during the shot; the handle must be held shorter, allowing the end to project beyond the pisiform. Particularly so in semi-Western grip and top spun forehand (Figs 19.6 and 19.7).

Comment

Not a common lesion, probably only reported in cyclists and occasionally racket games unless accompanied by trauma. Correction of the grip may be curative and surgery should not be considered until this has been corrected.

Pisi/hamate ligament strain

Findings

Localized pain over the pisiform when using a

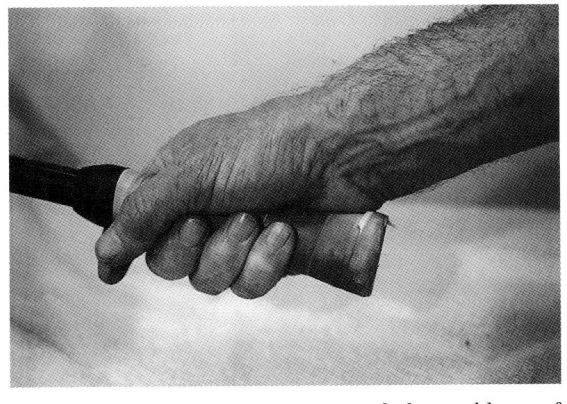

Figure 19.7 A correct grip to avoid the problems of Fig. 19.6.

racket or club and when gliding the pisiform on the hamate to strain the pisi/hamate ligament.

Cause
Pressure on the pisi/hamate ligaments from implements such as a tennis racket or golf club handle.

> **Caveat – Ulnar nerve compression through Guyon's canal (see *Ulnar neuritis*).**

Investigations
None clinically required, although possibly Hook of Hamate view on X-ray for a fracture if there is a history of trauma.

Treatment
(a) Electrotherapeutic modalities to settle inflammation, such as ultrasound and laser.
(b) Injection of pisi/hamate ligaments with cortisone.
(c) Correct the cause.
(d) Surgery.

Sports
(a) Mainly tennis, especially with semi-Western grip on the forehand shot with the racket held too near the end of the handle which therefore digs into the pisiform when rolling the top spun shot. Hold the handle shorter (see Figs 19.6 and 19.7).

(b) Golf. Same cause in the left hand but usually forcing the handle into the pisiform and then being acutely traumatized because the club is blocked, e.g. by a tuft of grass or tree root.

Comment
Physiotherapy does little and although an injection helps, avoidance of the cause is most important and may involve a lay off to allow the ligaments to settle, certainly before surgery is considered.

Extensor and flexor carpi ulnaris and radialis insertional strain

Pain at the wrist that is worse with extension and radial deviation (extensor carpi radialis), ulnar deviation (extensor carpi ulnaris) and flexion and radial deviation (flexor carpi radialis), ulnar deviation (flexor carpi ulnaris) are usually part of a traumatic sprain of the wrist, rather than being produced by a poor technique. They will require standard management of a tendon injury.

(a) RICE but beware nearby nerves.
(b) NSAIDs.
(c) Local cortisone to settle inflammation.
(d) Electrotherapeutic modalities to settle inflammation, such as ultrasound and laser.
(e) Massage techniques to prevent scar tissue adhesions such as frictions.
(f) Isometric loads to organize and lengthen scar tissue plus maintain muscle strength.
(g) Isotonic and skill-orientated loads the principle of the general muscle ladder (see Chapter 20).
(h) Surgery.

Radial stress fracture

Findings
Gradual onset of pain in the wrist, particularly on the radial volar aspect which might be associated with a particular gymnastic movement. Often unilateral in girls and bilateral in boys. The wrist

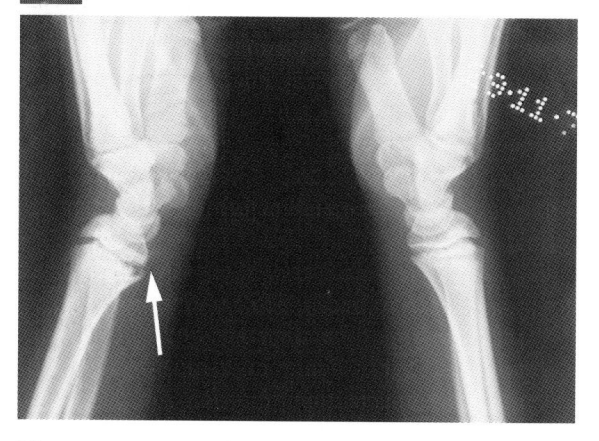

Figure 19.8 Lateral X-ray showing a hooked appearance of the radial metaphysis (arrow).

movement is often pain-free but tenderness is palpated over the volar and dorsal surface of distal radius. Volar pain over the distal radius should raise a high index of suspicion of a radial stress fracture.

Cause
A stress lesion of the radial epiphysis/metaphysis from repetitive compression and rotation across the wrist. Almost always confined to adolescent gymnasts and tumblers.

Investigations
(a) X-ray, AP and lateral (Figs. 19.8, 19.9).
(b) Bone scan may be difficult to interpret as the epiphysis is also hot on the scan.

Treatment
Rest from compressive exercises or all arm exercises for 7–12 weeks. Some have been successfully treated by permitting traction exercises such as the asymmetrical bars, beam, etc., but stopping compression exercises such as the floor and vault until healing has occurred [3].

Sports
Particularly gymnasts during vaults and floor work, perhaps twisting vaults such as the Tsuchahara, Diamadov on parallel bars and pommel horse for boys are causative.

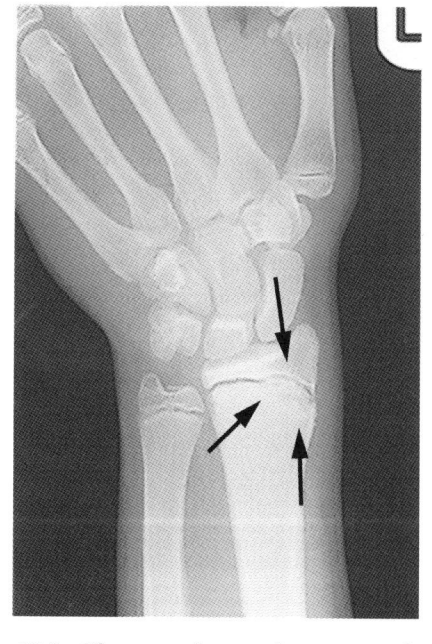

Figure 19.9 The more frequently seen 'moth eaten' early changes in the radial epiphysis (arrow).

> **Caveat** – Injury may produce premature fusion of the radial epiphysis and a long ulna (ulna congruence, ulnar variance) – effectively a short radius [4, 5].

Comment
Palpable pain over the volar radial surface must be investigated as a possible stress fracture in adolescent gymnasts or tumblers. A bone scan is difficult to interpret as it is normally 'hot' in a young child. The fuzzy, moth eaten appearance of the metaphysis is diagnostic (Fig. 19.9). All my cases have healed by just avoiding competitive and causative exercises until pain-free.

Trigger finger

Findings
A history of triggering of the finger which can sometimes be painful on holding a racket. There may be obvious triggering with a tender, mobile

nodule palpable on the palmar surface above the metacarpo-phalangeal joint.

Cause

A nodule on the flexor tendon of the finger catches through a stenosis in the flexor sheath, usually over the metacarpo-phalangeal joint.

> **Caveat** – Dupuytren's contracture.

Investigations

None clinically required.

Treatment

(a) Injection of the tendon sheath stenosis.
(b) Surgery.

Sports

Not commonly caused by sport, but too large a grip in racket games may effectively bow the flexors which then become irritated by the pressure of the grip. A reduction of handle size will treat the problem. However, once established then too small a grip may promote a tight flexion that maintains and irritates the flexor nodule, within the stenosis.

Comment

Many cases of trigger finger are functionally 'cured' without surgery so it is well worth trying cortisone in the early stages.

Finger splits

Findings

Common in implemental games when a painful persistent open linear wound on the pulp of the finger is found. Rock climbers produce an abrasive erosion of the skin at the tips of the fingers [6].

Cause

Frictional twisting of the finger on the handle splits the skin over the pulp of the finger.

Investigations

None clinically required.

Treatment

(a) Tape the fingers over the wound for games and keep clean.
(b) Try using gloves.
(c) Try another handle cover, possibly a soft rubber application, as toweling needs replacing frequently and dry worn towelling is often to blame.
(d) Embucrylate or Locktite® to 'stick' the split.

Sports

(a) Implemental games such as hockey and racket sports (e.g. tennis and badminton).
(b) Climbers.

Comment

Quite painful and occurring usually at the start of the season. Replaceable rubber taping to the handle seems to prevent this injury.

Lumbrical strain (shot putter's finger)

Findings

Pain whilst shot putting along the medial and lateral borders of the third and fourth fingers. Resisted flexion of the extended phalanges at the metacarpal phalangeal joint is painful.

Cause

A rare cause of pain in the lumbricals used to flex the fingers whilst putting the shot.

Investigations

None clinically required.

Treatment

Rest from shot putting; however, the inflammation may respond to local steroids. Taping may ease injury during practice but check the current rules as taping is severely limited for competition.

Comment
Very rare. Anabolic steroids may have an influence on tendon strength.

Interosseous muscle strain

Findings
Usually in racket players such as squash players. Pain and tenderness is palpated over the first interosseous muscle which is also sore on resisted adduction.

Cause
The index finger is held too far along the racket handle and the index finger applies constant excessive force to the grip which is opposed by a constant thumb force.

Investigations
None clinically required.

Treatment
(a) Electrotherapeutic modalities to settle inflammation, such as ultrasound and laser.
(b) NSAIDs.
(c) Alter the grip.

Sports
Racket games, particularly squash.

Comment
Some coaching manuals encourage the index finger grip to be laid along the racket handle, but someone always overdoes this grip and applies great force between the thumb and index finger. A simple adjustment in technique improves their squash and their injury.

Flexor injuries of the fingers

The forces applied by climbers by their flexor tendons is sufficient for the fibrous flexor sheath to be pulled away from the bone producing a bow string injury to the A2 pulley, usually of the fourth finger. Small tendon nodules suggesting old tears are present and collateral ligament sprains are chronic in climbers [7].

Ulnar stress fracture

An unusual stress fracture in the non-dominant arm with a double-handed backhand with only localized tenderness over the middle third of the ulnar to palpation and pain on resisted pronation. X-rays are negative and the bone scan positive. Tennis players using a double-handed backhand with these symptoms must be considered possible stress fractures [8]. It has also been reported in ten pin bowling [9], weightlifting and volleyball players and is seen in the tennis serve whilst cutting the serve.

Ulnar digital neuritis of the thumb

Reported in ten pin bowling as a neuropraxic injury to the ulnar digital nerve, with pain, hypersensitivity and a thickened palpable nerve, caused by rubbing of the thumb hole which produced fibrosis around the nerve [10].

Further reading

1. Braithwaite, I. J. (1992) Bilateral median nerve palsy in a cyclist. Br. J. Sports Med. **26**, 27–28.
2. Koga, Y., Seki, T. and Caro, L. D. (1993) Hypothenar hammer syndrome in a young female badminton player. A case report. Am. J. Sports Med. **21**, 890–892.
3. Read, M. T. F. (1981) Stress fractures of the distal radius in adolescent gymnasts. Br. J. Sports Med. **15**, 272–276.
4. DiFiori, J. P., Puffer, J. C., et al. (1997) Distal radial growth plate injury and positive ulnar variance in non elite gymnasts Am. J. Sports Med. **25**, 763–768.
5. De Smet, L., Claessens, A., et al. (1994) Gymnast's wrist: an epidemiological survey of ulnar variance and stress changes of the radial physis in elite female gymnasts. Am. J. Sports Med. **22**, 846–850.
6. Cole, A. T. (1990) Fingertip injuries in rock climbers. Br. J. Sports Med. **24**, 14.

7. Bollen, S. R. and Gunson, C. K. (1990) Hand injuries in competition climbers. *Br. J. Sports Med.* **24**, 16–18.

8. Bollen, S. R., Robinson, D. G., *et al.* (1993) Stress fractures of the ulna in tennis players using a double handed backhand stroke. *Am. J. Sports Med.* **21**, 751–752.

9. Escher, S. A., (1997) Ulnar diaphyseal stress fracture in a bowler. *Am. J. Sports Med.* **25**, 412–413.

10. Dobyns, J. H., O'Brien, E. T., Linscheid, R. L. and Farrow, G. M. (1989) Bowler's thumb: diagnosis and treatment. A review of seventeen cases. *Am. J. Bone Joint Surg.* **14**, 241–243.

Bruckner, P. and Khan, K. (1993) *Clinical Sports Medicine.* McGraw-Hill, New York.

Reid, D. (1992) *Sports Injury Assessment and Rehabilitation.* Churchill Livingstone, Edinburgh.

20

Rehabilitation and training with an injury

General principles of rehabilitation

(a) Rehabilitation needs to be performed little and often at least three to five times a day. Thirty minutes, three times a week is not sufficient.

(b) Develop exercises that train the uninjured parts of the body and maintain cardiovascular fitness, but rest the injured part until it can take controlled incremental loads.

(c) Athletes are target achievers and will use any method to achieve the goals set for them, and this will include 'cheating' by developing new skills. Watch for this in the early days, otherwise later they will have to stop rehabilitation and return to basics to reprogramme the correct skill.

(d) Rehabilitation of a skill that produces the best performance must not be sacrificed for a skill that enables a return to match play faster but has a less effective performance.

(e) Always be positive 'do this' rather than 'don't do that'.

(f) Overload injuries should not occur in training.

(g) Training must not delay or retard healing.

(h) Skill function and pain should control rehabilitation, not an arbitrary time scale.

It is better to delay a week or two to play at 100% than return and play all season at 90%.

How much training?

There is no perfect answer, but train so that the rhythm between contralateral sides or of the skill is correct and if this breaks down do not increase the speed or loading until the rhythm is corrected. Work up to the commencement of pain only, because rolling eyeballs and gritted teeth are for training, not rehabilitation. Within reason, whimping-out is permitted.

(a) If the pain stops immediately on cessation of the activity then continue at this level.

(b) If the pain continues for 20–30 seconds – stop! Start the exercise again at the next training session or the next day.

(c) If the injury does not hurt at the time but hurts later, use NSAIDs.

(d) If the pain has settled by the following morning, then training is within injury tolerance.

(e) If the pain is worse the following morning, but settles by midday, training is at the maximum, so reduce the load by 10%.

(f) If the pain is worse for the following 24–48 hours, then training has been well over the maximum recommended. Rest until the pain has settled. Start again with a considerable reduction in load, about 50%.

If good progress is being made, do not increase speed and distance, or weight and number, of repetitions at the same time. Build the training, by increasing the distance first, then build up the speed. When this reaches the speed required, slow down and increase the distance again. Repeat the cycle.

Similarly increase the number of repetitions first to 20–25, then add weights. Work until 20–25 repetitions are reached with the new weight and then increment weights again. Repeat this cycle until the desired weights are achieved.

Isokinetic training has the advantage of providing a fast angle of rotation which has a low resistance or a slow angle of rotation with a high resistance and the advantage that the machines will 'quit' when the patient 'quits', thus preventing muscle damage [1].

Always stretch properly before and after exercising – especially the injured part.

Open chain and closed chain exercises

Open chain exercises

Open chain exercises are those that fix the body and exercise the periphery but this will produce forces that can translate across the joint as well. Thus leg extension exercises, with the weight on the foot, will produce a translatory force across the knee, as well as through the articular surfaces. This can cause problems for the cruciate deficient knee. These exercises do not train coordination at the same time.

Closed chain exercises

Closed chain exercises in principle fix the periphery, and work the proximal joints and muscles. Thus leg presses are closed chain, and the forces travel through the joint and not across it. This is developed further by doing exercises balancing on one leg and using squats or hopping and jumping exercises. These have the advantage of training the mechanoreceptors in the joints and the proprioceptive coordination required to balance and move properly, at the same time as building strength.

How to increment loads

Non-committal loads

These are exercises that can be aborted at any stage without further damage or harm to the injury and they may be performed as isometrics, closed chain exercises, counter-balanced weights or resistance elastic bands.

The 'Rule of 7'

This should be used for these exercises when inviting patients to build them into their normal day, but can be pushed to a 'Rule of 10' for full training sessions.

The 'Rule of 7' is: 7 seconds work, 7 seconds rest, repeat seven times, preferably seven times a day, but three to five will do and is more achievable for the amateur.

Committal loads

These are movements that once initiated cannot be stopped or cannot be stopped without damage, such as running, jumping, throwing, hitting and using free weights.

Early stages of rehabilitation

Should use non-committal loads and non-committal exercises, and isometrics should be used with the muscle short, progressing to mid length and then long.

Middle stages of rehabilitation

Add committal loads at low speed and slow acceleration.

Later stages of rehabilitation

Build the endurance of the committal movement then increment speed and acceleration.

(a) Weights. Use body weight and build up repetitions until the patient can handle 25–30 repetitions and then increase the weight by, for instance, 2 kg until the patient can manage 25–30 repetitions, etc., until the desired weight is reached.

(b) Running. Run 1 mile at 10 minute mile pace. If no reaction to this then increase the speed in stages such as 9, 8 and 7:30 minute mile running pace until the desired running pace is reached. Run each speed on two occasions without problems before increasing the speed. When the desired running speed is reached then increase the distance but drop the speed down to 10 minute mile pace and repeat as above, until the desired speed and distance are again reached. The distance should be incremented more slowly, probably in mile steps after the first 2 miles.

(c) Hitting, throwing and kicking. These should be performed at slow speed, over short distance until 25–30 repetitions produce no reaction, and then increase the distance of the throw, kick, or hit, still at a slow speed until the limit of easy movement is reached, and then reduce distance and increase the speed or force, gradually moving out the distance. Finally return to a short distance to increase speed and force up to the desired power.

Final stages of rehabilitation

Add pliometrics such as bounding and depth jumping and use the rehabilitation ladders (see *Rehabilitation ladders*).

Principles of the training ladders

The ladders are designed to increment loads on the target muscles but also to give time for the skills to be redeveloped, as a trick movement may have been incorporated previously to get round the problem, but this movement is not the most efficient to achieve the end-point skill and must be eliminated, and the correct movement skill reintroduced. The stop points for moving up the ladder are pain lasting 20–30 seconds (see *How much training?*) or failure to put together the correct rhythm. Rhythm, which is a way of checking movement skill and also that one leg is working as hard as the other, is a vital ingredient of rehabilitation. Some people may find counting can impose a flow of rhythm to the body. This counting should be to an odd number not lower than 9 so that a flow of rhythm is maintained. Whilst counting, the emphasis and concentration are with the odd number, and this counting is a trick to switch the odd number and thus the concentration between both legs. Do not let the patient be logical, but just make them pick up the rhythm from the good leg and try to match it on the bad leg. If they cannot put together the skills to maintain rhythm at the lower stages of the ladder, they certainly will not be able to put these skills together at the top end and although they return to the sporting field their ultimate skills will remain severely compromised. Each new training session should be started at the bottom of the ladder but once the higher stages are reached then the first stages can be reduced to warm up, i.e. only one or two repetitions. The ladders must be looked upon as skill training (running is a skill) and not fitness training, although they will take on both roles at the latter stages.

Cross-training

Aerobic fitness and to a certain extent anaerobic fitness may be maintained by removing impact or by changing a technique so that the injury is rested but the heart and lungs are exercised – this is known as cross-training. For instance, pattering is impact cross-training and cycling is non-impact cross-training.

Patter routine

This simple exercise is effective in raising the pulse rate and building fitness without straining the knees or hips. It also takes up very little time. Quality, not quantity, is vital in fitness training. The secret is not lifting the feet far off the ground. A slow patter is more like a fast jog on the spot with the knees kept low. Feet must be lifted only 2.5–5 cm off the floor. A fast patter has the same low knee and foot lift, but pattering is done as fast as possible. It is testing, but simple.

Routine for an unfit athlete (3 minutes)

1 minute	slow patter
5 seconds	fast patter
50 seconds	slow patter
5 seconds	fast patter
50 seconds	slow patter
10 seconds	fast patter

Rest for 3 minutes whilst doing stretching exercises. Repeat the above routine at least twice, preferably four times.

Routine for a fairly fit athlete (5 minutes)

50 seconds	slow patter
10 seconds	fast patter
40 seconds	slow patter
20 seconds	fast patter
50 seconds	slow patter
10 seconds	fast patter
30 seconds	slow patter
10 seconds	fast patter
50 seconds	slow patter
30 seconds	fast patter

Then rest for 3 minutes whilst doing stretching exercises. Repeat the above training routine at least once, preferably three times.

Routine for a fit athlete (16 minutes)

Do the routine for the unfit athlete once, followed immediately by the routine for the fairly fit athlete, repeat.

Skipping routine

If the patient is good at skipping, use the same timing as for the patter routines. This gives the calf muscles a particularly good workout.

Swimming routine

Swimming is an excellent way to keep the muscles toned up, especially when the patient cannot 'run through' an injury. The water supports the body's weight but does not offer great resistance. Although less muscle power is required, the pulse rate is still raised by swimming. Running in water, using a flotation jacket for stability, may be used instead of actual swimming. The patient should not just run with a high knee lift but take large strides, really pulling with the hamstrings trying to mimic the running style.

Routine for a poor swimmer/non-swimmer

The athlete should jump in, swim or flounder across the width of the pool, climb out using the good leg and stand up, turn around and then repeat the routine for 3–5 minutes. After the exercise, they should rest for 3 minutes while doing stretching exercises. Repeat the above routine at least twice, preferably three times.

Routine for a good swimmer

As above but swim one length of the pool each time.

Rowing routine

A rowing or ergometric machine is required for this. It gives a thorough workout for legs, arms and abdominal muscles, and builds up stamina. Untrained rowers will find this much harder work than expected. Lying back at the end of each stroke will exercise the stomach muscles. The hand grip should be varied (either over the

top or underneath) if the arm muscles ache. Patients with knee problems should not throw the knees out to the side, but try and keep knees in line with the first and second toes as they move backward and forward. Drawing a mark over the midline of the knee caps will help to keep the knees on line. Make sure the athlete presses equally hard with both legs, trying to get both knees to travel at the same rate, especially when locking them straight.

Routine for patients doing long-distance/stamina events

The patient should be able to carry on a conversation, even if they are panting a bit. A least 10 minutes, although more than 30 minutes is preferable.

Routine for patients doing middle-distance events and running ball games

Should include aerobic and anaerobic training such as 2 minutes long distance, 1 minute sprint followed by a 3 minute rest. To be repeated as often as required.

Routine for sprint events and martial arts

At least 30 hard strokes per minute for 1–2 minutes. Rest for 5 minutes. Repeat as often as required.

Cycling routine

This removes impact from the ankle, knee and hips, and avoids jarring the back but still allows an excellent workout for heart and lungs. It may be done on a stationary exercise bike in a gym or on an ordinary pedal cycle out on the road. For stamina training athletes should use easy low gears at a pace where they are able to talk with only a slight pant, but for sprint training, harder, higher gears are used. Those with knee problems should keep the knees vertical over the first and second toes to avoid a varus or valgus action and try to take up pedal pressure at the top of the pedal cycle, not half way down, when it becomes easier. Count for rhythm.

Routine for long-distance running
The time on the bike should be equal to the time normally spent training on foot but over a much longer distance, preferably 2–2.5 times longer than they would usually run.

Routine for middle-distance running and ball games (5 minutes)
4.5 minutes   stamina training
0.5 minutes   sprint training

Rest for 3 minutes while doing stretching exercises. Repeat at least twice, preferably four times.

Routine for sprint events, strength events, volleyball, basketball, etc. (5 minutes)
2 minutes   stamina training
0.25 minutes   sprint training
1.75 minutes   stamina training
1 minute   sprint training

Rest for 4 minutes while doing stretching exercises. Repeat at least twice, preferably four times.

Change of direction training

(a) Karioke steps. A sideways step sequence crossing the feet in front and behind each other. This works the adductors and ligaments of the knees and the ankles.
(b) Side to side steps. Step sideways, draw the other leg up to the first and repeat with the first leg abducting sideways. This can be done at speed.
(c) Figure of '8' runs. Particularly stresses the ligaments of the knees and the ankles. The arc of the '8' can be reduced to increase the ligamentous stresses.
(d) Side stepping. Run in a straight line and add in side stepping.
(e) Shuttle or doggy runs. Sprint out to a mark and turn as fast as possible and sprint back.
(f) Kicking a ball against a wall. Kick the ball with the inside or outside of the foot. This stresses ankle and knee ligaments.

Stretching

(a) Stretching increases the number of sarcomeres.
(b) Stresses the stretch elastic component of the muscle/tendon complex.
(c) Can reset gamma efferents that control muscle tension allowing a fuller range of movement.
(d) Can prevent adhesions following injury.
(e) Provides a low load across the scar tissue helping to orientate healing fibroblasts.

Methods of stretching
General
Stretching is for the antagonist which is the muscle that resists the direction of movement, and should be done with a relaxed passive muscle which is achieved by breathing out and relaxing to reduce muscle tension whilst the stretch is employed.

Passive stretching
This type of stretching is limited by joint range and soft tissue abutment (Fig. 20.1).

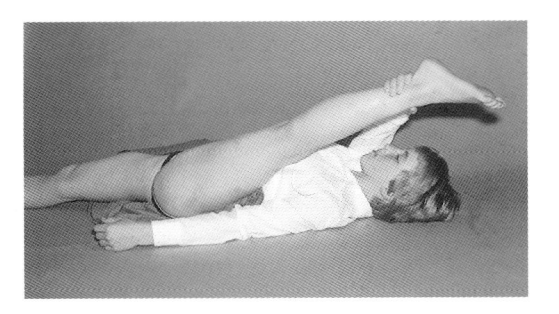

Figure 20.1 Passive stretching is only limited by joint range and soft tissue abutment!

Proprioceptive neuromuscular facilitation
This tries to enhance the relaxation for passive stretching by:

Method 1 Actively working the antagonist against the resistance of the therapist, then relaxing this muscle whilst it is stretched by the therapist.

Method 2 The antagonist should relax when the agonist is worked, so the therapist resists the agonist, the muscle that initiates the movement, whilst gradually stretching the antagonist at the same time [2].

Active stretching
This requires muscle work from the agonist and relaxation from the antagonist.

Yoga stretching
Allows the gamma efferents that control muscle tone to be reset producing long-term elongation, and does not habituate protective spasm from an injury.

Bounce stretching
Habituates protective spasm from an injury and does not permanently lengthen the tendon muscle complex, but increases teno osseous junction strength [3].

Ballistic stretching
Actively kicking a straight leg raise into the air with increasing rapidity will train the hamstrings, which are decelerating this movement, to decelerate the movement over a longer arc. EMG shows that the hamstring actively decelerates the swing phase of running so that the leg is braced ready for impact, and this combination of agonist and antagonist contracting together is known as co-activation [4]. If the hamstring is stretched forcibly it will encourage this mechanism to fire off, thus jump splits and hurdle stretches if forced may recruit active hamstring contraction at the very moment that relaxation is required, and therefore must be trained as a ballistic movement or done slowly with relaxation of the target muscle group at the end of range [4].

> **Caveat** – I have seen several avulsions of the ischeal tuberosity from forced intentional stretching of the hamstring (see Fig. 9.1).

Stretching pre-exercise
(a) Gently warm up first.
(b) Active yoga stretch for muscle relaxation for 15–20 seconds.
(c) Passive stretch using gravity or a partner for muscle relaxation of both agonist and antagonist [5, 6].
(d) Bounce stretch for teno osseous strength [3].
(e) Ballistic stretch for muscle co-activation [4].
(f) Slow mimic of sport activities.
(g) Stretch on warm down.

Stretching for injury
(a) Gently warm up.
(b) Active yoga stretch to stretch out scar tissue.
(c) Proprioceptive neuromuscular facilitation stretch for scar tissue.
(d) Ballistic stretch for scar tissue and muscle co-activation.
(e) Stretch on warm down.
(f) Warm up can slowly mimic activities required by the game which therefore encourages both active and ballistic stretching [3].

Useful simple stretches
• Calf stretches (Figs 20.2 and 20.3).
• Hamstrings (Fig. 20.4).
• Quadriceps (Fig. 20.5).
• Adductors (Fig. 20.6).
• Spine (Figs 20.7 and 20.8).
• Shoulders (Fig. 20.9).
• Hamstring quadriceps and adductors (Fig. 20.10).

Proprioception

Joint awareness and position sense are enhanced by balancing exercises. However, if the eyes can be removed from helping the balance then the various mechanoreceptors must do more. So balances may be done with the eyes shut or, on a busy day, by balancing whilst brushing one's hair or whilst talking on the telephone. Practising balancing whilst doing something else stops the

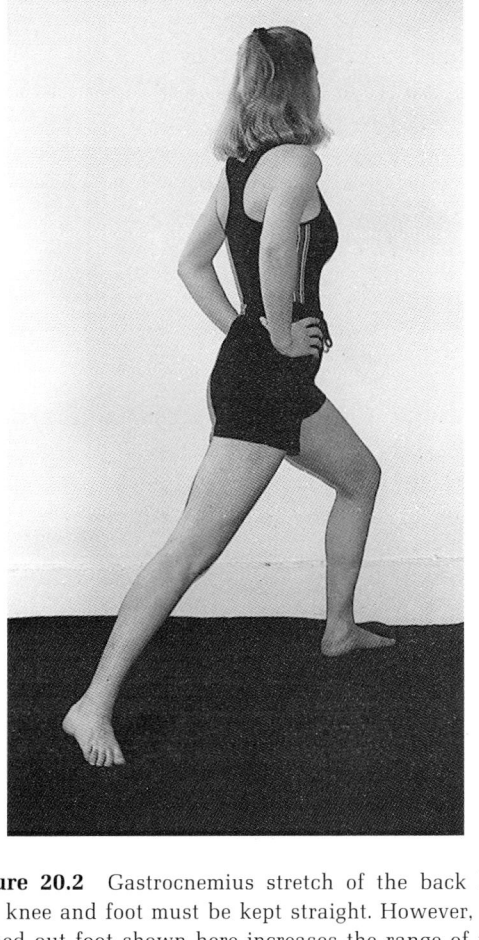

Figure 20.2 Gastrocnemius stretch of the back leg. The knee and foot must be kept straight. However, the turned out foot shown here increases the range of forward movement but achieves less stretch of the calf.

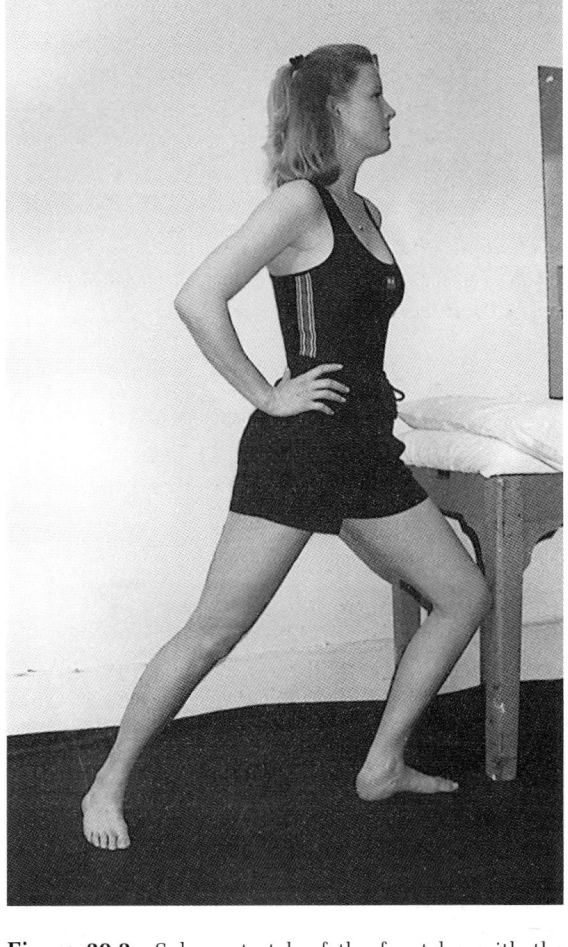

Figure 20.3 Soleus stretch of the front leg with the knee bent.

eyes and brain from helping the balance, thus making the mechanoreceptors contribute more, which is of course more representative of normal life. Proprioception can also be enhanced by support strapping which recruits the skin receptors into providing additional positional information [7].

Prophylactic strapping

Evidence from American basketball teams suggests that this does help reduce the number of ankle sprains; however, no increased protection from knee injury has been shown. Fingers and wrists seem to benefit, and thermoplastic splints for skiers' thumbs are invaluable. Sometimes strapping a muscle may be of help, possibly acting as an exoskeleton so that the muscle achieves purchase on the support and diminishes the loads being transferred to the attachments; a particular example may be the tennis elbow supports. Some prophylactic strapping requires 'undertape and meters of tape to be purchased and these may have been superseded by custom-made Velcro or lace-up supports [7].

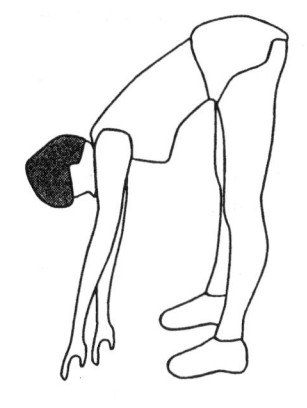

Figure 20.4 Hamstring stretch. Stand upright with feet wide apart and hands on hips. Push the bottom backwards, then pivot forwards from the hips with the back straight and the chest forward, and reach out towards the feet. Rolling the spine down the shoulders does not achieve a full hamstring stretch.

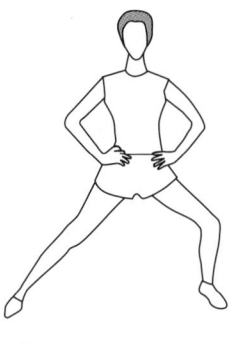

Figure 20.6 Adductor stretch. Stand with the feet wide apart, bend the left knee but keep the weight over the straight leg but do not lean forward. When a pull is felt in the groin of the straight leg, increase the stretch by leaning further over the straight leg, keep the bottom in and breathe out. Repeat exercise to the other side.

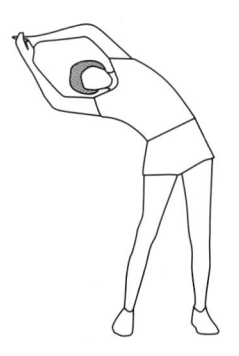

Figure 20.7 Stand comfortably and clasp the hands at full stretch above the head. Keep the trunk upright and lean sideways, not forwards, until a pull is felt down the opposite side. Breathe out. Repeat to the other side.

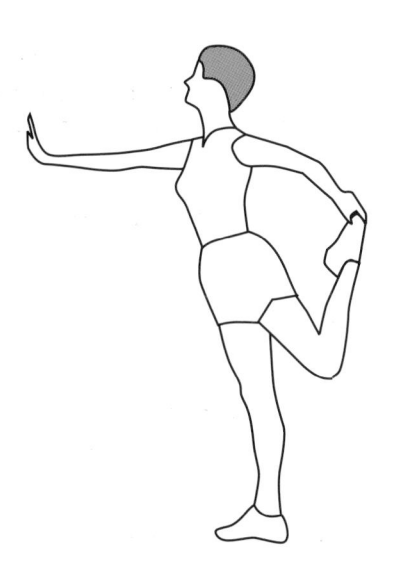

Figure 20.5 Quadriceps stretch. Stand on the right leg and hold the left foot in the left hand and pull the knee backwards, keep the back straight. When the pull is felt in front of the thigh, hold for 20 seconds, breathe out. Now stretch the knee away from the bottom. Keep the knee in line with the hips to stretch the quadriceps and the ilio-tibial band. Repeat exercise on the other side.

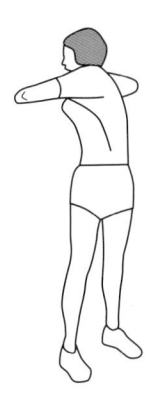

Figure 20.8 Stand comfortably with hands clasped in front of chest and slowly rotate the body to the right. Breathe out. Repeat to the other side.

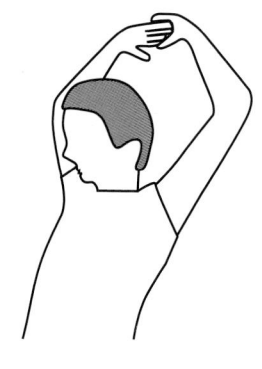

Figure 20.9 Clasp hands behind and slightly above the head. Press the shoulders and arms backwards. Breathe out.

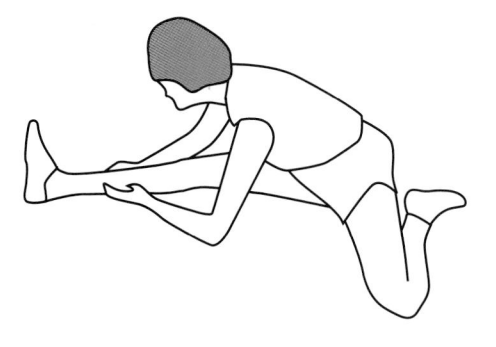

Figure 20.10 Hamstring, quadriceps and adductor stretch. Try to get the legs at right angles with the back leg bent, then keeping the back straight try to place the chest over the straight leg. When a pull is felt at the back of the knee, hold the stretch and breathe out. It is essential not to force this movement as this can damage the ischeal hamstring attachment. Leaning backwards in line with the straight leg will stretch the adductors and quadriceps of the bent leg. Repeat on the other side.

Convenient home rehabilitation

Most sportspeople are amateurs with jobs to hold down and exercises should be built into their working day if possible. They may attend two physiotherapy sessions a week for 15 minutes, which is hardly sufficient, but as they improve this will be rapidly abandoned. They will have to be given formal exercises at home, although some exercises can be designed to be done on the journey or at work and a few are given below.

General proprioceptive exercises for ankle, knee, hip and back

Balance on one leg whilst cleaning the teeth, brushing the hair, putting on clothes, answering the telephone or waiting for the train and indeed standing on the train.

Quadriceps and proprioceptive exercises

Balance whist holding a half knee squat on one leg whilst doing the general exercises above. Walk upstairs placing the whole foot flat on each tread, so that no additional thrust is obtained from the calf and propulsion is obtained only from the quadriceps. Walk slowly down stairs or slopes trying to hold the rhythm between both legs.

Calves

These should be trained one at a time by doing heel raises on one leg whilst waiting for a train, cleaning the teeth or answering the phone.

Isometrics using the 'Rule of 7' (see '*Rule of 7*')

(a) Peroneals. Cross ankles with plantar flexed foot and force outside of both feet against each other. Do not turn the foot so that the tibialis anterior is doing the work.

(b) Posterior tibialis. Push the big toe joint of the target foot against the inside heel of the other foot.

(c) Tibialis anterior and flexor hallucis. Pull the dorsum of the foot and great toe up into the sole of the other foot.

(d) Quadriceps and hamstrings. Sit on a desk, cross the ankles and push away with the back foot to extend the knee and work the quadriceps of that leg, whilst pulling back with the front leg heel into the ankle of the back foot to work the hamstrings of the other.

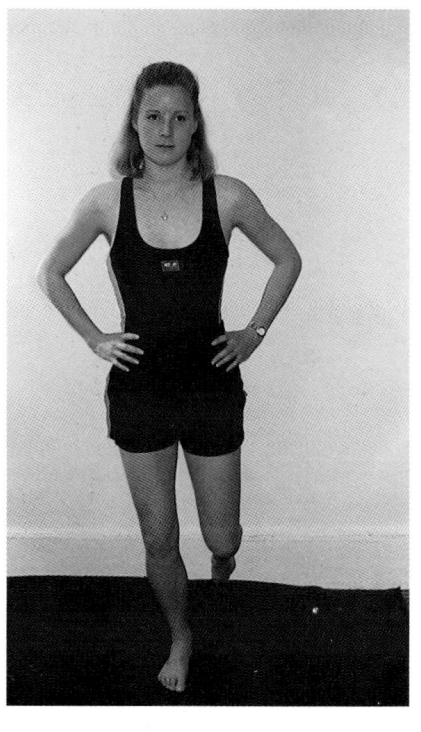

Figure 20.11 The half-knee squat. The pelvis is straight and the knee in line with the foot which works the hip stabilizers and external rotators.

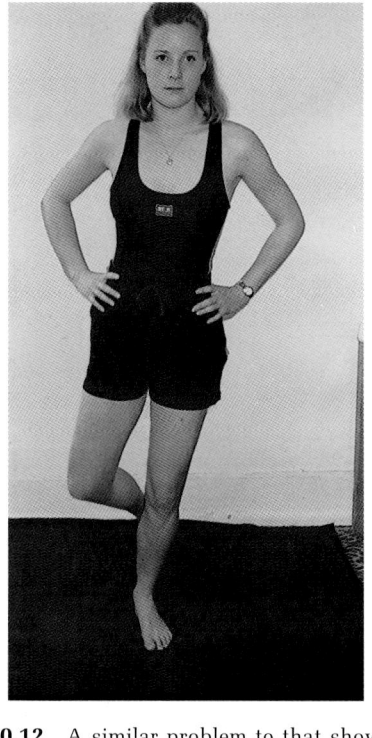

Figure 20.12 A similar problem to that shown above occurs when the pelvis swings forward to increase the external rotation of the hip.

This can be done sitting on the train if required.

(e) External hip rotators. Tighten the buttocks, drive the knees straight and externally rotate the knees (the movement comes from the hip but the patient often understands this phrase better). This then may be done one legged and a half squat balance on this leg added. However, the knee must not be allowed to drift into valgus, the foot of the unsupported leg swing behind the other leg nor the anterior superior iliac spine on the ipselateral side swing forward, all of which permit the external rotators not to work so hard (Figs 20.11–20.12).

(f) The rotator cuff may be given isometrics against the resistance of the restraining other hand. External rotation for infraspinatus, internal for subscapularis and elbow abduction from a position tucked in to the side for supraspinatus.

(g) For tennis elbow. Preferably with the elbow held straight, resisted extension of the wrist and as the pain settles then resist the extended fingers, against the other hand.

(h) For golfer's elbow. pressing the pulps of the fingers into the trapezius will work the flexors as will trying to pronate the target hand against the resistance of the other hand.

(i) Biceps isometrics pulling the forearm up to the shoulder can be done against the resistance of the contralateral hand.

Rehabilitation ladders

See following 12 pages.

General muscle ladder

At levels 7–8 of the general muscle ladder use closed chain work for the legs rather than open chain work.

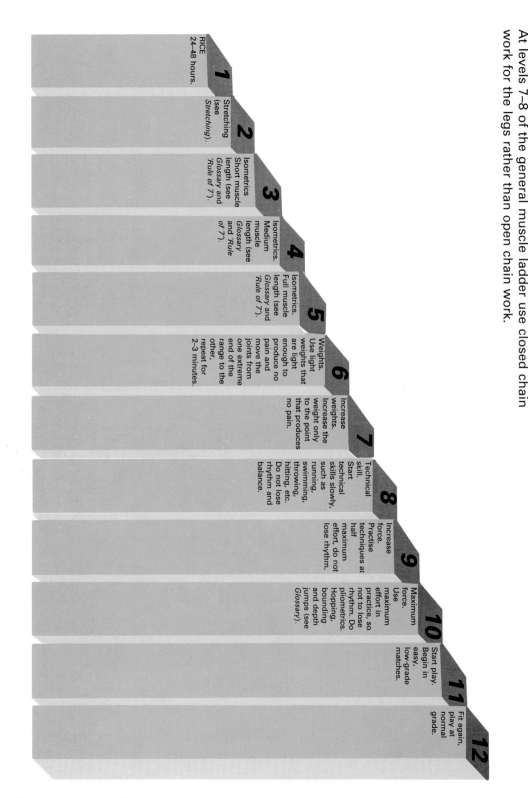

1 RICE 24–48 hours.

2 Stretching (see *Stretching*).

3 Isometrics. Short muscle length (see *Glossary* and *'Rule of 7'*).

4 Isometrics. Medium muscle length (see *Glossary* and *'Rule of 7'*).

5 Isometrics. Full muscle length (see *Glossary* and *'Rule of 7'*).

6 Weights. Use light weights that are light enough to produce no pain and that produces no pain. move the joints from one extreme end of the range to the other, repeat for 2–3 minutes.

7 Increase weights. Increase the weight only to the point that produces no pain.

8 Technical skill. Start technical skills slowly, such as running, swimming, throwing, hitting, etc. Do not lose rhythm and balance.

9 Increase force. Practise techniques at half maximum effort, do not lose rhythm.

10 Maximum force. Use maximum effort in practice, so not to lose rhythm. Do pliometrics. Hopping, bounding and depth jumps (see *Glossary*).

11 Start play. Begin in easy, low-grade matches.

12 Fit again, play at normal grade.

1 Stand up, lock knee into extension. Sit and cross heel of uninjured leg over ankle of injured leg and resist extension of injured leg. Use *'Rule of 7'*.

2 Knee extensions. Support upper leg of injured knee and straighten leg into extension, add a weight, e.g. 2 kg of sugar in a bag, and repeat extensions. Increase weights. (Not for anterior cruciate ligament.)

3 Balance on injured leg with half squat. Use *'Rule of 7'*. (Fig 20.11)

4 Slow step-ups. Step up onto a low bench or stair using alternate feet and the foot, flat of the foot, rather than the toes.

5 Leg press machine. If available use a leg press machine in a gym for closed chain work. Leg extensions, which are open chain, should not be used for anterior cruciate ligament injuries.

6 Squats. Sit with back against a wall with thighs parallel to the ground and hold for as long as possible. Move onto light weights, 'squatting' but not below 90° knee bend. Keep the knee vertically above the foot.

7 Bike routine. Use a gear as is comfortable with a low pedal rate, or a high pedal rate, continue until the muscle aches, rest 5–10 minutes, repeat as fitness allows. Try varying the seat height to make the knee work more flexed.

8 Depth jumps. Jump down from a low step 15–20 cm, then up and jump over a string or bar such as a high jump bar to compete with other recuperating athletes. The idea is to travel as far as one can and as measurable this is. Drop this height by 5 cm then repeat 10 times, then jump rhythmically with no bounce in between. Maintain rhythm and do not favour the injured leg. Eventually improve to single leg jumps, over weeks gradually raise the height of the step but not more than 40 cm high (see *Glossary; Pliometrics*).

9 Hop, step and jump. Start with right toe on a line, hop onto right foot, step onto left foot, jump from left foot, land on both feet, or hop, hop hop, etc. Measure distance travelled. Repeat starting from the left foot. Repeat five times on each side.

10 Weights. Resume normal weight training to level before injury.

Quadriceps ladder, heart and lungs

The heart and lung ladder builds up stamina. To rebuild muscle strength use the strength ladder. These two may be used in parallel. Competitors in power events should concentrate on strength, whilst speed and endurance competitors will find the heart and lungs ladder more appropriate. Competitors in most ball games will use both ladders.

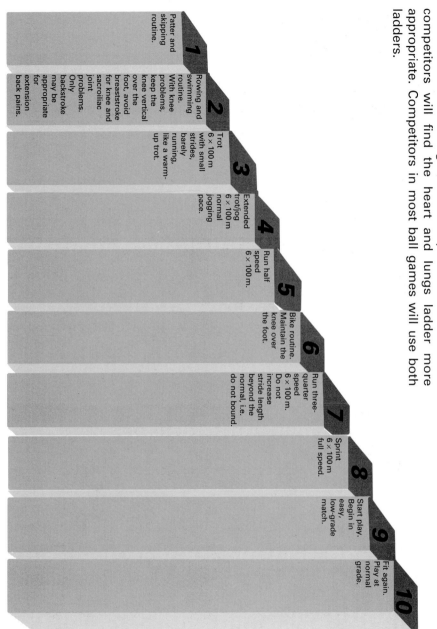

1 Patter and skipping routine.

2 Rowing and swimming routine. With knee problems, keep the foot, avoid knee and sacroiliac joint problems. Only backstroke may be appropriate for extension back pains.

3 Trot 6 × 100 m with small strides, barely running, like a warm-up trot.

4 Extended trot/jog 6 × 100 m normal jogging pace.

5 Run half speed 6 × 100 m.

6 Bike routine. Maintain the knee over the foot.

7 Run three-quarter speed 6 × 100 m. Do not increase stride length beyond the normal, i.e. do not bound.

8 Sprint 6 × 100 m full speed.

9 Start play. Begin in easy, low-grade match.

10 Fit again. Play at normal grade.

Knee ladder

The knee should be strapped or braced for the first 6 weeks of match play. This ladder should only be started after level 7 of the Achilles or hamstring top ladder has been reached. Kicking can start at the same time.

1 Using a soccer ball; 2 m away from a wall, use side foot and instep.
2 Move 6 m from the wall.
3 With a partner gradually move further apart.

Using a football or rugby ball:

4 Kick from the hand (caressing the ball).
5 Hard punt.
6 Hard kick from the ground.

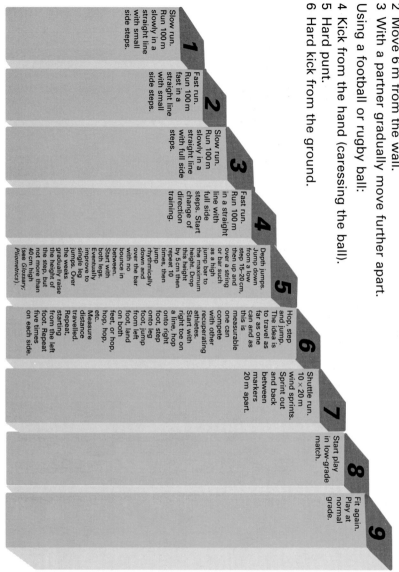

1 Slow run. Run 100 m slowly in a straight line with small side steps.

2 Fast run. Run 100 m fast in a straight line with small side steps.

3 Slow run. Run 100 m slowly in a straight line with full side steps. Start change of direction training.

4 Fast run. Run 100 m in a straight line with full side steps. Start jump bar to the maximum height. Drop from this height by 5 cm then repeat 10 times, then jump rhythmically down and over the bar with no bounce in between. Start with both legs. Eventually improve to single leg jumps. Over the weeks gradually raise the height of the step, but not more than 40 cm high (see Glossary; Pliometrics).

5 Depth jumps. Jump down from a low step 15–20 cm, then up and over a string or bar such as a high jump height. This is measurable so one can compete with other recuperating athletes. Start with right toe on right foot, step onto right foot, jump from left foot, land on both feet, or hop, hop, hop, etc. Measure distance travelled. Repeat, starting from the left foot. Repeat five times on each side.

6 Hop, step and jump. The idea is to travel as far as one can and as this is measurable one can compete with other recuperating athletes.

7 Shuttle run. 10 × 20 m wind sprints. Sprint out and back between markers 20 m apart.

8 Start play in low-grade match.

9 Fit again. Play at normal grade.

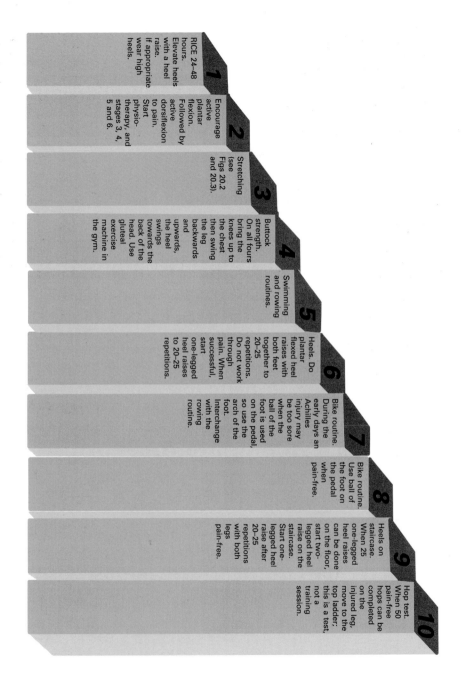

1 RICE 24-48 hours. Elevate heels with a heel raise. If appropriate wear high heels.

2 Encourage active plantar flexion. Followed by active dorsiflexion to pain. Start physiotherapy, and stages 3, 4, 5 and 6.

3 Stretching (see Figs 20.2 and 20.3).

4 Buttock strength. On all fours bring the knees up to the chest then swing the leg backwards and upwards, the heel swings towards the back of the head. Use gluteal exercise machine in the gym.

5 Swimming and rowing routines.

6 Heels. Do plantar flexed heel raises with both feet together to 20-25 repetitions. Do not work through pain. When successful, start one-legged heel raises to 20-25 repetitions.

7 Bike routine. During the early days an Achilles injury may be too sore when the ball of the foot is used on the pedal, so use the arch of the foot. Interchange with the rowing routine.

8 Bike routine. Use ball of the foot on the pedal when pain-free.

9 Heels on staircase. When 25 one-legged heel raises can be done on the floor, move to the top ladder; start two-legged heel raise on the staircase. Start one-legged heel raise after 20-25 repetitions with both legs pain-free.

10 Hop test. When 50 pain-free hops can be completed on the injured leg, start one-legged heel raise on the top ladder; this is a test, not a training session.

Calf and Achilles top ladder

Continue cross-training for fitness. Start each training session from the bottom of the ladder. Do six of stage 1 then six of stage 2, etc., until pain or loss of rhythm halt the training. Early ladder steps may be cut from six to two repetitions when working at the higher stages. Check that the leg rhythm is equal; do not gallop. One way to avoid favouring an injured leg is to count from 1 to 9 whilst running, which sets a rhythm for the legs to follow and allows concentration to move from one leg to the other. Match the feel of the bad leg to the good leg, counting 1, 2; 1, 2; tends to stress any limp. Do stretching exercises between each 100 m. Check heel pick up and knee lift are the same height. Stop if any pain last for more than 20–30 seconds and do not progress up the ladders if there is loss of rhythm.

1
Trot 6 × 100 m, small strides, barely running, like a warm up trot.

2
Extended trot/jog 6 × 100 m normal jogging.

3
High heels, 6 × 100 m, trot with the heels deliberately kicking the buttocks on each stride. This works the hamstring and increases the load on the calf.

4
Run half speed 6 × 100 m.

5
High knee trot 6 × 100 m. Keep stride length short, knees raised to horizontal or above. Non-sprinters can make do with 25–30 m.

6
6 × 100 m. Run three-quarter speed. Maintain normal stride length, do not bound.

7
Grade 1 sprint, 6 × 100 m. Accelerate over 25 m, sprint 50 m, slow down over 25 m.

8
Grade 2 sprint, 6 × 100 m. Accelerate over 25 m and decrease the distance required to stop over the six repetitions. Note: specialist runners should not use this stage, which is for stop/start games.

9
Grade 3 sprint, 6 × 100 m, increase rate of acceleration over six repetitions, sprint 50 m, fast stop 25 m.

10
Shuttle run, 10 × 20 m, wind sprints. Sprint out and back between markers 20 m apart.

11
Start play. Begin in easy, low-grade match.

12
Fit again. Play at normal grade.

Hamstring bottom ladder

An injured knee, particularly the ligaments, should be strapped or braced throughout all of this ladder work and for the first 6 weeks of match play.

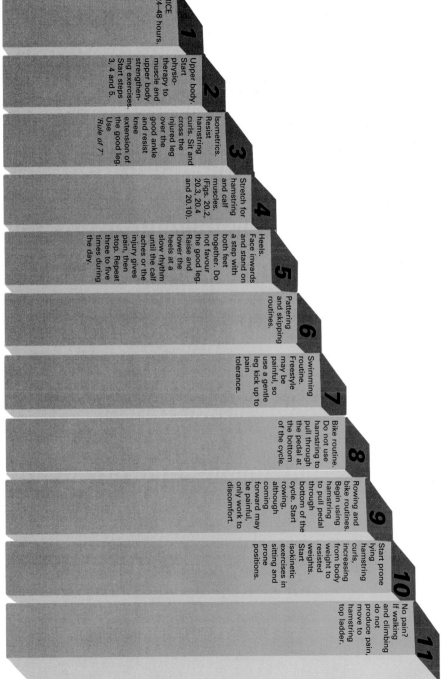

1 RICE 24–48 hours.

2 Upper body. Start physiotherapy to injured leg muscle and good body upper body strengthening exercises. Start steps 3, 4 and 5. Use 'Rule of 7'.

3 Isometrics. Resist hamstring curls. Sit and cross the injured leg over the good ankle and resist knee extension of the good leg. Use 'Rule of 7'.

4 Stretch for hamstring and calf muscles. (Figs. 20.2, 20.3, 20.4 and 20.10).

5 Heels. Face inwards and stand on a step with both feet together. Do not favour the good leg. Raise and lower the heels at a slow rhythm until the calf aches or the injury gives pain, then stop. Repeat three to five times during the day.

6 Pattering and skipping routines.

7 Swimming routine. Freestyle may be painful, so use a gentle leg kick up to pain tolerance.

8 Bike routine. Do not use hamstring to pull through bottom of the cycle. Start to pull pedal at the bottom of the cycle.

9 Rowing and bike routines. Begin using hamstring curls, increasing from body weight to resisted weights. Start isokinetic exercises in sitting and prone positions.

10 Start prone lying hamstring curls, move to hamstring top ladder.

11 No pain? If walking and climbing do not produce pain.

Hamstring top ladder

Continue cross-training for fitness. Start each training session from the bottom of the ladder. Do six of stage 1 then six of stage 2, etc., until pain or loss of rhythm halt the training. Early ladder steps may be cut from six to two repetitions when working at the higher stages. Check that the leg rhythm is equal; do not gallop. One way to avoid favouring an injured leg is to count from 1 to 9 whilst running, which sets a rhythm for the legs to follow and allows concentration to move from one leg to the other. Match the feel of the bad leg to the good leg, counting 1, 2; 1, 2; tends to stress any limp. Do stretching exercises between each 100 m. Check heel pick up and knee lift are the same height. Stop if any pain last for more than 20–30 seconds and do not progress up the ladders if there is loss of rhythm. Start using a ballistic stretch by swinging the leg into a high kick like a ballet dancer (see *Stretching*) slowly to the point of discomfort. As the injury improves build up the speed of swing, especially in kicking sports.

1
Trot 6 × 100 m, small strides, barely running, like a warm-up trot.

2
Extended trot/jog 6 × 100 m normal jogging.

3
High knee trot 6 × 100 m. Keep stride length short, knees raise to the horizontal or above. Non-sprinters can make do with 25–50 m.

4
Run half speed 6 × 100 m.

5
High heels, 6 × 100 m trot with heels kicking buttocks on each stride, start slowly, build up speed as pain permits.

6
Run three-quarter speed 6 × 100 m. Do not increase stride length beyond normal, do not bound.

7
Grade 1 sprint, 6 × 100 m. Accelerate over 25 m, sprint 50 m, slow down over 25 m.

8
Grade 2 sprint, 6 × 100 m. Accelerate over 25 m, sprint 50 m and decrease the distance required to stop over 25 m.

9
Grade 3 sprint, 6 × 100 m. Increase rate of acceleration over six repetitions, sprint 50 m, fast stop 25 m.
Note: specialist runners should not use this stage, which is for stop/start games.

10
Shuttle run. 10 × 20 m, wind sprints. Sprint out and back between markers 20 m apart.

11
Been bag shuttle. As stage 10, but incorporate bending to touch or pick up an object such as a bean bag from the floor.

12
Start play in easy, low-grade match, then play at normal grade.

Badminton ladder

This is for tennis elbow and shoulder injuries. Work with a willing partner for 5 minutes at each step, but start each training session from the beginning. Stop at the first sign of pain, but continue if the pain settles within 20 seconds. Otherwise stop, wait 24 hours then repeat from the first step (see *How much training?*). Concentrate grip on third, fourth and fifth fingers; relax second finger and thumb.

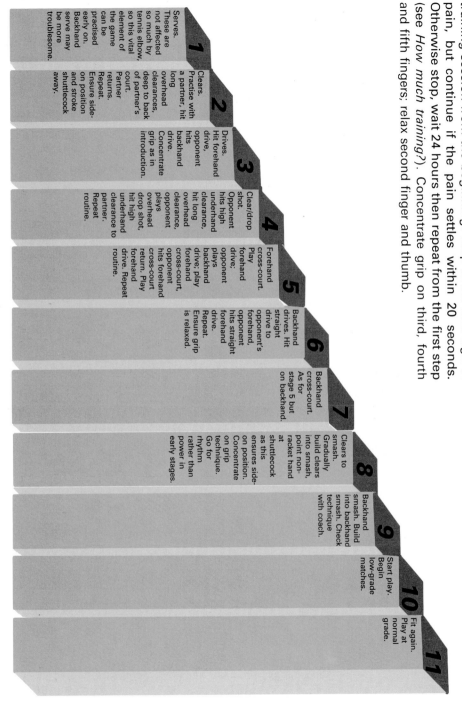

1 Serves. These are not affected so much by tennis elbow, so this vital element of the game can be practised early on. Backhand serve may be more troublesome.

2 Clears. Practise with a partner, hit overhead clearances, deep to back of partner's court. Concentrate grip as in introduction.

3 Drives. Hit forehand drive, opponent hits backhand drive. Concentrate grip as in introduction.

4 Clear/drop shot. Opponent hits high underhand clearance, hit long overhead clearance, opponent plays overhead drop shot, hit high underhand clearance to partner. Repeat routine.

5 Forehand cross-court. Play forehand drive; opponent hits high forehand drive; play backhand drive; play forehand cross-court, opponent hits forehand cross-court return. Play forehand drive. Repeat routine.

6 Backhand drives. Hit straight drive to opponent's forehand, opponent hits straight forehand drive. Repeat. Ensure grip is relaxed.

7 Backhand cross-court. As for stage 5 but on backhand.

8 Clears to smash. Gradually build clears into smash, point non-racket hand at shuttlecock as this ensures side-on position. Concentrate on grip technique. Go for rhythm rather than power in early stages.

9 Backhand smash. Build into backhand smash. Check technique with coach.

10 Start play. Begin low-grade matches.

11 Fit again. Play at normal grade.

Tennis ladder

This is good for tennis elbow, which is mainly suffered by those using the standard grip and single backhand. Semi-Western or Western grip is not often a cause of tennis elbow (see Figs 19.1–19.3. If it is, there may be too tight a grip with thumb and second finger. Semi-Western grip is most likely to cause golfer's elbow.

Work with a willing partner or a tennis machine. Concentrate on foot work and technique. When playing single handed backhand, make sure that the racket head stays above the wrist level (see Fig. 18.9). Do not lead with the elbow (see Figs. 18.7 and 18.8).

Work for 5 minutes at each level, stop at the first sign of pain. If the pain or ache goes away within 20 seconds, continue the exercises. If the ache or pain persists, stop, wait 24 hours, begin again from the first step (see *How much training?*). Do not grip racket too tightly with thumb and index finger.

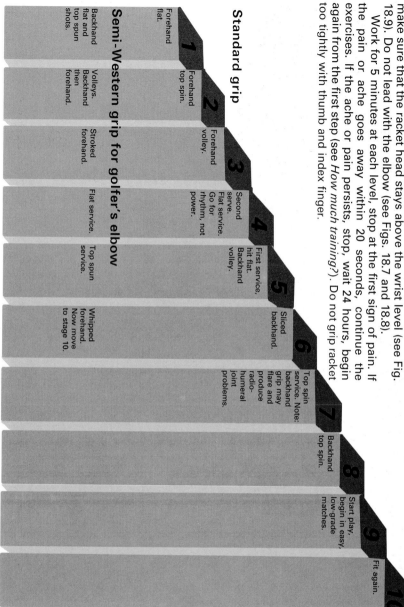

Standard grip

1 Forehand flat.

2 Forehand top spin.

3 Forehand volley.

4 Second serve. Flat service. Go for rhythm, not power.

5 First service, hit flat. Backhand volley.

6 Sliced backhand.

7 Top spin service. Note: backhand grip may produce radio-humeral joint problems.

8 Backhand top spin.

9 Start play, begin in easy, low-grade matches.

10 Fit again.

Semi-Western grip for golfer's elbow

1 Backhand flat and top spun shots.

2 Volleys. Backhand then forehand.

3 Stroked forehand.

4 Flat service.

5 Top spun forehand. Now move to stage 10.

Squash ladder

Useful for most injuries and particularly tennis elbow because the player can anticipate where the ball is going and will not be wrong footed. For golfer's elbow problems use the steps in different order, as follows: 5, 7, 6, 2, 3, 4, 8, 9 and 10.

Practise with a willing partner, work for 5 minutes at each level. Start each training session from the lower steps. Stop at the first sign of pain, but if the pain settles within 20 seconds, continue the exercises. Otherwise stop, wait 24 hours, begin from first step (see *How much training?*). Concentrate on gripping with third, fourth and fifth fingers, and releasing thumb and index finger.

1 Serves. These should be painless throughout training.

2 Forehand drives. Play for length down the side wall.

3 Forehand boasts. Hit forehand boast; partner hits backhand cross-court. Repeat, do not hit any other type of shot.

4 Forehand cross-court. Hit forehand cross-court; partner hits backhand boast. Do not hit any other type of shot.

5 Backhand drives. Practise drives for length down side wall.

6 Backhand cross-court. Hit backhand cross-court, partner hits forehand cross-court.

7 Backhand boast. Play backhand boast, partner plays forehand cross-court.

8 Paired boast and drive. Hit forehand boast, partner hits straight backhand drive. Hit backhand boast, partner hits straight forehand drive. Repeat. Swap position with partner.

9 Smash. Concentrate on holding racket with third, fourth and fifth fingers, relax thumb and index finger (see Fig. 18.5). Try to avoid playing a face-on position.

10 The long game. Use special rules where the ball must bounce over the half line but a hard drive bouncing to a good length is permitted. The player forced into playing a drop shot loses the point.

11 Start play. Begin in easy, low-grade matches.

12 Fit again. Play at normal grade.

Baseball or throwing ladder – for shoulder injuries

Work for 5 minutes at each level with a partner. Start each session from the bottom steps. At the first sign of pain, stop, but if the pain settles within 20 seconds, continue. If the pain persists, stop, wait 24 hours then begin again from the first step.

The shoulder muscles must build up strength not only to throw but also to stop the arm following the ball! It is easy to overdo this ladder.

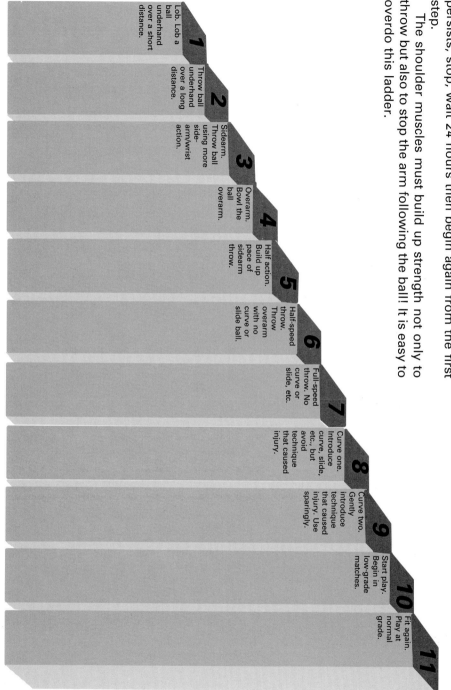

1 Lob. Lob a ball underhand over a short distance.

2 Throw ball underhand over a long distance.

3 Sidearm. Throw ball using more side-arm/wrist action.

4 Overarm. Bowl the ball overarm.

5 Half action. Build up pace of sidearm throw.

6 Half-speed throw. Throw overarm with no curve or slide ball.

7 Full-speed throw. No curve or slide, etc.

8 Curve one. Introduce curve, slide, etc., but avoid technique that caused injury.

9 Curve two. Gently introduce technique that caused injury. Use sparingly.

10 Start play. Begin in low-grade matches.

11 Fit again. Play at normal grade.

Further reading

1. Grimby, G. (1985) Progressive resistance exercise for injury rehabilitation. Special emphasis on isokinetic training. *Sports Med.* **2**, 309–315.
2. Wallin, D., Ekblom, B., Grah, R. and Nordenburg, T. (1985) Improvement of muscle flexibility. A comparison between two techniques. *Am. J. Sports Med.* **13**, 263–268.
3. Russell, K. (1985) Increasing joint range of movement in young athletes. Paper to *British Association of National Coaches*, Birmingham.
4. Osternig, L. J., Hamill, J., Lander, J. E. and Robertson, R. (1986) Co-activation of sprinter and distance runner muscles in isokinetic exercise. *Med. Sci. Sports Exercise* **18**, 431–435.
5. Smith, C. A. (1994) The warm-up procedure: to stretch or not to stretch. A brief review. *JOSPT* **19**, 12–17.
6. Murphy, D. R. (1991) A critical look at static stretching: are we doing our patients harm? *Chiro. Sports Med.* **5**, 67–70.
7. Robbins, S., Waked, E. and Rappel, R. (1995) Ankle taping improves proprioception before and after exercise in young men. *Br. J. Sports Med.* **29**, 242–247.

21
Team doctoring

Abdominal palpation and auscultation

A history of pain brought on by walking and relieved by rest suggests vascular and neurological claudication, and the older person especially with a history of vascular/cardiac problems should be checked for abdominal aortic aneurysm.

Aerobic training

Trains the oxygen transport mechanism through the lungs, heart and cellular mitochondria. It requires low-intensity endurance work for 30 minutes, three to five times a week, and trains the type 1 muscle fibres and does not produce much lactate.

Aeroplanes

Blow-up neck cushions are advised especially when sleeping on an aeroplane and the pillow provided should be used as a lumbar support. Walk around and do stretching exercises whenever possible. Medical staff travelling with teams will have to carry all their own equipment – do not expect too much help from the team or other staff. Either plan on a crate-sized container that is delivered to the venue or use several smaller cases as these stow more easily in the buses and you will have to manage them all by yourself! Be patient, take a good book or writing pad to infill time as travelling involves queuing and a big team cannot leave until the last person has collected their luggage off the travelator, it may as well be you, keep reading the book! See *Team travel.*

AIDS

Transmission during sport carries an extremely small risk. Transmission during sport is from blood, body fluids and other fluids containing blood. This weak virus is killed by soap and mild sterilizing solutions. Equipment, wrestling mats, diving boards, etc., should be wiped immediately with paper towels, and can be cleaned with bleach freshly prepared 1 : 10 with tap water but the dilution factor and chlorine of a swimming pool should prove sufficient to destroy the virus. Although those that sustain minor cuts or grazes may be left on the pitch, those who bleed must be removed from the pitch and blood-stained clothing changed. The wound should be sutured or steri-stripped and covered, sufficient for the competition. Embucrylate can seal the wound rapidly.

Latex gloves should be provided for all carers, and appropriate receptacles and disposal should be arranged for needles, syringes and surgical equipment, and soiled linen and uniforms. Post-event re-evaluation of the wound is required, and athletes should be responsible for proper treatment and covering of the wound before any competition. Confidentiality dictates that medical information is the property of the patient. Exceptions include medical conditions that are reportable by regulation and statute. The physician is not liable for failure to warn the uninfected opponent. That legal responsibility lies with the HIV-infected athlete. The uninfected assume some risk in sports activities because it cannot be assumed that other competitors are HIV or other blood-borne pathogens free. Hepatitis B and C are more virulent, and the above recommendations should suffice though vaccination is available for hepatitis B virus.

Exhaustive training regimens may compromise the immune system and already compromised HIV sufferers should not exercise to exhaustion. After an appropriate physical examination moderate exercise should be safe and beneficial to HIV sufferers. Education of athletes as to its infectivity should be undertaken and this should be emphasized to touring teams.

This information was abstracted from FIMS position statement on AIDS 1997 and therefore may change.

Alcohol

Alcohol causes peripheral dilatation and thus will hasten body cooling, and should not be used in the cold to apparently warm the patient. Alcohol can calm a nervous tremor and is sometimes used with those with an idiopathic tremor as beta-blockers are banned, but it does decrease hand/eye coordination and accuracy and balance. It is also banned in several sports such as modern pentathlon and shooting. The introduction of sports psychologists to teach stress management is perhaps more appropriate than knocking back the booze.

Altitude sickness

Usually occurs above 10 000 ft (3000 m). Presents with headache, fatigue and breathlessness. Increasing pulmonary oedema may be detected. Cerebral haemorrhage and thrombi and death may occur. Treatment consists of immediate oxygen and diuretics, plus a descent immediately 1000–2000 ft (300–600 m) lower.

Acclimatize by going in slowly and climbing up as opposed to flying straight in to base camp. Acetazolamide may help to prevent the episode but does leave 'zingy pins and needles' in the fingers, toes and circumorally. A fit person is just as likely to succumb as the unfit to altitude sickness.

Altitude training

Generally known to improve haematocrit which takes about 2–3 weeks to reach significant levels. Athletes often feel a little enervated on return and race best 7–14 days after returning to sea level. See *Erythropoietin*.

Amenorrhoea/oligomenorrhoea

See *Bone density*.

Anabolic steroids

Anabolic steroids are banned by almost every sporting federation. However they are available on the black market. Abusers tend to 'stack'

drugs to avoid side effects and thus take several different types one after the other. Abuse should be suspected with the triad of increased acne, striae, increased aggressive personality, often known as 'roid rage', but testicular atrophy and gynaecomastia may also be present. Premature fusion of the epiphyses produces a stunted growth. Females show increased androgenic effects, acne, male pattern hair growth, deepening voice, enlarged clitoris and suppression of menstruation, and both may have skin abscesses from infected needle wounds.

Investigations should include blood pressure for hypertension, urine for diabetes, and blood for liver and renal function as carcinomata are recorded. These drugs can be detected by gas chromatography and radioimmune assay. Testosterone is measured as a ratio to episterone when a positive test is a ratio of greater than $T:E\ 6:1$. High testosterone levels inhibit the stimulating hormone episterone. Therefore a high testosterone level should have a high stimulating episterone level, whereas extraneous testosterone will inhibit the episterone, increasing the normal ratio. Human growth hormone is known to be abused in sport but requires blood tests to detect. Probenicid has been used as a masking agent and to delay the excretion of steroids in the urine, and diuretics to dilute any excreted steroids, hoping to escape detection, and both are banned.

Anaerobic training

Trains the type 2 muscle fibres and requires high-intensity, short-duration work with longer recovery intervals (5 minutes), and it produces lactate. See *OBLA*.

Arthritis

Osteoarthritic joints are worse if totally rested or conversely overused. Ideally the joints should be moved but not impacted, thus rowing, cycling and swimming are preferable to running. Osteoarthritis hurts at the limit of joint range so a shortened walking pace, a thicker grip, etc., which alters the joint range can help. A thicker grip is not usually considered by golfers and yet it can make all the difference to the firmness of a pain-free grip. The explanation of a field surrounded by barbed wire, in which you can run around the field with no pain but when you try to extend that run you hit the barbed wire, can help the patients understand the pattern of arthritic pain.

Inflammatory arthritides require rest in the acute phase, isometrics for strength and mobilization when pain-free.

Asthma

Atopics are naturally worse around their allergies, e.g. horses, grass pollen, tree pollen, etc., so sports that avoid these contacts are recommended. However, note that high chlorine levels in a swimming pool can produce some surface irritant chlorine gas and thus irritation in an apparently allergen-free climate. Even though the asthmatic lungs may still have a problem with oxygen transfer, if the transport system to the muscles is improved by general training, so overall fitness will improve.

Exercise-induced asthma (EIA)

EIA is worse in the cold, running long distances and in dry conditions, and better in warm, moist air with interval games. Breathing warmer air through a mask or 'turbinator rebreather' may help. Interval games are handled better because of the refractory period of exercise-induced asthma. A beta-agonist, with or without an alpha-antagonist, should be taken 15–20 minutes before exercise, plus standard maintenance therapy such as sodium cromoglycate is beneficial. Steroid insufflation is permitted but parenteral steroids are banned.

Bending

Lifting increases intra-abdominal pressure but rather like a dam wall the spine counteracts this by a convex surface (lordosis) so that a neutral to lordotic spine is required. Strong abdominals will help to splint the spine in this position [2], but too many types of abdominal exercises will harm the spine, e.g. straight leg raises force extension. Flexion and rotation abdominals may well stress facet joints. Too many diagrams show the spine during lifting being splinted, and the knees and hips bent, but the buttocks tucked under the spine. Most people cannot lift from this position without flexing the spine and reaching into a cupboard to lift is impossible. So the bent position must have an extended or neutral back, but the buttocks should be pushed backwards, feet wide apart so that the forearms can be rested on the thighs (see Chapters 2 and 5). This is how weightlifters lift and how labourers in fields bend all day. This posture must be adopted for the slightest load, even cleaning the teeth, if the back is inclined towards flexion.

Bends

Scuba divers should have diving guidelines from BSAC or PADI for depth and time of dive and repressurization stops. However, divers presenting with joint pains, headaches, blurred vision and shortness of breath should be transferred immediately to the nearest depressurization chamber. Avascular necrosis from the bends will show on bone scans and MRI, and lung perfusion studies show bullae.

Beta-blockers

Beta-blockers reduce stress. In many sports this is undesirable but some sports do benefit, and shooters can also use the increased time of diastole in which to squeeze the trigger and obtain more accuracy! Familial idiopathic tremor is also helped by beta-blockers; however, as they are banned these players have to turn to alcohol, which is hardly a desirable substitute.

Blood doping

Blood doping is illegal! Between 0.5 and 1 litre of autologous blood is packed and freeze-dried, and after the athlete has replenished their own haematocrit, about 4 weeks later, prior to an event, the blood is retransfused. Even this illegal method has been reported to be abused at an Olympic Games, with the apparent transfusion in a hotel bedroom of heterologous blood.

Bone bank

A phrase used to express the amount of bone developed during growth that is available to dissipate against the advances of senile osteoporosis.

Bone density/osteoporosis

Exercises, even isometrics, improve bone density and thus the 'bone bank'. Post-menopausal osteoporosis is therefore delayed by exercise. Equally female hormones seem to be protective so that hormone replacement therapy may reduce post-menopausal osteoporosis and biphosphonates may delay or reverse this degradation. Oligo/amenorrhoeic athletes may diminish their bone bank. Exercise seems to delay menarche and can produce oligo/amenorrhoea in the heavily exercising adolescent, and this may be weight related, 7 stone/50 kg being the critical weight below which amenorrhoea seems to occur. However, delayed menarche may confer sporting ability. Some girls with a delayed menarche, who start their training after the onset of menarche, reach elite levels. Many animals are oestrus and do not ovulate under stress, and it may be that humans alter from the menstrual to the oestral cycle if stress is high, and therefore stop or delay their menstruation. Management should consist of:

(a) Checking dietary calcium levels as these are often low.

(b) Beware of true anorexics using exercise as an excuse for their under nourished body image – a good dietary assessment is required.

(c) Beware of unusual stress fractures such as the femur, pubic ramus or sacrum.

(d) Advise middle-distance runners that a power/weight ratio does not mean reducing the weight by dieting, because the subsequent reduction in muscle glycogen from the dieting will result in a reduction of muscle strength and endurance.

(e) Check pituitary and ovarian function.

Bone growth

Children mature at different rates, and should be matched in sport in both natal and developmental age. Monitoring of the Tanner Scale for secondary sexual characteristics, though helpful, may be socially embarrassing [3]. Skeletal growth rates may be monitored radiologically. Parental morphology may indicate the future adult developmental status and the child's growth hormones may be monitored.

Children may be selected into sports by maturing early, but this maturation may be inappropriate for that sporting position or sport at a later date or age. Reassessment of physical development vis-a-vis the sport and position played must be maintained throughout the teens. A 10 st, 5 ft 8 in 12-year-old may be ideal for the rugby scrum, but at 17 may still be 11 st, 5 ft 8 in and in fact should be playing in the backs (Fig. 21.1). During increased growth rate the epiphyses are most at risk and flexibility is reduced because the muscle tendon complex does not seem to lengthen at the same rate as the bone. Thus avulsion apophysitides are common and training should in fact be reduced during the growth phase. Broad-based training is required until apophyseal fusion when specific event training and weight training may be increased. Management should be directed towards a fit healthy adult rather than a child prodigy. See *Children*.

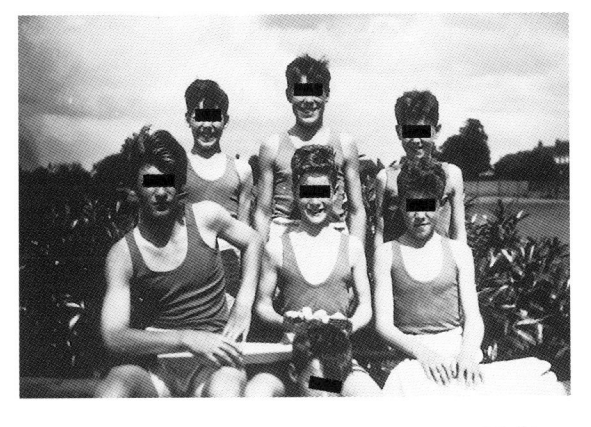

Figure 21.1 A group of 11–12-year-old schoolchildren showing different rates of growth. These may be even more diverse between 13 and 17 years.

Brain damage

Although the 'punch drunk' syndrome dementia pugilistica is well recognized, there have been suggestions that heading a soccer ball can produce long-term damage to the brain. Evidence suggests that this might be more related to acute injuries rather than from repetitive heading [1].

Breasts

Unsupported breasts may stretch and pull on the stroma and ligaments of Ashley Cooper and cause discomfort during exercise. Sports bras do provide the support and firmness for comfort. Protective plastic cups may be added in sports where trauma is expected. Nipples, both male and female, can be chaffed by the running vest, especially when it is roughened with sweat, which causes cracking and bleeding of the nipples. Cover with petroleum jelly or preferably second skin gels or sleek plaster to prevent this chaffing. When traumatized, breast fat may become tender and lumpy for several weeks raising the possibility of cancer – reassurance is required.

Bunny hops

Hopping routines into a full squat can produce meniscal tears – indeed the duck waddle (see *Glossary*) is used to test for meniscal tears. Virtually no sport requires strength in the full squat position and thus this training method should be abandoned.

Calcium

Dietary assessment of oligo/amenorrhoeics shows a lack of calcium intake either in the form of milk with its supplementary calcium or generally within the diet. Added calcium is advisable. Treatment of osteoporosis includes calcium supplements [2].

Check-ups

Should include all standard medical assessments but for exercise must contain auscultation for cardiac murmurs and an exercise electrocardiogram (ECG). Pre- and postexercise spirometry or FEV_1 for asthma. Fainting or dizzyness during exercise requires further investigation including echocardiogram. An assessment of the back and peripheral joints for biomechanical faults, and particularly for runners correction of overpronation perhaps with orthotics. Assessment of ligamentous laxity using the Beighton–Horan score (see Glossary) may suggest avoidance of some sports or the use of prophylactic bracing, and an indication of Marfan's syndrome will not prevent activities but will raise the index of suspicion to any chest pains for aortic dissection. Routine scanning for hypertrophic cardiomyopathy and spinal X-rays for congenital problems including spina bifida occulta with its increased association with spondylolisis in gymnasts is probably not cost-effective, although the previous East German regime would have excluded these congenital abnormalities from training [5]. However, there is a low yield per number of check-ups that makes this not very cost-effective for the standard athlete or child [6]. See *Exercise prescription*.

Chewing gum

Can cause airway obstruction if inhaled and should be banned during sporting activity.

Children

Should be trained on a broad basis until epiphyseal fusion has occurred when specialized event and weight training may be increased. During the growth spurt the bones grow faster and are weaker at the epiphyses than the muscles and tendons. This promotes a stiffness from the muscle tendon complex trying to catch up and stresses appear in the epiphysis rather than as a muscle or tendon lesion (see *Bone growth*). More time and information is required to guide coaches and doctors in developing high earning potential sportspeople and at the same time keeping the rest of the school population fit and actively enjoying sport [7]. Ruttenfranz' statement shows vision and understanding; 'children involved in elite sport can be considered participants in an uncontrolled experiment... Ethics committees to control training procedures of gifted children and to propose higher age limits for participants, especially in international sports events, seem to be needed. The basic ethical consideration is not to harm or alienate children by using them as objects for sports organizations, spectators or nationalists' [8]. Think on the East German regime and let us always watch the ethics of our involvement in sport.

Circadian rhythm

Circadian rhythm is the natural body basal metabolic rate that alters throughout the 24 hour cycle. This appears to adjust at approximately 1 hour per 24 hours of the time shift and the importance is avoiding participation during time zones that are equivalent to the current body basal metabolic rate (BMR) running at its lowest rate. Travel in time for this adjustment to have taken place at

competition, but an alteration say from 10.00 a.m. to 10.00 p.m. is not likely to have an effect. Melatonin may help [9] and travelling westward can have a faster adaptation than eastward [10]. See *Travelling with a team*.

Coffee/caffeine

May help fat metabolism and can therefore improve muscle endurance by delaying utilization of muscle glycogen. Above 12 parts per million coffee is considered dope positive, but the average level in the normal population of coffee drinkers is only 2 parts per million, suggesting anyone over the accepted level is definitely doping and not addicted to coffee!

Collapse

Collapse during, as opposed to after, exercise should be taken very seriously. Look for temperature disturbance and cardiac or respiratory problems in particular. Collapse after an event is more likely to be cessation of the calf muscle pump returning blood to the heart, in which case keeping the athlete on the move or lying them with their legs elevated, and even possibly cycling the legs, will be of benefit.

Corticosteroids

Corticosteroids are banned orally or parenterally, but are permitted as a topical application, insufflation and for local soft tissue or intra-articular injections as long as this is reported in writing, precompetition, to the doping control officer. Enteral steroids are permitted in special cases when application to the governing body is approved, e.g. coeliac disease.

Diabetics

Diabetics must be advised to wear a MediAlert style disc and increase their glucose intake and or reduce their insulin before exercise, and carry glucose and glucagon with them at competition besides their usual equipment. The team doctor and event doctor should be informed.

Diarrhoea

Travellers
Teams should be instructed and advised on going abroad:

(a) Gassy drinks on aeroplanes cause gastric distension.
(b) Air conditioning causes dehydration.
(c) Beware of food outside the hotel, especially shellfish, reheated foods, ice and ice cream.
(d) Check that bottled water has a sealed cap as this may be presented as bottled water but filled from the nearest local tap. Note bottled water may be stored in ice blocks which have been known to be a source of contamination.
(e) Avoid salad.
(f) Peel all fruit.
(g) Clean teeth with bottled water.

Treatment
Pre-check the prevalence of causative factors in the area, especially *Shigella*, *Giardiasis*, *E. coli* and Enterovirus so you are aware of the most likely infection. It is generally thought that pro-phylactic antibiotics are unnecessary unless in a particularly endemic area. Antidiarrhoeal treatment is with Imodium. Note that atropine-containing drugs affect performance. If possible culture stools, prescribe an appropriate antibiotic if required and maintain fluid replacement.

Runner's diarrhoea
Many sportspeople have precompetition gastric hurry caused by anxiety but long-distance runners may produce diarrhoea and even melaena, possibly from splanchnic ischaemia. Many a long-distance runner has to take toilet paper and spot the whereabouts of public toilets. It does appear to be runners rather than cyclists or swimmers who suffer and rarely ball games players, perhaps backing up the caecal slap theory. Appropriate fluid replacement is required later but precompetition 'gassy' drinks, available free at many venues, may also be causative [11].

Dehydration

Warn athletes that they do not have a thirst equivalent to their dehydration in the first 3–4 days before acclimatization [12]. A 5% dehydration can produce a 25% drop in performance. Make up an isotonic drink in a 5 gallon container and leave out near the exit to the team's accommodation. Also leave scales nearby and get the athletes to weigh themselves before and after training, and remind them that most of the weight loss will be fluid. Athletes must also check the colour of their urine, if it is dark they are dehydrated. Urine should be clear or straw coloured. Regular fluid replacement must be taken during performance. Sodium and potassium ions may be of benefit, but especially aid absorption of water which is vital. Five percent glucose or glucose polymers increase water absorption and if muscle energy is required at the same time then increase the glucose content. It is easier to drink from a squeeze bottle whilst running but the athlete should practise this whilst training to find which technique suits them the best. Gassy drinks should be poured out early and the addition of a sugar lump will decarbonate the drink, often violently. Alcohol causes dehydration.

Caveat – The following pitfalls have been recorded in international competition:

(a) Officially supplied water for the marathon was gassy.
(b) Supplied water was put out too soon in the sun so that when the runners came to drink it was hot and undrinkable.
(c) Ice to cool the bottled water has been found to be contaminated.
(d) The seals on the bottles were found to be broken and the bottles had been filled from the local tap.
(e) Athletes have been known to drink too much. The urine is clear but the athlete is passing water far too frequently and performance is thus also affected.

Caveat – Beware of the player that appears quite nervous and is noted not to be eating. High adrenaline levels will burn up the glucose and this athlete's performance will suffer. If the athlete cannot eat because of nervous tension then push high glucose fluids or glucose polymers such as drinks, chocolate and fruit during the prematch time available.

Diet

Carbohydrate loading

To increase muscle glycogen, light training only should be undertaken during the last week prior to an endurance event and the diet switched to high carbohydrates, especially during the last 2 days when training should be suspended. Glycogen depletion beforehand as originally described is not required [13].

Tournament diet

Muscle glycogen is replaced fasted when carbohydrate is taken within 30 minutes of the end of the game and certainly within a 2 hour window, either as food or as a high glucose drink. The evening meal may have steak to add flavour and creatinine but must have carbohydrates such as potatoes and rice. They do not have to be pastas for the main course, for puddings may be used equally effectively as carbohydrate loaders. Gastronomic boredom is debilitating especially on tour. Breakfast should be continental. Coffee may aid fat metabolism but caffeine at high levels is banned (see *Coffee/caffeine*).

General diet

Many athletes eat badly – not getting their fat and carbohydrate balance correct. Fatigued athletes should have a dietary revue and all athletes should be instructed how a rest day can restore their muscle glycogen. Power/weight ratios are often misunderstood, athletes losing weight but forgetting that power (type 2) fibres are heavy and that consequently their power goes down as well. Thus many one paced oligomenorrhoeic athletes will lose out on the sprint at the end of the race because they have not developed the muscle bulk of the fast twitch fibre and will require dietary advice, often to put on weight and making it carbohydrate orientated. Long-distance running has permitted the true anorexic to maintain their perceived body image without criticism and as these athletes' performance improves so they are often prepared, with dietary advice, to accept the requirements of training rather than the requirements of body image. Percentage body fat measurements are therefore much more vital than just actual weight.

Diuretics

Diuretics have been used to dilute the urine to escape detection of banned substances but they have also been used to 'make the weights'. Here it can be particularly dangerous as dehydration reduces performance and can promote hyperthermia and collapse under competition situations. Athletes self-medicating have the 'if one helps, four will help four times better' mentality. They can be responsible for gynaecomastia and are banned in sport.

DOMS

Delayed onset of muscle soreness (DOMS) has been experienced by most of us as the tender aching muscle that appears 24 hours after unaccustomed activity. It is more apparent after eccentric exercise and after long endurance exercise such as the marathon. It may be displayed on a bone scan when the muscles show increased uptake as well as the bones. Creatinine phosphokinase will be raised for 3–5 days, and T2-weighted or STIR sequence MRI shows an increased signal. This increased signal has been recorded as lasting nearly 3 months after eccentric exercise – an important point when managing soft tissue pain [14].

Drugs

Doctors prescribing for common illnesses must remember that some regularly prescribed drugs contain banned drugs in a sporting situation. See the current International Olympic Committee (IOC) list of banned drugs. The drug testing laboratories will probably be able to give you a list of drugs that you can use as well as those that are banned.

IOC list of doping classes and methods
Banned classes of drugs:

(a) Stimulants.
(b) Narcotics.
(c) Anabolic steroids.
(d) Beta-blockers.
(e) Diuretics.
(f) Peptide hormones and analogues.

Banned doping methods:

(a) Blood doping.
(b) Pharmacological, chemical and physical manipulation.

Classes of drugs subject to certain restrictions:

(a) Alcohol.
(b) Marijuana.
(c) Local anaesthetics.
(d) Corticosteroids.

Some International Federations have asked the IOC to test for marijuana, but not all, and snow boarding seems to permit its use.

Athletes not deliberately cheating are caught out by preparations in cough and cold mixtures, and by impure ginseng preparations that contain ephedrine or phenylpropanolamine, often in spite of labels of contents showing only permitted ingredients. Those positive on the 'A' test will have the 'B' sample tested by another technician and may have their own expert present during the second test.

Many charges of drug abuse are defended around the failure to handle the sample procedures correctly rather than the results of the tests. See *Drug/dope testing*.

Drug/dope testing

Who will be tested?
(1) An official decision will be made on the event or game to be tested by the body running the meeting. Notify the testing laboratory of the date of this event and the turn around time for results required, i.e. 24 hours, longer, shorter.
(2) An official decision on which place(s) in a race are to be tested or whether a random draw of players from teams by numbers will be required.
(3) Records will only be ratified after a negative dope test done at the time.

Notification of athlete
The athlete will be notified by an official with an appropriate document noting that a random position has been selected. The official will fill in the name of this athlete in the athlete's presence. The athlete will sign to confirm that (s)he is the relevant athlete and that they understand they must

attend at the dope control centre within a given time which is specified, usually 30–45 minutes. The time of notification is recorded. A copy of this document is kept by the official and collected by the doping control officer. This need only be kept if the athlete does not attend on time and may be destroyed once the test is declared negative.

Site

Signpost directions must be displayed that are visible from all conceivable routes and at all conceivable corners, turns, etc. The use of lines on the floor to direct athletes to the testing centre can be helpful. There must be no possible excuse that the athlete could not find where to go. Place a map in the official programme.

Waiting area

Admit access to the athlete with a test form and one team official (doctor/manager) but exclude all others. The time of attendance at the centre should be recorded on the notification sheet and notified to the test officer for recording on the documents. Seating and reading material are to be available. Drinks (non-alcoholic) must be from sealed cans or bottles and clean disposable cups must be used. The athlete must take and pour their own drinks.

Testing area

An official should check the identification of the athlete. The athlete selects a testing pack and must always have at least a choice of two. The athlete opens the pack, breaking the seal. The official points out A sample and B sample bottles that are engraved with a unique code. The official points out that in the event of sample A being positive, sample B will be tested by another laboratory technician, and the athlete and professional representatives may be present. The athlete unscrews the top of the bottle, and takes the top and bottle to the toilet with them. The athlete is accompanied to the toilet by an official of the same sex and is observed to pass preferably 100 ml of urine into bottle A. In practical terms 75 ml is acceptable.

Females may require a collecting slipper which should be sterile and sealed in protective wrapping, and this again should be selected from a choice of at least two by the athlete and opened by the athlete. The athlete is observed by the official decanting 25 ml of urine from sample A into the bottle sample B. The athlete screws the tops on both bottles and places them in the testing pack. The athlete seals the testing pack and is offered a selection of coded sealant tags for this pack (some systems use a coded outer container, not a tag). This code is recorded on the athlete's form and the athlete is required to check that this code is the same as that on the pack. The official will fill in the documentation.

Sheet 1 should contain:

- Name, sex, country, event.
- Drugs currently being taken.
- Time of notification, time of arrival at testing centre, time of test.
- Event code, pack sealant number.
- Athlete's signature.

To be handed to the athlete.

Sheet 2 will be a copy of Sheet 1 and kept by the organizers in event of a positive test to identify the individual from the pack number.

Sheet 3 will only record:

- Event code, pack code number.
- Drugs currently being taken.

This sheet will be sent with the sample. The athlete signs the top form which imprints the second but not the third and these facts are displayed to the athlete.

The pack is stored in a fridge until all the day's samples are collected and then these packs are placed in a large container sealed with a further coded sealant, or uniquely labelled outer bag, and transported to the testing laboratory within 24 hours.

Problems

(a) Pack seal numbers are not recorded properly at the test or in the laboratory, or not checked by athlete – **double check!**
(b) The athlete cannot pass urine before the end of the meeting. As long as the official in charge approves, the athlete may leave, but always in the company of a test official until the sample

has been collected. Thus the athlete may return to the hotel.

Random testing
This is usually on a voluntary code, and the athlete's home, work and training addresses are recorded; plus a photograph of the athlete. Notification should be given that they will be banned if they fail the test under IOC laws or they are consistently unavailable for testing. Notification of testing within 24 hours is reasonable when a convenient address (the athlete's home) may be agreed, plus a leaflet outlining the procedures for sample collecting should be sent to the athlete. However, testing at training may have short or no notice. The athlete signs to confirm the venue, date and time of collection, and the name of the athlete and the collector are printed out. The testing procedures are the same as in competition.

Some recorded or apocryphal methods of cheating
(a) A tube strapped to the penis passing urine from a bag. The athlete is asked to hold up his shirt and drop his shorts.
(b) Urine left by another source in the toilet. The athlete must be observed and the urine must be warm at body temperature.
(c) The athlete is catheterized with someone else's urine after emptying their own bladder. Two athletes were found to have an exactly similar chemical make up of urine as each other after gas chromatographic testing.
(d) Remember most cases go to court on the technique of the testing procedure not the drug analysis.

ECG
ECG evidence of large left ventricles and raised ST segments may be normal in an athlete.

Epilepsy
Controlled epileptics may take part in sport avoiding contact games where the head is at risk and situations such as climbing or sub aqua where a fit may prove fatal. They should wear MediAlert discs and inform team doctors. Check with the relevant sports authorities who have their own guidelines.

Erythropoietin (EPO)
EPO has now reached the athletic market and is being abused to increase the haematocrit. It seems that blood testing, as opposed to testing urine, will have to become the next move to detect this type of abuse.

Ethics in sports medicine
Various countries have made some attempts to establish a code of ethics and some suggestions are made below.

For the purpose of this code, sports medicine shall mean medicine practised by a physician in the field of competitive and recreational sports, whether by advising on how to avoid illness and injury or by administering treatment.

Medical practice
(1) The same rules that apply to general medical ethics shall apply to sports medicine.
(2) A physician who regularly treats or advises athletes shall possess the special knowledge of sports medicine, including the special physical and psychological demands of a sportsperson.
(3) Physicians shall not keep to themselves treatment methods for ill or injured athletes nor restrict this knowledge to a select group.
(4) Physicians shall not keep to themselves any testing or training methods with a curative or injury preventative effect.

(5) Physicians shall not conceal harmful side effects of training or therapeutic strategies.

(6) Physicians must at all times consider the long-term health of the patient and the natural healing of the injury to be the prime objective but recognize that sport practice has short-term goals. If these two requirements conflict then full and adequate explanation of possible risks and rewards shall be discussed between physician and athlete and any other party of consequence to the decision. The physician shall apply no duress to influence the athlete's decision. For those under the legal age of consent the physician shall only take consideration of long-term health and natural healing.

(7) The grounds for infusion therapy are no different for an athlete than for the general population.

(8) With the exception of the contraceptive hormones, hormone supplement is only acceptable if, compared to a norm, there is an abnormal decrease of hormone level, which in modern accepted practice is related to an increased threat to the athlete's health.

(9) A team physician has a duty to the team and the individual, but his prime concern is to the health and confidentiality of the individual. However, if this confidentiality is detrimental to the well-being and performance of the team then the physician shall attempt to persuade the individual to inform team management, but if this fails shall be permitted to advise team management of the likely short- and long-term problems for the team. Notifiable diseases shall be notified and the team management informed.

(10) If athlete and/or team management wish to partake of activities that the physician considers deleterious to the athlete's health then the physician has a duty to point this out, but will respect the personal responsibility of the athlete to control their own destiny. An exception to this guideline occurs if health risks for third parties are involved or the decision follows a medical emergency to the athlete.

(11) A team physician shall not prevent an athlete from taking a second opinion, but shall not be obliged to oversee nor be held responsible for the practice of this second opinion.

Publicity

(12) Physicians shall refrain from publicly criticizing fellow professionals.

(13) Case studies may be presented in research papers, books and lectures, but the athlete may not be named without express permission from the athlete. Some athletes are so high profile that their case will still be recognizable, but the presentation must still not name the athlete and will confine itself to the medical and psychological incidents that have direct bearing on the management problem.

(14) Physicians shall only release statements for publicity about an athlete's well-being in a format agreed with the athlete.

Banned drugs

(15) Physicians who are approached by athletes to prescribe medication listed on the banned list as defined by the National Body for the participant's sport and/or to physicians confronted by the use of medication listed on the banned list as defined above which were prescribed by another physician on medical grounds is obliged to advise the athlete and his medical advisor of non-banned therapies that will achieve the same therapeutic affect. Physicians confronted by the use of banned medication which the athlete is using on non-therapeutic grounds with the object of enhancing their performance shall advise against further use of this medication. If after the warning the athlete continues the physician shall advise the athlete that further persistence will be reported to the relevant Governing Body. If the transgression persists then the physician shall report the offender to the Governing Body.

(16) If the medication is listed on the banned list and has no alternative medication and its withdrawal will have a deleterious effect on the well-being of the athlete, then the physician shall inform the National Governing body to request dispensation for this individual.

(17) The physician will cooperate in performing or arranging to be performed compulsory anti-doping tests for athletes laid down in the sports regulations.

(18) The physician may express opinion on doping problems regardless as to whether this opinion is for or against the medication on the banned list.

Children

(19) Physicians responsible for the medical supervision of athletes under the legal age of consent will take due regard of the excesses of sports practice on the well-being of the developing child.

(20) Physicians will not artificially alter the growing rate of the child.

Third parties

(21) Physicians who perform examinations at the request of a third party will on request show the answers to the athlete before sending them to the third party. The objections of the athlete to release of this information shall be respected, but the physician shall inform the athlete of an obligation to advise the third party as to the fitness, unfitness or fitness under certain defined conditions, of this athlete.

Monies

(22) Physicians shall not accept any financial reward or gifts incommensurate with the usual fee.

Records

(23) Physicians will record medical notes of consultations and these records will be kept for the required legal time.

(24) These records will be kept in the usual confidential filing system accepted for standard medical practice. If for sake of continuity the records are housed at team headquarters then due diligence to security and confidentiality shall be ensured.

Exercise prescription

It is important to consider advice on exercise as a prescription, so the advice should only be given after a diagnosis has been made of the problems and the requirements of the patient understood. The type of exercise, the dose of exercise and the frequency of exercise must be defined. Many taking exercise after a long lay off will in fact break down their musculoskeletal system before they overstress their cardiovascular system. Do not target set, allow the body to give information. Start slowly at a speed where the patient can talk but has a catch in the breath. Weights should be low, building to 25–30 repetitions before incrementing the weight. Stop if the muscles feel fatigued or ache. Build to a distance slowly then increase the speed in gentle increments until the desired running speed has been obtained. Step up the distance but slow down the speed again. Once the increased distance has been obtained without muscle discomfort, then gradually increase the speed until the desired distance and speed are reached.

An easy guideline is:

(a) No reaction to exercise on two occasions – increase.

(b) Ache after exercise but better by the morning – maintain but do not increase.

(c) Ache after and lasting through the next morning to mid day – reduce by 10%.

(d) Ache after and all next day – rest that day and reduce by 50%.

Fainting

See *Collapse* and *Fatigue*.

Fatigue

(a) Anaemia. Sportspeople may have physiological anaemia from a greater circulating volume and serum ferritin should thus also be measured.

(b) Post-infective. The ubiquitous virus that is never proven seems to exist. Investigations should include viral antibodies, monospot and Epstein–Barr, but as the athlete usually presents some weeks after the problem there will be no rising titre to establish the diagnosis.

(c) Diet. Carbohydrate stores as muscle glycogen are depleted by a poor diet, but more usually because no rest day is programmed into the training so that muscle glycogen can be replenished. See *Diet*.

(d) Muscle damage. Muscle breakdown is shown by a high raised creatinine phosphokinase. The muscles are tender to palpation, and a history of direct muscle trauma, eccentric exercises and DOMS or extreme endurance exercise are obtained. This normally settles in 3–5 days.

(e) Overtraining. Physiologically not well understood, but the immune mechanism may show alterations in T cell ratios, and viral antibodies show titres for coxsacie B, toxoplasma, cytomegalovirus, Epstein–Barr, etc., but not suggestive of current infection [15]. The athlete seems to underperform and OBLA shows a shift to the left (see *OBLA*). Branch chain amino acids [16] may be altered, and some athletes have thicker tenuous bronchial mucus and altered hormonal ratios. Three weeks' rest in the early stage is curative [17] but when established it is similar to a chronic fatigue state when exercise must be severely curtailed into tolerance; 100 m may be tolerated but 101 m produces 4 days' fatigue. Short distances with rest are required. Viral protein one (VP1) may be positive. During incremental training runners should be moved onto ball games and exercises that they have not done before, because they try to monitor themselves on a previous training diary, which of course bears no relation to their current fitness but by their failure to achieve previous goals provokes a reactive depression, complicating the whole assessment of the situation.

Femininity check

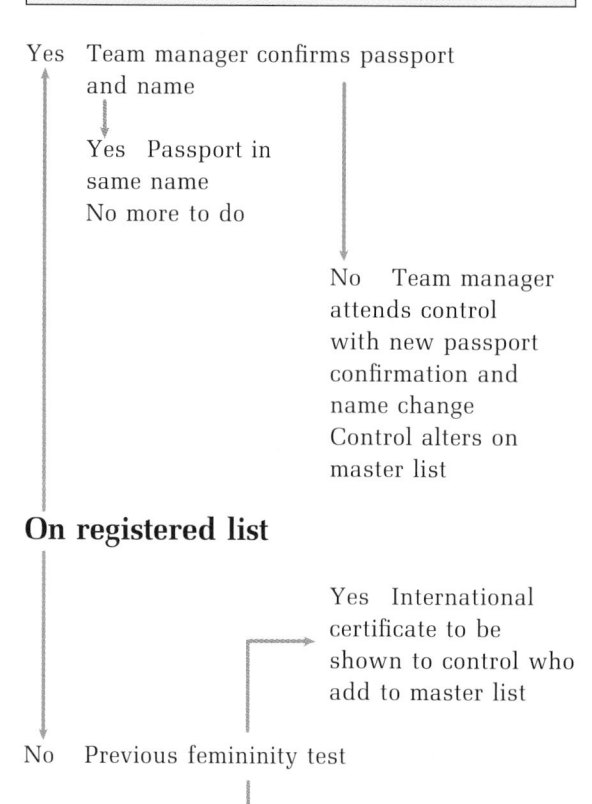

Yes   Team manager confirms passport and name

Yes   Passport in same name
No more to do

No   Team manager attends control with new passport confirmation and name change Control alters on master list

On registered list

Yes   International certificate to be shown to control who add to master list

No   Previous femininity test

No   Bring passport sized photo to test

Example test establishment

Room 1   Waiting.

Room 2   Check those who have certificate – may then leave. Check passport and entry list from those with passport photo. Photograph those without photo (Polaroid camera) and fill in femininity document.

Room 3   Cups and mouthwash. Bucal smears by trained staff. Clip smear slide to official femininity document.

Room 4   Cytologist – two to six in number. Examine slides. Sign documents when passed as correct.

Room 2 or 5   Record on list for forwarding to master list. Official stamp and date on official certificate. Record on entry list.

Everyone on entry list must have been checked that they are:

(a) Already on master list.
(b) New (married) name recorded.
(c) Not on master list but official certificate already issued and checked.
(d) Tested today and approved.

Failed tests must be counselled by the team doctor and must have blood tests with full chromosomal analysis.

Whether or not they should be performed is a debatable matter [18].

Flexibility

See Chapter 20 (*Stretching*) and Glossary (*Beighton–Horan score*).

Growth rate

See *Bone growth*.

Gumshields

Gumshields can be made from moulds but really should be cast made for the upper teeth and mainly prevent fractures of the teeth and perhaps reduce some impaction to the skull from a blow through the jaw. Trimming of the palateal portion may be required for easier respiration.

Haematuria

Frank haematuria may occur after marathon or ultra-marathon runs, often associated with melaena. Possibly associated with splanchnic and renal ischaemia and dehydration. Settles with appropriate rest but further investigation should be undertaken to exclude disease. Check with haemastick as haemoglobinuria or myo-globinuria may occur which are negative on testing.

Haemoglobinuria

Haemoglobinuria produces a red urine but is negative to haemasticks. Caused in sensitive people by fragility of vessels, particularly in the inferior calcaneal fat pad, and may be cured by shock absorbent soles.

Hay fever

Systemic corticosteroids are banned and antihistamines can be too sedative so Cromoglyconate and/or nasal steroid insufflation and menthol containing drops such as Synex are permitted.

Headaches

The standard infective causes and referred cervical pain (see Chapter 3) must be excluded. Exercise-induced migraines are reported but are difficult to diagnose and a neurological opinion should be sought. Acute post traumatic headaches must be seen urgently (see Chapter 1).

Headcolds

Menthol crystals or nasal sprays such as Synex are permitted. Anything containing ephedrine or pseudoephedrine is banned. Codeine is now permitted; however, do not allow training or competition if:

(a) The temperature is raised.
(b) There is a generalized myositis.
(c) If the resting pulse is raised 10 beats per minute, but if the resting pulse is raised 5–10 beats per minute, then complete a medical examination before making a decision.

Headguards

Headguards are designed to prevent cuts as in boxing, or to decelerate impact as in motorcycling, ice hockey, etc. The hard outer shell may appear intact after an accident but the polystyrene inside can be damaged and the helmet thus defective, so these types of helmet must be changed after each accident. There is an argument that the face guards prevent cuts and lacerations but increase the rotational force of head blows and thus the likelihood of concussion or tentorial tear.

Hepatitis

See *AIDS*.

Hyperthermia

Hyperthermia at rest and pre-exercise is a contra-indication to exercise. The temperature should be monitored rectally after exercise (aural/oral thermometers read low). If hyperthermic, then cool with spray or ice pack particularly over the groin and neck. If the mental state is normal and the athlete sweating, then observe, but there is probably no problem. If confused and dry, then rehydrate and cool but take the temperature regularly as this should return to 40°C in 10 minutes. If not or the patient remains confused and rigors, then admit. Beware, the onset of neurological signs is indicative of severe problems. Early rehydration essential – usually orally but many require intravenous fluids.

Hypothermia

Advise patients on prophylaxis, especially the effect of wind chill on top of being wet. Particularly advise about heat loss from the head, hands and feet and the legs, especially those that wear jeans. Be prepared – take waterproofs on mountains even in fine weather and carry a thermal blanket or a plastic bag to act as whole body protector. Do not drink alcohol, it dilates the periphery increasing temperature loss. Curl in a ball to reduce exposed surface area. Stay still in water and if possible float rather than swim. Reheat the body core with warm drinks and body blankets but do not massage or exercise the periphery until the core temperature is above 35°C. If mentally confused or the temperature below 35°C, then admit.

Isotonic drinks

Quite what they are isotonic to is debatable, but the principle is for the drinks to contain sodium, potassium and chloride, to replace loss in sweat, and also glucose or glucose polymers for energy whilst trying to be iso-osmolar to normal plasma. If dehydration is the problem then water must be replaced and these solutions may be diluted. If glycogen depletion accompanies the dehydration then the proportion of glucose or glucose polymer is increased. Pure glucose in high concentration can be sickly and be absorbed so rapidly that it produces an insulin oversecretion and hypoglycaemia – possibly this is more experimental than practical. If caught without any commercial replacements then a pinch of salt and a tablespoon of sugar in a pint of water will be suitable.

Jet lag

See *Team travel*.

Jogger's nipple

See *Breasts*.

Melaena

See *Haematuria*.

Menstruation

It is generally accepted that normal athletic performance can be achieved during menstruation but some have perimenstrual problems of water retention which cannot be controlled by the banned diuretics. Hormonal adjustment (contraceptive pill) can be of benefit and bleeding during competition can be prevented by shortening or lengthening the cycle as a planned exercise. Some athletes have weight/exercise-induced oligo/amenorrhoea, but these athletes that weigh above 50–55 kg should have a hormonal assay. The bone density may be lowered (see *Bone density*).

Muscle fibre

Type 1   Aerobic oxidative metabolism of glycogen with CO_2 as a waste product.
Type 2b   Anaerobic glycolytic with lactate as a waste product.
Type 2a   Perhaps an intermediate with some aerobic capacity.

Muscle imbalance

Muscle function requires a balance of strength between agonist and antagonist, and this balance may alter with speed. When this is upset, muscle damage may occur. However, it must also be noted that one side of the body should have a balanced relationship to the other one. Sometimes the weak side is the side to be damaged but the damaged side is not necessarily the weak side as the strong side may have to work disproportionately hard to make up for the weak side and thus become damaged. Racket sports may produce disproportionate shoulder strength that can produce a scoliosis. Exercises should be given to the non-dominant side.

Myoglobinuria

Local trauma or excessive exercise may produce muscle breakdown with the appearance of myoglobin in the urine.

OBLA

Onset of blood lactic acid (OBLA). This is monitored during exercise and the 2 or 4 level plotted against the work done. The fitter one gets the more work one can do at these levels and the curve is said to move to the right. Loss of fitness moves the curve to the left.

Physical maturity

See *Bone growth*.

Resting pulse

The resting pulse should be taken first thing in the morning on wakening and before rising. The athlete should be taught to take this pulse as it may be used as a rough and ready guide to fitness for competition or training. It can be used to monitor an aerobic training effect when the improved fitness will show as a slowing of the resting pulse. It may also be used to monitor stress and illness, where a pulse raised 10 beats per minute probably reflects illness or an incipient illness and suggests physical activity should be curtailed. Pulse increases of 5–10 beats per minute should see the doctor who will check for illness and signs of stress. This player should be watched. The anxiety may prevent eating and will also deplete muscle glycogen. Invariably it is this player who is substituted. High glucose energy drinks can be a way to top up the muscle glycogen in this type of player.

Sunburn

Many athletes enjoy bronzing whilst on tour but must be warned against sunburn, especially head, neck, nose, ears, and tops of feet and knees, as well as the usual torso, shoulders and arms. Sunglasses should always be worn around water and snow, and protective sun creams must be advised.

Tanner scale

An assessment of physical maturity based on the development of secondary sexual characters; breast buds, pubic hair, etc. See *Bone growth* and *Children*.

Team talk

The team talk will be run by the coach and the doctor may have to spend long nights listening to the coach rehearsing this talk. Some coaches will deliberately raise the level of stress; however, to some players, who are already tense, this is not to the best advantage, and during the talk the doctor should observe the team for individual signs of stress and anxiety that may inhibit the player from eating and thus loading the prematch carbohydrates. Glucose energy drinks may be the best substitute to food for these players.

Team travel

Arrange a pretour medical or questionnaire to obtain the basic medical history and check inoculation requirements, then inoculate the probables and possibles. Check time zone difference and allow approximately 24 hours per hour of time zone difference for an adjustment in circadian rhythm.

(a) Advise management of optimum acclimatization time.

(b) Start sleep routines at home or on the plane to fit with the host country. Sleeping tablets and melatonin may help.

(c) Plan training times as near to match times as can be obtained, but training abroad at the home time equivalent to a low body biorhythm should be light.

If uniform is worn take loose clothes and shoes to change into on the plane. Arrange analgesia, antacids, antiemetics, antihistamine, antidiarrhoeals and sleeping tablets to be in your cabin baggage, not in the hold. Most countries do not require a licence to practise if you only treat team members. Most countries allow your relevant drugs to be carried whilst travelling with the team. Advise on dehydration from alcohol, coffee and the air-conditioning, and gastric distension from decompression and from gassy drinks. This is important if flying out to compete that same day. Administer sleeping tablets if appropriate – not to yourself! Recommend regular walks and stretching exercises to the legs during long journeys.

At the accommodation

Take the largest room available as it will have to be both a consulting and a bedroom. Post the doctor's room number on the team notice board and leave a notice on your door when you are out and when you are expected back and where you are. Arrange surgery times – but you will still end up consulting *ad hoc* as well. Obtain a print-out of competition times and travelling times to and from the venue as:

(a) Management often forget to inform the medical staff.

(b) In track and field, for instance, you can prioritize consultations to those still in the competition.

Arrange to review your patients at the training or to be with those that have a known problem during their event. Arrange and organize training for the injured as the coach has too much to think about with the fit team and those left out through injury get depressed unless physically worked. Liaise daily with the physiotherapist over all injury problems and inform the coach of injury problems, actual and potential. Put out scales in the team corridor to monitor:

(a) Weight gain. Food on tour can be fantastic and when bored eating becomes a communal habit.
(b) Weight loss. Especially suggestive of dehydration or stress.

Make available daily fluid drinks in the team corridor as this encourages athletes to drink and observe their urine colour for dehydration (see *Dehydration*).

Know where the polyclinic is in the village and other medical services that are available as they may be of value. Record telephone numbers of the venue and village in your medical case. Do not forget your pass – hang it on the door handle at night. If appropriate, have at least two pairs of spectacles – leave one at the venue and one at the village. Make accurate notes and arrange with management where they will be kept for the intervening legally required years.

At the venue (Fig. 21.2)
Reconnoitre as soon as possible to find:

(a) The shortest distance from the team changing or warm-up area to the competition area and finishing line.
(b) Locate the stadium medical room and meet the stadium medical officers if possible.

(c) Locate the source of ice.
(d) Locate the source of drinks.
(e) Locate the dope testing room.

Try and meet the stadium manager to discuss:

(a) Medical track clearance – to where will they be taken – especially events such as the marathon, time trials, walks and triathlon.
(b) The nearest stretcher and type of stretcher.
(c) The nearest first aid team and where others are stationed.
(d) The nearest hospital and telephone number.

Take down a sticky label with the team name on it and put it on the best changing room you can find; however, you may have to get up early on the day of competition to bag this room, but once you have it, most other teams will treat it as sacrosanct.

Medical requirements at a venue
Team doctor, crowd doctor with advanced life-saving training, ambulance/St John's/paramedics stationed around the venue, drug testing team, track or playing area clearance team trained in first aid and stretchering. A communication system which may require vibrating as opposed to ringing call system at golf and a map of designated grid areas so that the problem can be located easily. Fluorescent jackets with title inscribed. The major hospital should be informed of the date and type of event, especially the casualty consultant, and the telephone numbers of this hospital and relevant doctors recorded.

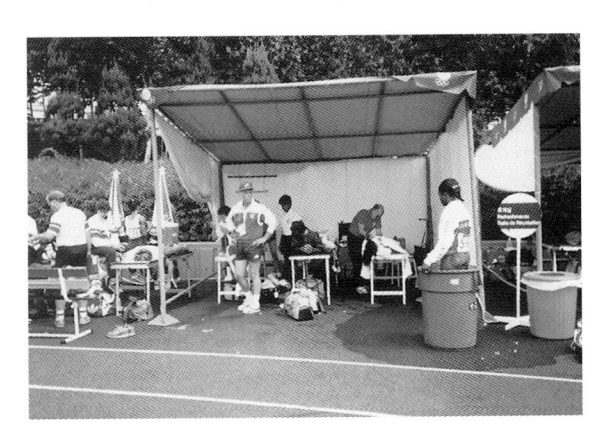

Figure 21.2 Millions are spent on Olympic games but facilities for medical care are appalling. Pictured are the facilities for two Olympic track and field squads.

Further reading

1. Jordan, S. E., Gary, A. *et al.* (1996) Acute and chronic brain injury to United States National Team soccer players. *Am. J. Sports Med.* **24**, 205–210.
2. Mottram, S. and Comerford, M. (1998) Stability dysfunction and lower back pain. *J. Orthop. Med.* **20**, 13–18.
3. Caine, D. J. and Broekhoff, J. (1987) Maturity assessment: a viable preventative measure against physical and psychological insult in the young athlete? *Physician Sports Med.* **15**, 67–802.

4. O'Brien, M. (1996) Osteoporosis and exercise. Editorial. *Br. J. Sports Med.* **30**, 191.

5. Donath, R. GDR (1985) Sports-medical care for walkers. Abstract from lecture to the Amateur Athletics Association seminar for coaches in walking, Birmingham.

6. Rowland, T. H. (1986) Preparticipation sports examination of the child and adolescent athlete: changing views of an old ritual. *Pediatrician* **13**, 3–9.

7. Caine, D. J. and Lindner, K. (1990) Preventing injury to young athletes Parts 1 and 2. *J. de l'ACSEPL* Part I, Mais/Avril, 30–35; Part II Septembre, 24–30.

8. Rutenfranz, J. (1986) Ethical considerations: the participation of children in elite sports. *Pediatrician* **13**, 14–17.

9. Arendt, J. and Marks, V. (1982) Physiological changes underlying jet lag. *Br. Med. J.* **284**, 144–146.

10. Winget, C. M., DiRoshia, C. W. and Holley, D. C. (1985) Circadian rhythms and athletic performance. *Med. Sci. Sports Exercise* **17**, 498–516.

11. Brouns, F., Saris W. H. M. and Rehrer, N. J. (1987) Abdominal complaints and gastrointestinal function during long lasting exercise. *Int. J. Sports Med.* **8**, 175–189.

12. Greenleaf, J. E. (1966) Exercise and waterelectrolyte balance. Special Publication, **110**, 47–58.

13. Fogelholm, G. M., Tikkanen, H. D., *et al.* (1991) Carbohydrate loading in practice: high muscle glycogen concentration is not certain. *Br. J. Sports Med.* **25**, 41–44.

14. Stoller, D. W. (1994) *Magnetic Resonance Imaging in Orthopaedic and Sports Medicine*, 2nd edn, p. 1352. California: Lippincott Williams and Wilkins.

15. Shephard, R. J. and Sheck, P. N. (1994) Potential impact of physical activity and sport on the immune system – a brief review. *Br. J. Sports Med.* **28**, 247–255.

16. Blomstrand, E., Cesling, F. and Newsholme, E. (1988) Changes in plasma concentrations of aromatic and branched chain amino acids during sustained exercise in man and their possible role in fatigue. *Acta. Physiol. Scand.* **133**, 115–121.

17. Koutedakis, Y., Budgett, R. and Faulmann, L. (1990) Rest in underperforming elite competitors. *Br. J. Sports Med.* **24**, 248–252.

18. Fox, J. S. (1993) Gender verification – what purpose? what price? *Br. J. Sports Med.* **27**, 148–149.

Bruckner, P. and Khan, K. (1993) *Clinical Sports Medicine*. McGraw-Hill, New York.

22
Glossary

Accessory navicular or os tibialis externum

An accessory ossification centre of the navicular which when fixed and large is referred to as a cornuated navicular. About 10% of young have an accessory ossification centre, but only about 2% in adults remain uncoalesced. It may produce symptoms due to its prominence, when it rubs on the shoes or because of its tibialis posterior attachment enthesitis. See Chapter 13 (Fig. 13.12) and Chapter 14.

Acromio-clavicular joint

Grade 1   Superior ligament damage or sprain.
Grade 2   Superior and inferior ligament tear.
Grade 3   Superior and inferior ligament tear with disruption of the conoid and trapezoid ligaments.

There may be a more chronic onset causing degenerative changes within the joint and showing osteophytic lipping. See Chapter 17.

Active compression test

A test to display intra-articular shoulder lesions or acromio-clavicular joint problems. The standing patient forward flexes the arm to 90° with the elbow in full extension and then adducts the arm 10–15° medial to the sagittal plane of the body and internally rotates it to point the thumb downwards. The examiner applies uniform downward pressure on the arm. The manoeuvre is repeated with the palm upwards. The test is positive if pain is elicited in the first manoeuvre and reduced in the second. The acromio-clavicular joint 'points' to the top of the shoulder, and the labral tear produces pain and clicking 'inside' the shoulder [1].

Adson's manoeuvre

For arm pain. Abduct the elbow to 90° with the shoulder and add external rotation of the arm. Pain reproduced on looking toward the painful arm equals a possible disc. Pain on looking away or pulse decreases equals a possible thoracic outlet syndrome.

Adverse neural tensioning

Nerves must be capable of moving as a joint is flexed and extended. The spinal cord similarly moves within the spine. If the nerve is trapped by a disc, adhesions or tumour then free movement cannot occur and pain is produced. The classic example would be the straight leg raise test, made worse by stretching the sciatic nerve (Lasegue's) and then adding stretch of the spinal cord (Kernig's) so that the slump test becomes the combination of these tests. Gently stretching just into pain over a long time may free up these adhesions or possibly encourage growth of the neurovascular bundle to produce adequate length. Therapeutic adverse neural tension uses gentle stretching techniques to stretch the nerve, perhaps releasing the restraining compressive areas. However, the Iliserov technique to lengthen bone has to be accompanied by lengthening of the neurovascular bundle and perhaps this stretching of 2 mm per day is produced by adverse neural tension techniques, so that the adhesion remains but the nerve develops enough length to cope with the movement required functionally [2].

Adverse neural tension is used clinically for nerve root adhesions in the arm and leg, and peripheral adhesions such as the piriformis and hamstring syndrome. See Chapter 9.

Allen's test

Pressure on both the radial and ulnar arteries at the wrist to exclude the blood flow and with the release of one at a time, a flush of the hand, as the blood flow returns indicates whether each **artery is patent**.

Anderson's test

A grinding test for **meniscal lesions**.

Anterior apprehension test of the shoulder

Standing behind the patient, flex the shoulder to 90°, externally rotate as fully as possible and then press on the posterior aspect of humeral head to increase the anterior translation. Apprehension or pain is a positive test for a **subluxing** or **unstable shoulder**.

Anterior draw test

The knee is flexed to 90° and the tibia is rotated internally. Sitting on the foot fixes the distal tibia. The tibia is then drawn anteriorly when increased translation is permitted by a torn or ruptured **anterior cruciate ligament**. The starting position must be noted as any sag caused by a posterior rupture will then allow increased apparent anterior gliding and a false positive. Comparison must be made with the other leg.

Apley's test

For the **knee**. Compression and distraction manoeuvres of the tibia performed on a flexed knee at 90° through to 180° with the patient lying prone. Pain only on distraction suggests a **ligamentous** cause, whereas pain and grinding on compression and rotation suggests **meniscal** or **articular surface** damage.

Apprehension test

See *Anterior apprehension test of the shoulder* and *Patella apprehension test* in the **knee**.

Arcade of Frohse

A ligamentous band over the posterior interosseous nerve as it enters between the two heads of the supinator. A tight band can cause **radial nerve entrapment**.

Ballottement

See *Bulge test*.

Bankart lesion

Fracture defect in the inferior glenoid labrum caused by **shoulder** dislocation. Visible on X-ray, but an MRI may show an inferior labral defect with no bony lesion. See Fig. 17.11.

Bankart's repair

Surgical repair of the glenoid labrum and Bankart lesion in a dislocated or recurrent **dislocating shoulder**.

Bayonette sign

A sign indicative of possible **patellar maltracking**. The patella tendon insertion lies well lateral on the tibia, thus producing a valgus alignment of the patella tendon from the lower patellar pole to its insertion on the tibia, giving the appearance of a bayonette on a rifle.

Beighton–Horan score

A score for **ligamentous laxity**. Score 1 point for right and 1 point for left side:

- Little finger extending to 90°.
- Hyper-extension of the elbow beyond 15°.
- Hyper-extension of the knee.
- An ability to touch the back of the thumb onto the front of the forearm.

Score 1 point for:

- Touching flat of hands onto the floor.

Total score = 9.

Bennett's fracture

For the **thumb**. Fracture dislocation of the proximal end of first metacarpal. See Fig. 19.5.

Blocked movement

It is easiest to consider this in a kick of the football. The kicker subconsciously prepares the whole movement pattern into the 'follow through', but if an opponent stops the ball from moving then the kicker's movement is 'blocked'. Because the programmed musculo-skeletal action was completion of the kick, there is no preparatory deceleration and the muscle contraction continues on after the leg has been stopped from moving and this produces an acute **resistance to contraction** which often ruptures the muscle. Clinically the expression can be used for describing a resisted muscle test, e.g. 'block external rotation'.

Bone scan

Radioactive technetium-99, given intravenously, is taken up by active bone and when this radioactivity is scanned early stress lesions in bone will be displayed. When these are accompanied by pain

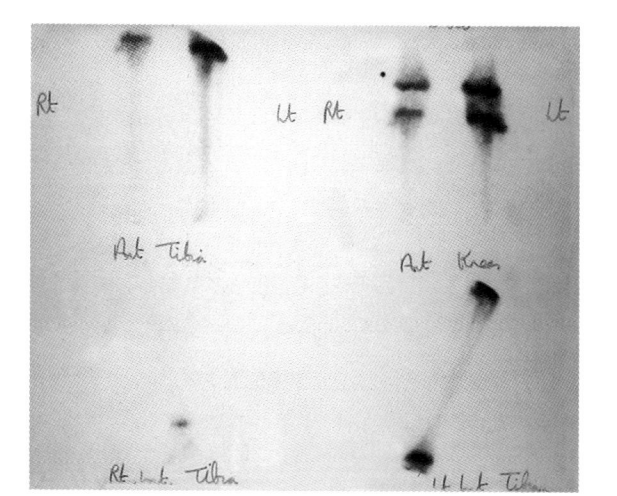

Figure 22.1 Bone scan shows reduction in uptake in the right leg of an adolescent gymnast with reflex sympathetic dystrophy. She was stretching her hamstrings on a partner's shoulder when her foot slipped off.

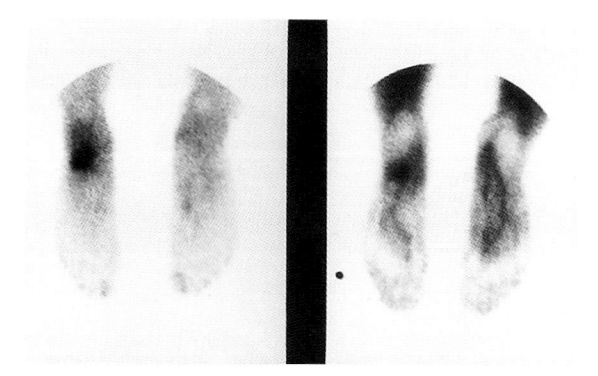

Figure 22.2 A bone scan in its blood phase showing increased uptake in the right ankle with soft tissue inflammation.

they are defined as stress fractures. Increased blood supply will be displayed by an increased radioactivity count, but only during the phase when technetium is in the blood. A count taken during the injection phase and monitored over 2 min will display areas of poor **blood supply** (reflex sympathetic dystrophy) (Fig. 22.1) and increased blood supply as in an inflammatory lesion (Fig. 22.2). The three-phase bone scan reports the early and late blood phase, and then the bone phase 2–4 h later (Fig. 22.3). Muscle damage as in **DOMS** can have an increased count.

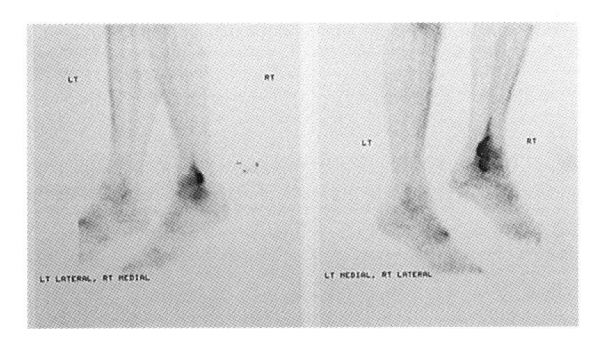

Figure 22.3   Increased uptake in the bone phase of the right ankle.

Bowstring sign

The bowstring sign attempts to differentiate between a **hamstring lesion** and **sciatica**. The straight leg raise is taken to the onset of pain, then the knee is allowed to flex until the pain disappears, at which stage pressure is applied to the popliteal fossa to restretch the sciatic nerve. A recurrence of pain suggests sciatica.

Brachial nerve tensioning tests

Neural stretch tests for the brachial, ulnar, median and radial nerves, respectively. See *Adverse neural tensioning*.

Bristow repair

For recurrent **dislocation of the shoulder**. The tip of the coracoid containing its attachments, short head of biceps and coraco-brachialis, is screwed to the neck of the scapula and produces a dynamic sling antero-inferiorly.

Brostrom repair

Surgical repair of ruptured **lateral ligaments of the ankle** – resuturing the ruptured ligaments.

Bulge test

A small amount of **fluid in the knee** may be displayed by compressing one side of the knee to move all the fluid to the other side. The suprapatella pouch is compressed during this manoeuvre and then the opposite side of the knee is stroked. Fluid will return again to the first side and is seen as an increasing bulge. Too much fluid, 20 ml or so, will not empty from one side to the other and is palpated by ballotting the fluid with one hand and feeling the impulse with the other. A volume of 30 ml or more will show as a patella tap, because increased fluid lifts the patella off the femur from where it may be pressed down onto the femur and springs out again when the pressure is removed.

Burner/stinger

Transient irritation of a **cervical nerve root** where temporary paralysis, often C6 distribution, plus lancinating pain into shoulder and arm; may only last 10–15 min but traces of a neurological deficit may last months.

Calcaneo-tibial compression test

Because standing on tip toe can load the Achilles or compress the posterior structures of the ankle, this test is used to differentiate **Achilles lesions** from **posterior ankle and talar/subtalar lesions**. With the patient lying prone the foot is whipped into passive plantar flexion to impinge the superior surface of the calcaneum against the posterior structures of the ankle. No pain occurs with Achilles lesions but does if structures at the back of the ankle are damaged. See Fig. 13.14.

Camber running

Many **roads are domed** to run off water to the sides and this produces a slope or camber. Running on the same side of the road all the time will produce a functional long and short leg. This inequality may stress ligaments throughout the lower limb, especially in knees and ankles. Runners must vary the side of the road on which they run.

Checking shoes

The most important aspect of a shoe is the **integrity of the uppers**. The heel cups must be capable of holding the heel and must not lean in or out. Their attachment must be solid and the heel tag must be soft and the sides not too high. See *Shoes*.

Clarke's sign

A compression test of the patella to display **patello-femoral pain**. Compress the patella in a distal direction and then the patient contracts the quadriceps – this may produce total inhibition, pain and/or grating. An indicative test rather than an absolute positive test and one that should be compared to the other side.

Claw hand

When the **median nerve** is involved as well as the **ulnar**, all the fingers claw.

Clunk test

Circumduction of the **shoulder** in full abduction. A clunk or grinding suggests internal derangement.

Compartment pressures

Are measured by a split catheter with a pressure transducer that is inserted into a **muscle compartment**. These are read before and after exer-

cise or monitored continuously. A rise in pressure beyond a certain level either at rest or after exercise may be pathological. Various levels are recorded as abnormal in the calf with continuous monitoring: above 30 mmHg in the relaxation phase and above 50 mmHg in the contraction phase, although some accept above 85 mmHg in the contraction phase. Patients should be tested by repeating the exercise that brings on their pain as a patient may not bring on the problem by just running. Sometimes a patient has rested for some weeks before the test and the pressures record as normal, probably because the chronic increase in pressure of the compartment builds up as a result of the effects of one training session not being allowed to settle before the next is started.

Concentric muscle contraction

The muscle force elongates the stretch elastic component before shortening occurs. The mechanical force is positive and the muscle contraction occurs together with shortening such as the biceps lifting a weight up towards the shoulder. It is an acceleratory force. See *Eccentric muscle contraction*.

Congruence angles

An angle on X-ray between the patella and femoral condyles at 45° of flexion which is used to assess **malalignment of the patella**.

Cortisone

Depomedrone should not be used with epidurals, particularly translumbar, as the dilutant/preservative is irritable to the meninges if the dura is penetrated. Hydrocortisone acetate produces less subcutaneous atrophy and should be used in superficial injections such as for the Achilles peritendon and tennis elbow, but triamcinolone remains active locally for longer.

Cram test

Pressure on the **sciatic nerve** at the popliteal fossa to exacerbate the straight leg raise. See *Bowstring sign*.

Crank test

The circumducted arm is moved backwards and forwards between external and internal rotation and pressure exerted through the arm towards the joint. Pain and clunking suggest possible internal ligamentous disruption such as a slap lesion.

CRP

C-reactive protein. An early blood marker of some systemic diseases.

CT

Computed tomography of X-rays to produce 'slices' through body tissues displaying both soft tissue and bone.

Depth jumping

See *Pliometrics*.

Disc probe

The annulus has nerve ends and some annular discs probably only represent increased nucleus pulposus pressure on the annulus without herniation. It may be treated by an intradiscal injection of hydrocortisone. The disc can be destroyed with chymopapaine but the occasional complication of transverse myelitis makes the less destructive microdiscectomy a better procedure. With neuroleptic analgesia this technique of disc probe may be used for the **diagnosis of vertebral** pain when the facet and sacro-iliac joints are also stimulated.

DISH

Disseminated idiopathic skeletal hypertrophy with its tendency to produce traction spurs at many apophyses.

DOMS

Delayed onset muscle soreness. Endurance events, eccentric work and muscle overtraining cause muscle stiffness and pain some 24–48 hours after the exercise that may last 5–7 days. During this time creatinine kinase is raised, technetium bone scan may be positive over the muscle concerned and T2-weighted scans show an increased signal. At its severest may even last 2–3 months with the changes visible on T2-weighted MRI. See Fig. 22.4.

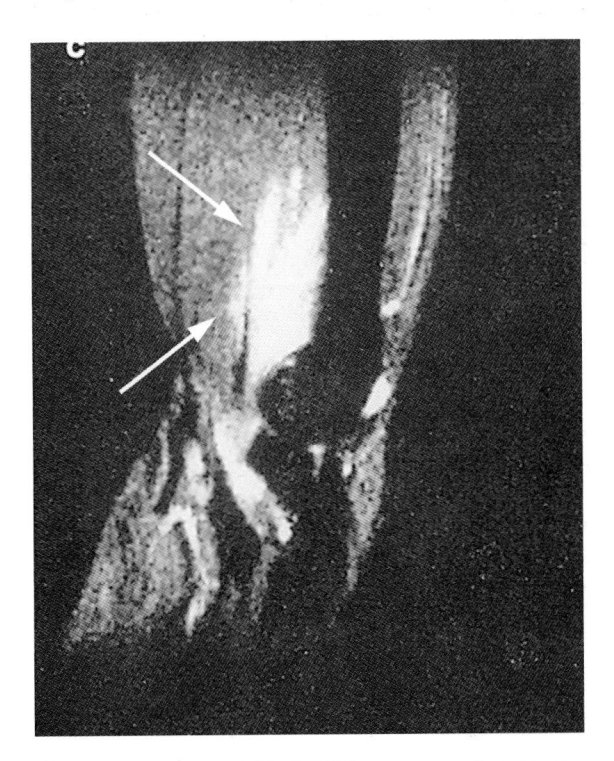

Figure 22.4 T2-weighted MRI sequence showing increased signal in the biceps following eccentric muscle exercise.

Downing's sign

The supine leg is flexed at the hip, externally rotated and then straightened. An apparent lengthening of the medial maleolus indicates the **sacro-iliac joint** is mobile. This apparent lengthening reduces with hip flexion, adduction and straightening of the leg. It is not an accurate test but may help to decide when a sacro-iliac joint should be manipulated or sclerosed. The mobile joint does not need manipulating.

Drop jumping

See *Pliometrics*.

Duck waddle

For subtle **meniscal** pathology. Moving forward in a full squat position is painful but an effusion, lack of full extension, pain on full flexion and patello-femoral problems may complicate this test. See Fig. 22.5.

Dural stress tests

Straight leg raise, slump, Kernig's, brachial nerve tensioning, arm raising, Valsalva and Lhermitte's will all stress the dura, and if the dura is prevented from moving will produce pain. The straight leg raise and slump tests will be variably positive in herniated discs and adhesions of the nerve root or dura, and blowing a Valsalva may also produce lumbar pain with acute dural irritation. See *Adverse neural tensioning*.

Dye strapping

A strapping technique to squeeze the subcutaneous fat of the heel, preventing its spreading

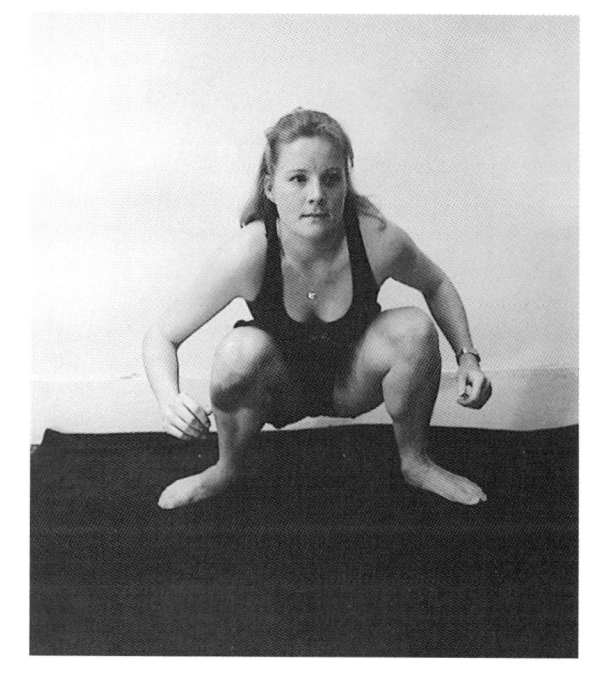

Figure 22.5   The 'duck waddle'.

sideways on heel impact, and thus increasing the thickness of the heel pad and maintaining support for the stroma in between the fat globules. This is the mechanism that has been copied by the 'air soles' in running shoes. Used for type 1 **plantar fasciitis**.

Eburnation

A description in degenerative joints when the articular cartilage is destroyed and bone is articulating with bone.

Eccentric muscle contraction

The load lengthens the stretch elastic component first and then the muscle lengthens during contraction. The mechanical force is negative and is a deceleratory force. Less motor fibres per Newton are required. This movement is more prone to muscle damage and a raised creatinine phosphokinase may be measured for 3–5 days after heavy eccentric work, e.g. the biceps lowering weight onto a table (see Fig. 22.4). See *Concentric muscle contraction*.

ECG

Electrocardiogram. Recording of the heart's electrical activity. A large left ventricle and raised ST segment may be normal in athletes.

Effort thrombosis

Paget–von Schroetter syndrome with distended veins and oedema which is usually found in the arm and requires a venogram and possible anticoagulate. It is a rare syndrome.

EMG

Electromyogram. Checks how well nerve muscle complex is working by measuring conduction rate of peripheral nerves.

Enthesis/enthesopathy

The enthesis is the cellular transition zone where the **tendon becomes bone**, i.e. the attachment of tendon to bone. An enthesopathy is an inflammation or damage of this area.

Epidural injections

May be given by the caudal or translumbar approach. The caudal with 0.5% procaine allows the patient to walk away and be treated as an outpatient. A stronger solution may be given for intense pain giving some short-term analgesia, but the motor effects of this must be considered. The 'caine anaesthetics possibly may close the S or H gates within the myelin sheath, so that a continued sodium leak which produces a continued ionic-induced noci stimulus is aborted. Certainly there appears to be a desensitization occurring over a few days rather than a short-term analgesic effect from epidural therapy. In the acute prolapsed disc there will be accompanying oedema which increases the pressure on the dura and nerve root, increasing the damage and neuropraxia, so that the addition of a steroid to the solution will reduce the increased inflammation and swelling, and therefore reduce the subsequent pressure and pain. It may also help to prevent long-term adhesions. The epidural does not reduce a herniated disc and in the presence of increasing disc herniation when a nerve palsy is developing will not appear to help as the mechanical pressure from the disc is too great for the reduction in swelling to make any difference. The **reasons for epidural therapy** are:

(a) Night pain.
(b) Neurological signs. Note S3 and 4 which require immediate surgery.
(c) Too acute to give any other treatment, bar rest.
(d) Sciatica uncontrolled by other analgesics.
(e) Chronic sciatica when the cause is ionic root irritation.
(f) As a diagnostic test when there is a suggestion of dural irritation.

ESR

Erythrocyte sedimentation rate raised in older age but particularly with systemic disease. Slower onset than CRP.

Faber test

Flexion, abduction and external rotation of the **hip** while the ankle is placed on the opposite knee. Groin pain and limited abduction suggest hip or ilio-psoas problems. Back pain may be from the **sacro-iliac joint**.

Facet joint and sacro-iliac joint stress tests

Examination of the facet joint and sacro-iliac joint dysfunction is only indicative rather than absolutely diagnostic, as stress tests almost certainly impinge on both elements. One must also remember that with even a minor disc disturbance there may well be associated disturbance of the other articular structures, such as the facet joints.

(a) **Facet joint rocking**. With the patient prone the ileum is pulled posteriorly whilst the butt of the other hand holds down the transverse process of the L5 thus allowing the facet of the sacrum to be impinged onto the facet of the adjacent L5. This is repeated rocking L5 into L4, etc. The examiner tests each segment at a time and then the other side.

(b) **Facet joint rolling**. If there are no signs of dural tensioning, then rolling the supine patient into a ball and taking both legs towards first one shoulder and then the other will gap the facet joints – if there is capsular irritation then this will produce pain.

(c) **Local palpation**. The facet joints lie level with the gaps between the spinous processes and local pressure about 2 cm out may be tender. Rocking the spinous process only shows the dysfunctional level, not the underlying cause.

Facet joint injections

Perifacetal injections of corticosteroid will relieve the acute episode and may, when combined with local anaesthetic, provide for earlier manipulation. Chronic osteoarthritis of the facet joints will be improved on the same basis as injections of any osteoarthritis joint, i.e. if there is capsular inflammation, then there will be benefit; however, if the source of the pain is bony, then there is less improvement. In these cases it is important to know that the facet joint has been injected and facetal injections should be done under X-ray control.

Femoral stretch

A dural tensioning test for the **femoral nerve** where the patient is laid on their side with straight legs. The straight leg is taken into extension; however, as this extends the lumbar spine, pain produced at this stage is from the lumbar spine. Then the knee is flexed to stretch the femoral nerve and pain produced in the back or down the front of the thigh that is similar to the patient's pain is a positive test. See *Adverse neural tensioning* and *PLKF*.

Figure of '4' sign

For **popliteal muscle strain**. Flex the knee and externally rotate the hip, whilst resting the ankle on the contralateral thigh. The appearance is of a figure '4'. See Fig. 22.6.

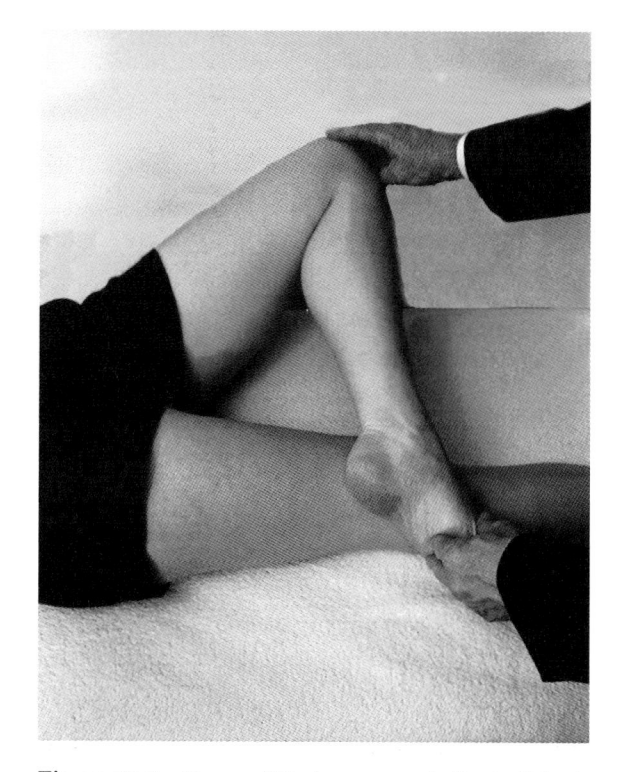

Figure 22.6   Figure of '4' sign – very similar to Faber's test.

Finklestein's test

For extensor **tenosynovitis of the thumb** (de Quervain's) where the wrist is ulnar flexed and the thumb passively flexed across the palm. Pain on this manoeuvre over the dorsum of the wrist is a positive test.

Fitch catch

Lean backwards trying to grab the back of one Achilles with the opposite hand. This test provokes greater extension and, plus the one-legged hyperextension test, may be the only tests to hurt with facet joint or **pars interarticularis lesions**. See Fig. 22.7.

Flamingo view

See *Stork view.*

Forrestier's disease

See *DISH.*

Freiberg's infraction (Kohler's second disease)

Osteochondral necrosis of usually the second or third **metatarsal head** of the metatarsophalangeal joint. See Fig. 16.2.

Freiberg's sign

Passive internal rotation of the **hip** causes pain. Possibly diagnostic for piriformis syndrome; however, the hip joint, sacro-iliac joint and trochanteric bursa may also cause pain.

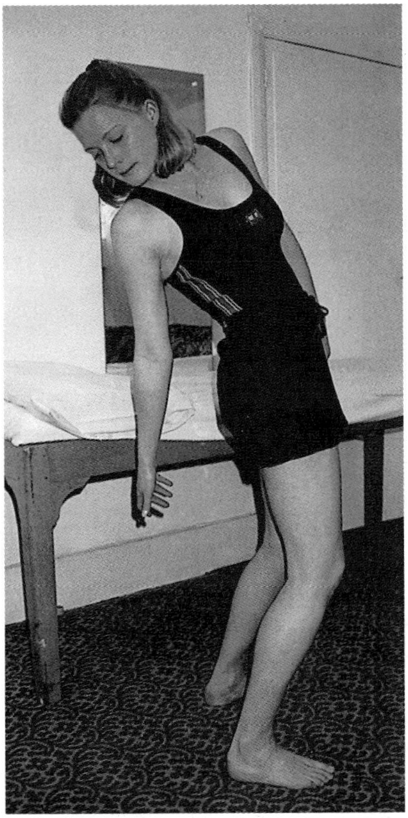

Figure 22.7 Fitch catch.

Froment's sign

A test for **ulnar nerve** damage where a piece of paper is gripped between the straight thumb and index finger – if the adductor policis does not work then the long flexors help and the thumb bends at the PIP joint to maintain grip. The damage must be proximal to Guyon's canal to involve the motor branches. Damage at Guyon's canal at the wrist (sensory branch) will not produce this sign.

Fowler's position

See *Traction.*

Gadalinium

A contrast dye used with **MRI** to differentiate scar or fibrous tissue, especially from a disc lesion.

Gilmore's groin

See Chapter 8 (*Conjoined tendon*).

Glasgow Coma Scale

A standardized chart to record levels of conscioness.

Godfrey test

See *Sag sign*.

Golfer's elbow

Medial epicondylitis of the **elbow**.

Gurney's tubercle

Insertion of the lateral collateral ligament and iliotibial tract on to the **tibia**.

Guyon's canal

The pisi hamate tunnel at the wrist for the ulnar nerve.

Haembursitis

Bleeding within a bursa from trauma or bleeding diathesis which can be treated by aspiration but may need ultrasound control and pressure bandage. It tends to recur and frequently needs repeating several times. Hydrocortisone into the bursa probably does not reduce recurrence. It is theoretically a potent site for infection so possibly cover the aspiration with 48 hours antibiotics.

Haglund's syndrome

Heel pain. Superficial Achilles bursa, retro Achilles bursa and enlarged posterior calcaneal boss. Large 'pump bumps'.

Half squat test

Gives an indication of whether there is a functional **valgus of the knees** and functional **over-pronation of the feet**. See Figs 22.8 and 22.9.

Haswell's lesion

Defect of the **patella**, typically superior lateral quadrant of either necrotic or vascular fibrous tissue. Benign progressive lesion – observe. Possibly biopsy if it is hot on bone scan.

Hawkins' sign

An impingement sign for the subacromial bursa. The arm is circumducted and internally rotated (Fig. 22.10). See *Impingement test* for the shoulder.

Hill–Sach's lesion

Recurrent dislocation of the shoulder. X-ray change in the superior humeral articular surface from chronic subluxation, caused by impingement into the acromion. See Fig. 17.12.

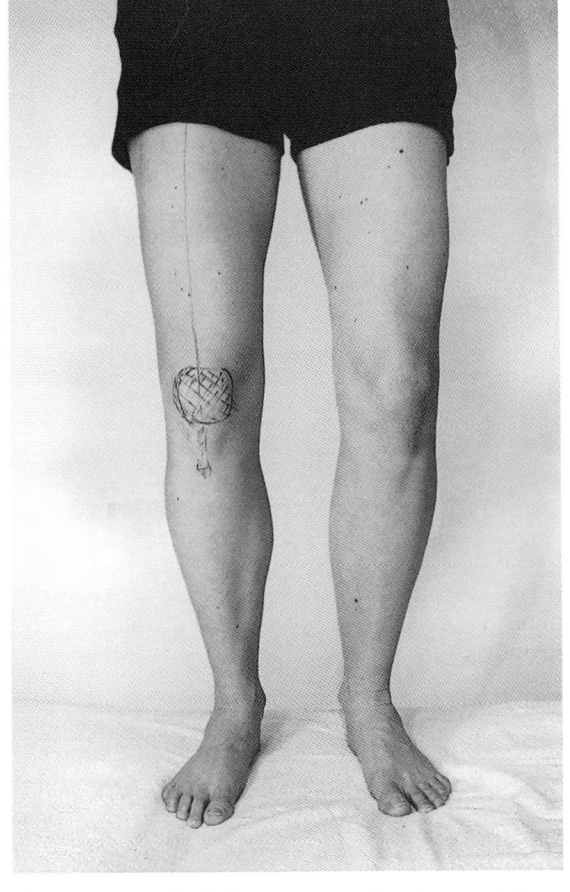

Figure 22.8 The half squat test showing good function with the knees half bent over the first and second toes and good maintenance of the long arch of the foot.

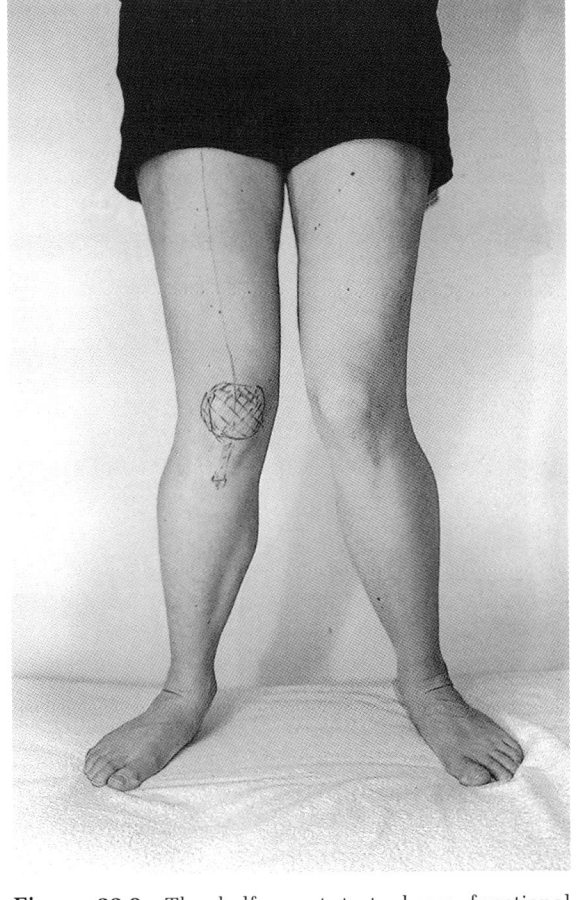

Figure 22.9 The half squat test shows functional valgus with the knees dropped inside the feet and pronation that in this case follows this movement rather than causes it.

Hoffa's fat pads

Extra-articular fat at the front of the **knee** that functions as shock absorbers.

Hughstan's jerk test

See *Jerk test* and *Reverse pivot shift*.

Hoover test

A test to check whether a patient is trying or volitionally showing **rectus femoris** weakness. Resisted contraction of the rectus femoris will provoke downward pressure onto the couch or testing hand of the contralateral leg.

Hypermobility

This is usually measured by the **Beighton–Horan** score and usually has a congenital link. These hypermobile people are more prone to ligamentous injuries. Elastic supports and taping may help, but these should be reinforced with postural exercises that set the gamma efferents to balance between

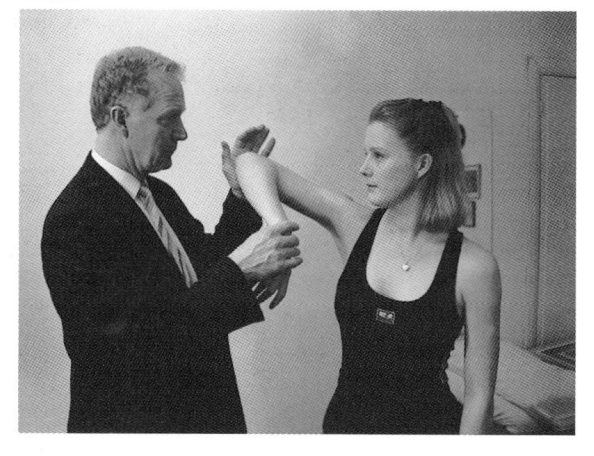

Figure 22.10   An impingement test for the subacromial bursa.

agonist and antagonists, so that joint control is maintained – this is especially so with anterior knee pain, sway back knees and elbows. Suppleness has advantages but may not take the heavy strain of some sports so that four piece gymnasts with sway back elbows may have to be pushed towards rhythmic gymnastics instead. Congenital problems like Marfan's and Erb–Duchenne are particularly prone, and may have added complications such as aortic dissection.

Impingement test

For **subacromial bursa** and **rotator cuff**. Shoulder pain on internally rotating the circumducted humerus (see Fig. 22.10). See *Hawkins' sign* and *Neer's sign*.

Interferential

Short electromagnetic waves are therapeutic but do not penetrate body tissues. Two fast waves say 1045 Hz and 1050 Hz will penetrate but interfere with each other to leave a residual wave of 5 Hz.

Various wave lengths are said to heat muscles

and joints and can also stimulate muscles and control pain.

Iselin's disease

Traction apophysitis of the proximal **fifth metatarsal** (rare).

Isokinetic muscle contraction

At the same speed tested through angular rotation, maybe eccentric or concentric. Peak torque occurs at different angles. Used both in rehabilitation and in testing to record muscle balance such as between quadriceps and hamstrings. The strength diminishes with increased speed.

Isostatic muscle contraction

Force applied without movement and therefore the mechanical movement is zero. The training effect is angle specific and is a differential training of type two muscle fibres (white).

Isotonic muscle contraction

A contraction involving the same muscle tone throughout its length of contraction. Cam pulleys are required as otherwise peak torque changes through the angles of movement. The mechanical force may be positive or negative, concentric or eccentric.

Jerk test

For **anterior cruciate ligament tear** where the patient lies supine, with the hip flexed to 90° and tibia in internal rotation with valgus stress across knee. Slowly extend knee. Tibial subluxation and relocation is felt as a jerk. This fails in subtle anterior cruciate ligament tears.

Jones' fracture

Fracture of the proximal shaft of the fifth **metatarsal**. Prone to non-union.

Jump sign

For **anterior cruciate ligaments** when during movement of extension and flexion the femur may ride up on the posterior horn of the meniscus and then 'jump' back into place – suggests anterior cruciate ligament instability.

Kager's triangle

X-ray appearance to describe the area of fat subtended between the anterior surface of the **Achilles** and soleus and the posterior surface of the tibia and flexor hallucis longus and the calcaneum inferiorly. Soft tissue swellings that distort this area may be visualized.

Keinbok's disease

Idiopathic avascular necrosis of the **lunate**. Initially cold on bone scan, hot during revascularization. See Fig. 19.4.

Kernig's test

Neck flexion to stretch the proximal elements of the **dura** which is also used to diagnose menin-

gism. Pain is produced if the dura is tethered, and this test is often added to straight leg raise and Lasegue's to constitute the slump test. See *Adverse neural tensioning* and *Dural stress tests*.

Kohler's disease

Idiopathic osteochondrosis or avascular necrosis of the **tarsal navicular**. The average age of diagnosis is 6 years. The child walks on the outside of the foot and it is symptomatic for 3–9 months. X-ray changes evolve over 2–4 years, but it is not associated with long-term osteoarthritis. Also Kohler's second disease (see *Freiberg's infraction*; Chapter 16).

Lachman test

Test for **anterior cruciate ligament** instability where the basic principle is to relax the restraining posterior pull of the hamstrings on the tibia, thus allowing easier anterior translation. This may be done by supporting the femur in the hand, on one's own leg or the edge of the examination couch [3] when the tibia is drawn anteriorly, whilst the femur is held downwards. See Figs 22.11 and 22.12.

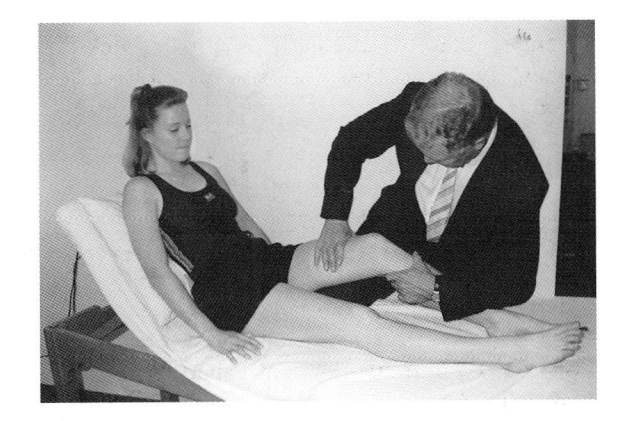

Figure 22.11 The Lachman test with the hamstring relaxed and supported on the examiner's thigh.

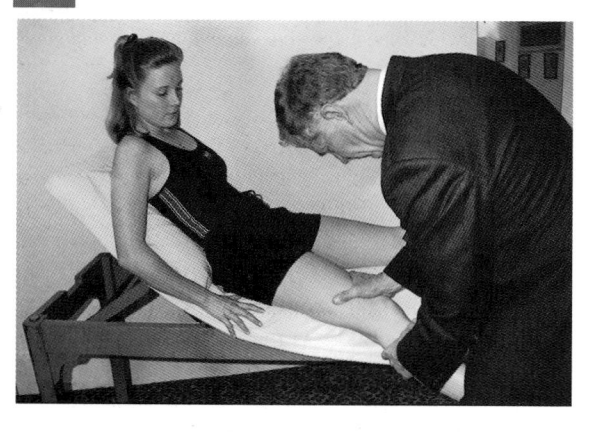

Figure 22.12 The femur is supported on the couch, the ankle between the examiner's legs. Then with the femur stabilized by one hand, anterior draw is applied to the lower leg.

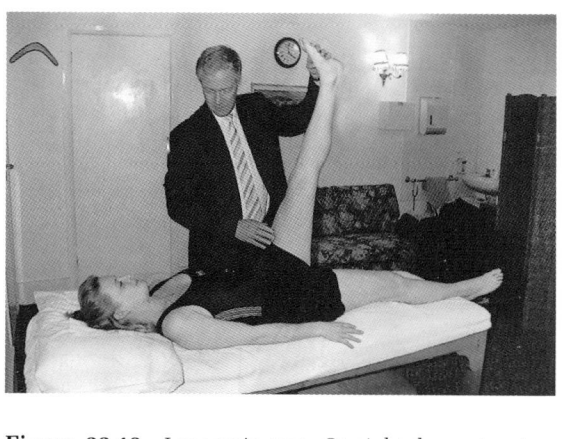

Figure 22.13 Lasegue's test. Straight leg raise tensions the sciatic nerve and this pull is increased by adding dorsiflexion of the ankle in this position.

Lasegue's test

Dorsiflexion of the foot is added to the straight leg raise to stretch the sciatic nerve further. This is a **nerve root or sciatic nerve test** rather than a dural stress test. Thus hamstring and piriformis entrapment of the sciatic nerve has a positive straight leg raise and Lasegue's, but a negative slump test (Fig. 22.13). See *Adverse neural tensioning*.

Laser

(a) **Surgical**. Higher frequency laser light is used as a surgical tool to vaporize and cauterize.
(b) **Medical**. Laser is applied to soft tissues where it seems to have a similar effect as **ultrasound**. However, its effect does seem to reach a maximum over four sessions and an increase in intensity and length of treatment does not produce further benefit. The higher wavelengths over 800 Hz do not seem to be effective and variations in wavelength may benefit different types of tissue. Laser light is no longer columnated after contact with the skin and it may be that multiple light wavelengths are of similar benefit though not so accurately directed at the tissue [10].

Leg length

Osteopaths are taught to call rotations of the ileum (anterior spine – anterior or posterior) as leg length discrepancies, so that often their phrase of a short leg does not reflect a true short leg but a possible functional short leg. The only true measurement of leg length is by X-raying the patient standing against a graded screen. Clinically assessing the levels of the iliac crests to check leg length is usually sufficient and by getting the patient to stand with supinated feet the inequality caused by pronation will be eliminated. Most patients have adjusted to 1–2 cm of shortening and do not require treatment. However, bigger discrepancies may cause back problems and will benefit from a partial correction. In this case clinically measuring from the umbilicus, and anterior superior iliac spine to the inferior border of the medial maleolus, checking the medial malleoli remain the same length when the patient sits from lying and when the pelvis is raised and dropped on the couch, must all register the same leg as being shorter before a leg length discrepancy should be diagnosed. Within 2 cm is within tolerance. However, if symptoms persist then correction with a heel raise at first inside the shoe may help. If this helps, then the raise may be moved to the exterior of the shoe heel and, if necessary, a further raise introduced inside the shoe as a trial, which again would be attached to the exterior of the shoe heel if successful. Note camber running and pronation can produce an apparent short leg.

L'hermitte's sign

A **dural stress test** where neck flexion or extension produce symptoms in the back and legs. See *Dural stress tests*.

Lisfranc joint

The **second tarso metatarsal** joint which may be inflamed in dancers.

Lombard's paradox

A muscle that crosses two joints may have to contract at one end whilst relaxing at the other, i.e. contraction of the hamstring should flex the knee and extend the hip, but some movements produce a paradoxical flexion at the hip and flexion at the knee.

Losee's subluxation test

See *Reverse pivot shift*.

Ludloff's sign

Inability to actively flex the hip whilst sitting is indicative of **psoas** weakness.

Magnuson stack

Repair of **anterior dislocation of the shoulder** – strengthening of the anterior inferior margin with subscapularis, capsule and rotator cuff.

Manipulation of the spine

There are various manipulative techniques, e.g. Cyriax, Maitland, osteopathic, chiropractic, Mulligan's, etc., all of which may prove successful with some problems whilst only some of which will prove useful in others. However, probably, a disc lesion does not respond well to manipulation, whereas a facet joint or the facetal element of a disc problem will. Sacro-iliac joint manipulation can also be successful. There is discussion as to when mobilization, which is a gentle rocking of a joint, finishes and manipulation which has an end-point thrust begins, but in practical terms this will inevitably depend on the patient who will either be too sensitive to allow the joints to reach end-point, and thus only permit mobilization, or will relax enough to permit manipulation. Treatment of the soft tissues can be given at the same time, by massage [4] and heat, and the improved healing time with ultrasound or laser [5] treatment may also be beneficial.

March fracture

Stress fracture of **metatarsal** bone, usually the second, third or fourth. See Fig. 16.1.

Massage

A variety of stroking, rubbing, pummelling or slapping techniques to remove oedema, encourage an increased blood supply, and organize scar tissue and prevent adhesions [4].

McConnell strapping regimen

Used for **anterior knee pain**. An assessment of patella glide, tilt and rotation with a strapping technique to control patella maltracking. Vastus medialis obliquus coordinated work with biofeedback and coordinated control of external rotation of the hip is also trained.

McKenzie extension exercises

May be done lying or standing, straight or with a side flexion, but should be used for **flexion-orientated disc** problems. They should not be used for extension-orientated problems and a trial of extension should be done to see if the pain peripheralizes down the leg or leg pain is produced. This exercise can make the collar stud L5 S1 disc positively worse, but as the disc improves, and the collar stud deformity settles into the more normal hernial configuration of the disc, so extension exercises may be added. Facet joint, sacro-iliac joint, and lateral canal entrapments will be made worse. See Fig. 22.14.

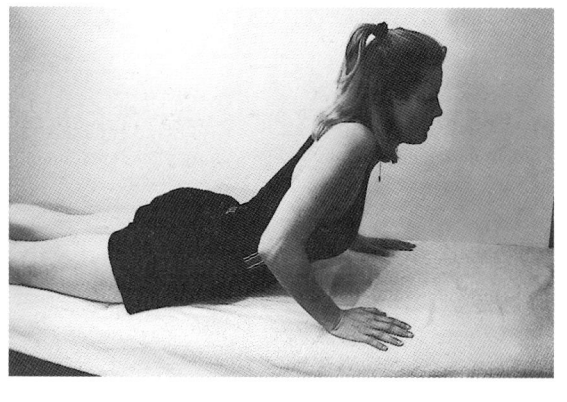

Figure 22.14 McKenzie extension exercises. Breathing out allows the muscle tension to relax and the extension to be applied more directly to the vertebrae. Its acute angle should be directed towards the problem level.

McKenzie flexion exercises

Pulling the knees to the chest and stretching the low back into flexion will aid extension-orientated spinal problems such as facet joints and L5 S1 collar stud. The addition of gapping rotations (rolling knees to one side or hanging one leg over the other) will help the facet joint, lateral canal and sacro-iliac joint. Creeping unstable flexion-orientated discs will be made worse. See Fig. 22.15.

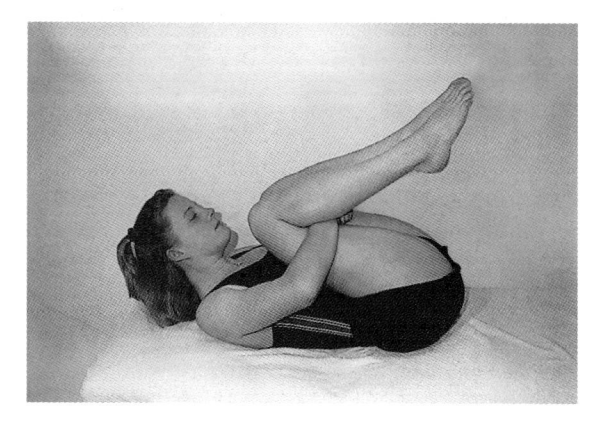

Figure 22.15 McKenzie flexion exercises. Good for extension-orientated problems.

McMurray's test

A test for **meniscal lesions**, but impossible to perform with moderately tense effusions as this prevents the full knee flexion required for the test. A grinding test of the tibia on to the femur with the patient lying supine. Forced internal and external rotation of the knee through flexion into extension with varus and valgus stress. About 60% positive, 5% false positives. A clunk and pain is the classical positive sign – menisco-collateral ligaments are painful without the clunk.

Meniscal cyst

Lateral **meniscus** more frequent than medial – usually accompanied by a radial tear of the meniscus. More prominent in extension of the knee. Can occur as an anterior cyst.

Mill's manipulation

For chronic **tennis elbow** to free up adhesions on the lateral condyle, but the radio-humeral joint

Morton's neuroma

Inter-digital neuroma of the foot, classically adjacent to third or fourth metatarso-phalangeal joint. Can produce interdigital neuritis, but all interdigital neuritis is not produced by neuroma.

Mumford procedure

Operation for chronic **acromio-clavicular joint** arthrosis or arthritis which removes the distal clavicle and sometimes part of the acromion. Good results in sport, although 3 months' healing are required before increasing loads. Weightlifters may still have problems.

MRI

Magnetic resonance imaging. Body scan for bone, disc, brain and soft tissue. Body tissues polarize along the magnetic lines and the relative rates of return to normal differentiates various tissues giving good but not perfect pictures of body parts.

Nage's test

Another test for assessment of **anterior cruciate ligament** instability.

Neer's sign

An impingement test for the **shoulder**, which is passively flexed and internally rotated. See *Impingement test*.

Noble's sign

For **ilio-tibial tract syndrome**. The ilio-tibial band flicks over the lateral femoral condyle at

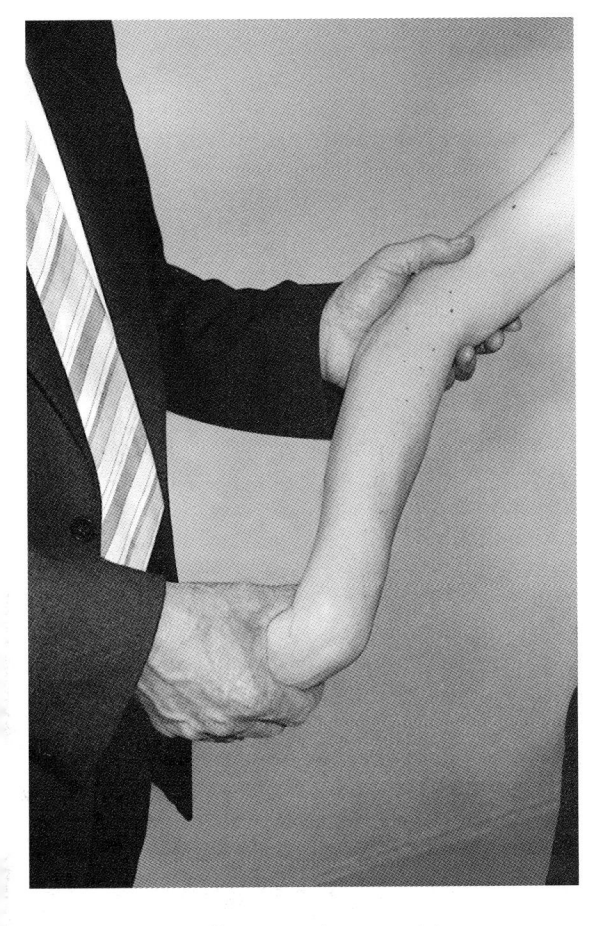

Figure 22.16   Mill's manipulation position.

must be exculpated first. The wrist is fully pronated and then flexed at which stage the elbow is jerked into full extension. See Fig. 22.16.

MJO

Milton J. Ongley's stress test for the **sacro-iliac joint**. See *Sacro-iliac stress tests*.

Morton's foot

Present in about 50% of the population. The first metatarsal is shorter than the second giving a longer second toe.

about 30° of knee flexion and this may be palpated. Pressure over this condyle whilst the knee is moved produces pain at about 30° of flexion.

Noye's flexion rotation draw test

A test for **anterior cruciate ligament** tears. This is a gentle pivot shift. The 10–15° flexed knee is supported at the tibia. This allows the femur to drop back and externally rotate. Increased flexion with downward pressure on the tibia to drop the knee backwards reduces the subluxation

NSAIDs

Non-steroidal anti-inflammatory drugs to counter and inhibit inflammatory prostaglandins.

Ober's test

To display tightness of the **ilio-tibial band** the patient lies on their side, knee slightly flexed, hip is flexed, abducted and externally rotated, and then taken into extension. A tight ilio-tibial tract does not allow the knee to drop down level with or below the hip.

O'Donaghue's triad

Trauma to the knee resulting in damage to the tibio-collateral ligament, the meniscus (usually medial) and the anterior cruciate ligament.

One-legged hyperextension test

A test for spondylolisis and **extension-orientated back pain** wherein the patient stands on one leg, raises the contra-lateral knee towards the chest and leans backwards (Fig. 22.17). See *Fitch catch*.

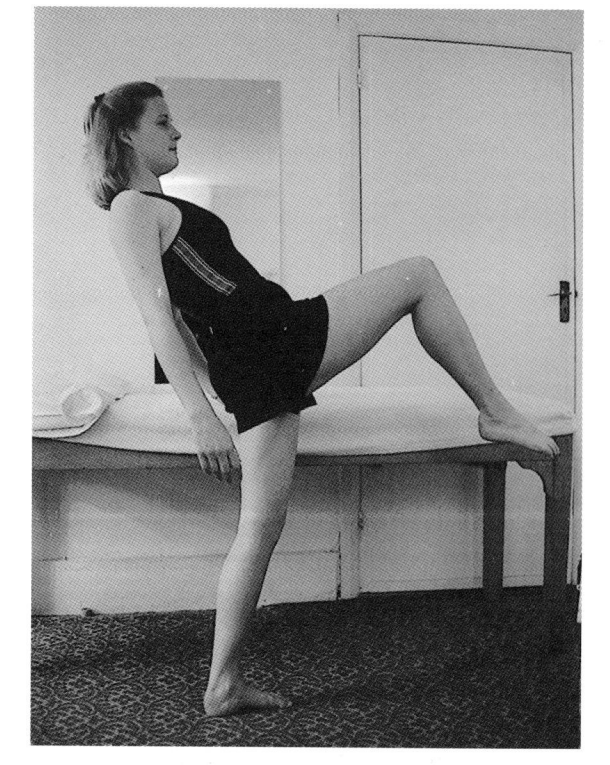

Figure 22.17   The one-legged hyperextension test.

Os acetabulare

An accessory ossicle around the **hip** from the acetabulum which may limit the range of hip movement, and thus become a problem in gymnastics and martial arts (see Fig. 8.1). See Chapter 8.

Osgood–Schlatter disease

Apophysitis of the patella tendon attachment at the **tibial tubercle** (see Fig. 11.15).

Osteoarthritis

A degenerative condition of articular cartilage that may follow trauma or attrition through age and wear and tear. Articular cartilage is nourished by the synovial fluid but movement is required to massage the fluid into the nutrient cannaliculi. Thus total rest in a cast brace makes osteoarthritis worse, but because the thickness of the articular cartilage is reduced, so impact also stresses the subchondral bone. Therefore non-impact exercise of low loads, high repetitions are best for osteoarthritis.

Os trigonum

Separate ossification centre of the **talus** that may impinge between the calcaneum and posterior surface of the tibia during plantar flexion (see Fig. 13.22). See *Calcaneo-tibial compression test*.

Overpronation

The overpronated foot cannot achieve supination in time for impact or lift off. This may come from calcaneo valgus and a collapsed mid foot, or forefoot varus. Posterior tibialis weakness and ligamentous laxity contribute. See *Supination/pronation*.

Paget–von Schroetter syndrome

See *Effort thrombosis*. See Chapter 12.

Panner's disease

An osteochondritis of the capitulum in the **elbow joint**, possibly from an avascular or traumatic cause. The incidence is 90% males and 5% bilateral. Loose bodies are more frequent over the age of 8, and pain from joint, locking, clicking and swelling are found clinically.

Paravertebral blocks

Lateral canal entrapment of the nerve root, by enlarged facets, narrowed lateral canal from disc collapse, and lateral disc prolapse, may irritate the nerve. The patient often has discomfort standing and walking around, and may relieve the discomfort by sitting or drawing the knees up to the chest. They tend to perch on table edges and may be eased by using a shooting stick if they are on their feet for a long time. An epidural will not reach the root as it is mechanically blocked; however, an injection of hydrocortisone and local anaesthetic into the lateral canal may be achieved by a paravertebral approach.

Patella apprehension test

With the patient sitting, knees extended and relaxed, the patella is pulled laterally by the examiner. The patient with the **dislocating or subluxing patella** will be worried that it might dislocate or may experience discomfort in the maltracking patella and this shows on the patient's face which should be watched throughout this test.

Patella alta

High riding patella which may have the camel sign – two lumps, the patella and fat pads. Patella alta is associated with patella maltracking.

Patella beja

Low placed patella. At 30° angle, the patella to patella tendon length should be a ratio of 1. More than 20% is abnormal. Patella beja is associated with maltracking problems of the patella causing anterior knee pain.

Patella tap

See *Bulge test*.

Patrick's test

See *Faber test*.

Pellegrini–Stieda syndrome

This is a type of myositis ossificans or bone formation that may complicate tibio-collateral ligament or adductor tendon lesions over the **femoral condyle**. See Fig. 11.17.

Pelvic spring

A test for the **sacro-iliac joint** stability. See *Sacro-iliac stress tests*.

Perthe's disease (Legg–Perthe)

Avascular necrosis of the **femoral head** which appears between the ages 5 and 10 with disturbance and flattening of the femoral head leaving this deformity and a restricted hip range into adult life. May be more prone to eventual osteoarthritis. See Fig. 22.18.

Pes anserine bursa

The bursa alongside the **knee** lying on the medial side beneath the semitendinosus and semimembranosus as these extend to their insertions.

Phalen's test

Tingling within first, second and third fingers with the wrist held in flexion for 60 seconds is produced with a **carpal tunnel syndrome**.

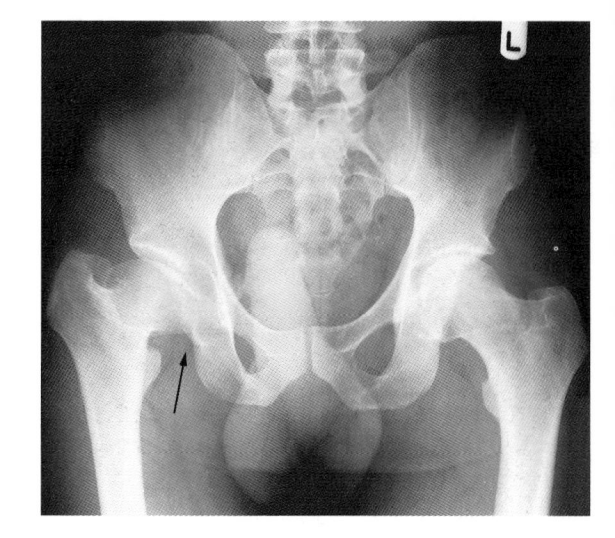

Figure 22.18   Old Perthe's disease of the hip.

Piedallu sign

The examiner places their thumbs on the posterior inferior iliac spines (piis) and asks the patient to raise a knee towards the chest. The piis should move downwards on that side and in the abnormal the fixed sacro-iliac joint may elevate. Fixation and elevation of the posterior inferior iliac spines may indicate **sacro-iliac joint** dysfunction. However, one must be careful when assuming than we humans are absolutely symmetrical creatures, as too many manipulations to correct a non-painful, probably non-pathological asymmetry, can produce ligamentous laxity and further problems.

Pivot shift

A test for **cruciate ligament** instability. The 20° flexed knee is internally rotated and a valgus force is applied. In the cruciate-deficient knee, the lateral side of the tibial plateau subluxes anteriorly and this is increased by thumb pressure, but as the knee is extended the ilio-tibial band pulls this backwards into place with an appreciable jump [6]. A patient who has pain with this

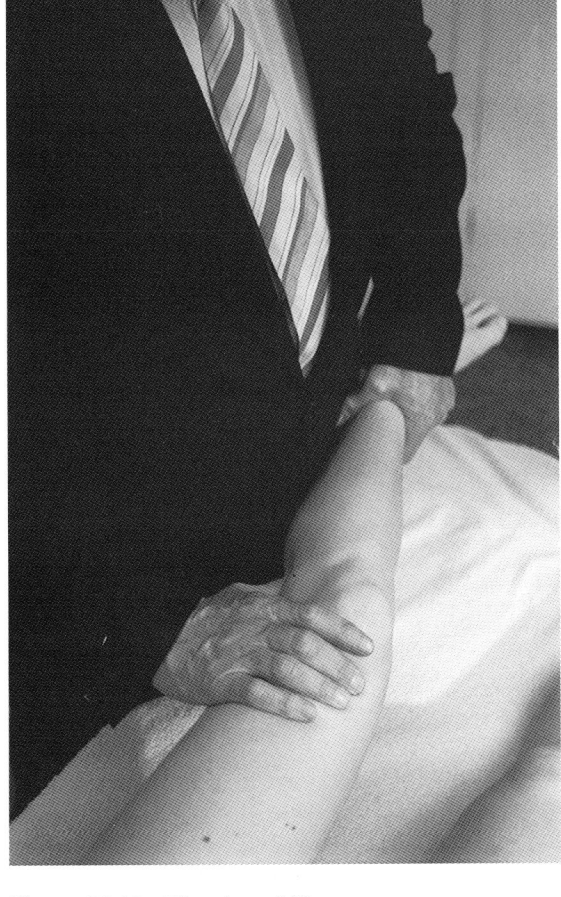

Figure 22.19   The pivot shift.

movement may resist and then this sign can only be exposed under anaesthetic. See Fig. 22.19.

Pliometrics

A **training method** that involves landing and taking off again immediately, so that eccentric and concentric muscle work is cycled as in running. Usually done by depth jumping, jumping down from maximum height of 20–40 cm and then jumping as high as one can. Hop step jump routines and bounding are pliometrics [7, 8]. See Chapter 20.

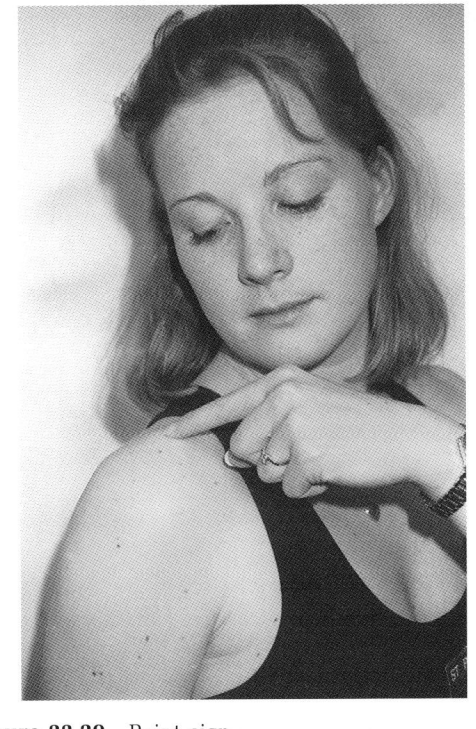

Figure 22.20   Point sign

Point sign

When the acromio-clavicular joint is involved the patient points directly at the joint to indicate the source of pain. See Fig. 22.20.

Pope's sign

Flexion contracture of fourth and fifth fingers due to **ulnar nerve palsy**.

Posterior apprehension test

For **posterior subluxation of the shoulder** when with patient lying supine, flex the humerus to 90° and add axial pressure through the elbow to force the humeral head posteriorly. If this produces a click or apprehension and is relieved by external rotation of humerus and a feeling of anterior shift of the humeral head when the posterior aspect of the joint is palpated, it is a positive test.

Posterior calcaneal compression test

See *Calcaneo-tibial compression test*.

Power

Power is **speed times strength**. Slow speeds generate more strength, high speeds less strength, but the power may be equal. This principle may be seen in the karate chop or in the rugby scrum when the slow application of more force is less effective than the concerted timed shove, when force is applied with speed. The essence of power is timing.

Pronation

See *Overpronation* and *Supination/pronation*.

Prone lying knee flexion (PLKF)

A **femoral nerve** stretch test when the patient lies prone and the knee is bent passively. Increased pain in the thigh or particularly the back is a positive test, whilst flexing the hip as well will increase any neural tension. See *Adverse neural tensioning* and *Dural stress tests*.

Pulled elbow

Swinging a child by the arm can sublux the proximal **radial head**. Flexion and rotation of the forearm usually reduces this subluxation.

Putti Platt

A type of repair for recurrent **shoulder dislocation** which shortens and plicates the subscapularis. Repaired shoulders have limited external rotation.

Q angle

The **knee**. The Q angle is the angle whilst standing or lying supine that is subtended by a line from the femoral head to the centre of the patella and a line from the central patella to the tibial tuberosity. Generally accepted that $15°$ or less of valgus is normal (see Fig. 11.8). See Chapter 11.

Referred pain

Is generally thought of as nerve in origin and the distribution may suggest the level of the problem. However, not all referred pain is from a nerve origin, and may also be from facet joints, the sacro-iliac joint, myofascial trigger points, and ligaments and joints. Thus not all pain referred down the leg is sciatic nerve in origin, for experiments and clinical experience of injecting various sites will produce referred pain as well, but this usually does not radiate into the foot. Sciatica is leg pain from the sciatic nerve, but not all leg pain is sciatica.

Reflex sympathetic dystrophy

The cause is not fully known but guanethidine works on the sympathetic sites within the arterioles and may have a curative effect.

Stage 1   Raised circulation. Oedema. Hot dry skin. Livid colour. Burning, everlasting pain worse to touch. Not in dermatomal distribution.

Treatment Intravascular sympathetic blockade with guanethidine. Sympathetic ganglion block. Peripheral nerve block. Epidural or spinal block with an indwelling catheter. Elevate. NSAIDs. Exercise but no massage. Neuroleptics. See Fig. 22.1.

Stage 2   Pale cold cyanotic skin. Vasospasms. Sweating. Atrophy of skin and muscle. Contraction of joint.

Treatment   Treat pain as in stage 1 but the therapy is less effective.

Stage 3   Irreversible atrophy of bones, muscle and connective tissue. Joint contractures. Skin is cold, pale and dry. X-ray osteoporosis, particularly around the joint. Pain may ease at rest but movement causes terrible pain. Sympathetic blockade may not work.

Treatment   Epidural or plexus block to try and obtain movement. TENS. Neuroleptics.

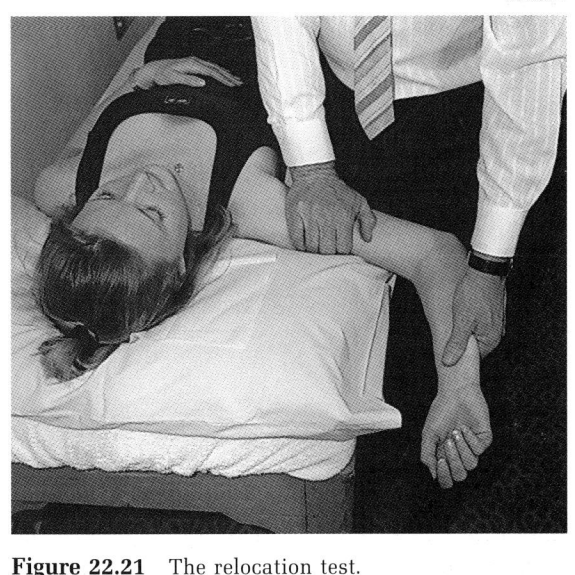

Figure 22.21   The relocation test.

Reiter's syndrome

Urethritis, arthritis and conjunctivitis. May have a venereal link, but it is also part of the inflammatory spondylarthropathies.

Relocation test

For the **anterior subluxing shoulder**. Whilst lying supine the arm is taken into 90° circumduction, the elbow is flexed to 90° and the arm taken into increasing external rotation. If the pain produced is reduced by pressure on the anterior humeral head, but worse on release of this pressure, then it is a positive test for subluxation. When the pain is relieved the shoulder may be taken a little further into external rotation and on release of the restraining hand on the humeral head will sublux forward producing sudden pain. See Fig. 22.21.

Renne test

For **ilio-tibial tract syndrome**. Stand on the painful leg with knee bent to 30–40°. Pain at the lateral femoral condyle is indicative. Hopping may accentuate the problem. It should be noted that the external rotators of the hip will also be affected by this manoeuvre at the hip.

Resting pulse

The pulse taken first thing in the morning before getting out of bed. See Chapter 21.

Reverse pivot shift

For the **anterior cruciate ligaments**. Start with the patient supine and relaxed, the knee bent and tibia externally rotated. Straightening takes the knee into subluxation (near the end of extension) and back to location in full extension.

Rhizotomy

Chronic facetal osteoarthritis may be helped by ablation of the sinu-vertebral nerve. The ablation may be cryo- or radiorhyzotomy. See Chapters 2 and 5.

RICE

Rest, Ice, Compression, Elevation
The first-line principle for treating an acute injury.

(a) Rest for 24–48 hours to prevent the clot spreading and an increase of inflammatory exudate. Mobilization too soon produces thicker scar tissue which is not easily penetrated by fibroblasts and it may provoke continued bleeding.
(b) Ice will cool the periphery and shut down local vessels to decrease bleeding. Ice straight from the fridge may be less than 0°C and will produce an ice burn unless separated from the skin by a cloth. Melting ice may be used as a bath for 20 minutes but locally applied ice for 5–10 minutes can have an effect [9]. Reusable cold packs that may be stored in the fridge are available, as are some chemicals that freeze on mixing, but the frozen packet of peas that moulds to the shape of the body may prove most cost-effective. Be careful around nerves as they can suffer cold-induced neuropraxia.
(c) Compression is again designed to reduce inflammatory exudate and the spread of haemorrhage.
(d) Elevation prevents tracking of inflammatory products to the periphery thus requiring less effort to return these products centrally.

Rock onto heels test

An individual displays an inability to perform this manoeuvre when weakness of the tibialis anterior, extensor hallucis and extensor digitorum exist, usually from an L4 or L5 **nerve root palsy**. See Chapter 5.

Sacro-iliac joint

The sacro-iliac joint has an auricular shape, and although it has articular cartilage it has an irregular surface and ligamentous attachments within its joint. It moves in an antero-postero plane by a few millimetres. The movement of the sacrum within the iliac wings is nutation, a nodding movement. In particular, it transmits impact loads up from the legs to the spine and is crossed by only the psoas muscle. Sacro-iliac dysfunction is often seen during pregnancy and around menstruation, perhaps because the hormone relaxin levels are higher. Dysfunction can often be reduced by sacral manipulative techniques and sclerosant therapy. See Chapters 2 and 5.

Sacro-iliac stress tests

(a) Pelvic spring. Distracting or compressing the anterior wing of the ileum will produce the opposite effect on the posterior structures. This is thought to be a test for the sacro-iliac joint but quite obviously when one can reduce some types of the pain from this test by supporting the L4/5 segments on the patient's hand, then other structures must be involved as well.
(b) MJO. With the patient supine the hip is flexed and a posterior compression and internal rotation force is applied. Pain over the sacro-iliac joint is indicative. With the hip in full flexion and the force directed from the opposite shoulder the stress is thought to be sacro-tuberous, mid range, sacro-iliac and with the knee being tensioned from mid opposite thigh, ilio-lumbar.
(c) Direct compression of the sacro-iliac joint may be painful.

See *Piedallu* and *Facet joint and sacro-iliac stress tests*.

Sag sign

Appearance of the tibia sliding backwards under the femur when the knee is flexed at 90° and the patient lying supine. This indicates a **posterior cruciate ligament tear**. Note that this starting position may therefore produce a false-positive anterior draw sign (see Fig. 22.11).

Salter classification of epiphyseal fracture

Type 1 Through the zone of hypertrophy and is treated by closed reduction with good results.

Type 2 As type 1 but with metaphyseal involvement which is treated by closed reduction with a few complications.

Type 3 A fracture through the zone of hypertrophy and epiphyseal plate where open reduction is complicated by joint incongruity.

Type 4 Through the epiphysis and metaphyseal plate which is treated by open reduction but has a high complication rate.

Type 5 Crushing of the zone of hypertrophy treated by closed reduction with a high complication rate.

Scheuermann's disease

Osteochondritis of the ring epiphysis of the **vertebrae** which can produce altered growth in the thoracic spine of adolescents, especially in 12–13-year-olds. Changes may allow herniation of the disc into the vertebral body. There is a girl:boy ratio of 2:1 boys. Treat by modifying activity. There may possibly be an increased incidence in gymnasts (see Fig. 2.2). See Chapter 2.

Schmorl's nodes

Herniation of disc into the **vertebral body**, usually pain-free. Diagnosed on X-ray.

Schober's test

For **ankylosis of the spine**.
(a) **Dorsal vertebrae**. A measuring tape is placed on the vertebral prominence, and 30 cm measured off and marked on the skin, full vertebral flexion should increase this distance by 3 cm.
(b) **Lumbar vertebrae**. Mark up 10 cm from the spinal dimples. Full flexion should increase this distance by 5 cm or mark up 10 cm and down 5 cm from the dimples when full flexion should be 20 cm plus.

Sclerosant injections

A solution of dextrose sclerosant diluted with equal parts anaesthetic may be injected into the posterior lumbar ligaments and sacro-iliac joint. It is particularly useful for ligamentous pain and the unstable pelvis with pelvic spring positive, and has a lesser but definite benefit in helping to stabilize the spondylolisthesis and unstable vertebral segment. It is known in USA as prolotherapy as it has a fibro proliferative effect. Sclerosants may be used for ligament laxity, pelvic spring positive patients, sacro-iliac joint stress test positive patients, and the unstable disc, plus spondylolisthesis, chronic facet joint dysfunction and post surgery to the posterior lumbar ligaments.

Scoliosis

Primary scoliosis does not correct when the patient bends forward so that the asymmetry and fullness in the paravertebral muscles remains. The anterior chest wall may also show this asymmetry. Progressive increase in the distortion of a scoliosis should be referred onto a specialist scoliosis clinic for possible surgical correction. Secondary scoliosis does correct with forward bending. It may be due to leg length difference and can later promote facet joint dysfunction.

Segond's sign

Avulsion of the lateral collateral ligament of the **knee** leaves a small flake of avulsed bone visible on X-ray. See Fig. 11.18.

Shaving test

An **anterior interosseus nerve neuropathy** where the individual cannot put tips of first and second fingers together, only pulps, due to weak flexor digitoris profundus and flexor policis longus.

Shoes

What to look for:
(a) A curved last is for supinated feet.
(b) A straight last is for pronating feet.
(c) Thick soles with shock absorbancy are for straight line sports.
(d) Lower soles are for twisting, turning sports as the high sole is too unstable.
(e) The first indicators of a broken shoe are distorted or loose heel cups rather than worn soles (Figs 22.22 and 22.23).
(f) The so-called Achilles protector is just for appearance and if anything may cause Achilles peritendinitis (Fig. 22.24). The cut away area is as high as a plain Achilles tag and the higher elements, even higher, and sometimes rub under the malleoli causing pain. The tag should be soft and pull easily away from the Achilles with light finger pressure. At the slightest indication of Achilles

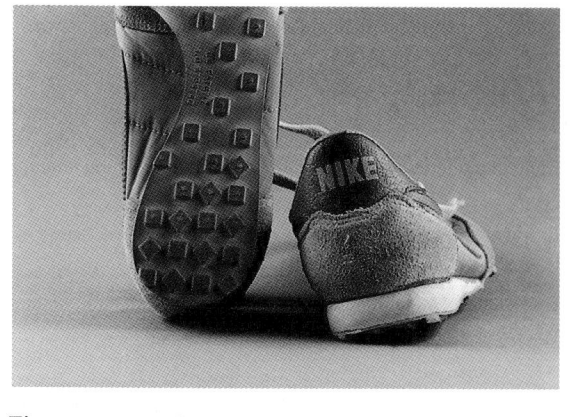

Figure 22.22   These shoes are new enough to have the nipples on the studs, but the right shoe is rolling into pronation by itself and will cause the foot to follow.

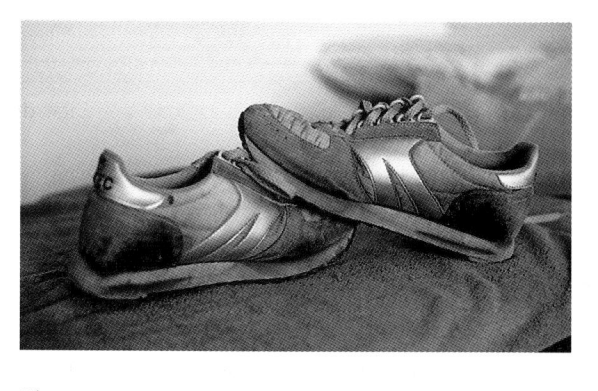

Figure 22.23   The line of mud on the soles with a clear area above shows that during use the heel cups crush over the sole and are in fact broken.

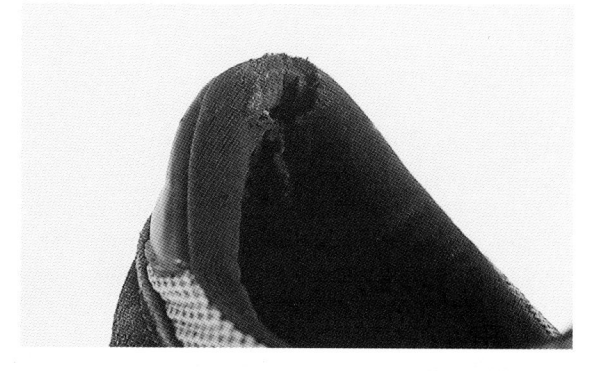

Figure 22.24   This stiff Achilles protector has been rubbed away by the Achilles causing peritendinitis.

problems or before, the heel tags should be cut off or cuts made wide out on either side down to the heel cup.

(g) Eye holes for laces that are placed further back along the shoe tighten the Achilles tag.

(h) Cut away arches remove support from the foot and can precipitate overpronation (see Fig. 22.22).

(i) Sprint spikes with no heel raise should not be used for endurance training. Middle distance spikes with heel raise are required.

(j) Worn studs alter foot balance.

(k) Track spikes with spikes that come over the outside of the ball of the foot can produce a Ben Hur effect and lacerate other runners.

Short wave diathermy

An electromagnetic wave length to produce deep tissue heating.

Shoulder–hand syndrome

The hand and wrist on the ipsilateral side of a **frozen shoulder** may swell, possibly from postural disuse oedema, but possibly from a reflex sympathetic dystrophy.

Simmond's test

For **Achilles rupture**. Simmonds reported this test first but it seems to be known generally as Thomson's test. See *Thomson's test*.

Sinding Larson Johannson syndrome

Apophysitis of the inferior pole of the **patella** in those with an accessory ossification centre at the lower pole. See Fig. 11.14.

Slipped capital femoral epiphysis

Follows trauma, an immature Frohlich type, and a tall for age group and presents at the age 10–15 years, often as thigh/knee pain.

Slocum's test

A test for rotatory instability of the **knee** in large heavy legs. Positive anterior draw fails to tighten in 25° of external rotation.

Slump test

Flexion of the neck and spine added to a straight leg raise and Lasegue's in the sitting position (Fig. 22.25). See *Adverse neural tensioning* and *Dural stress tests*.

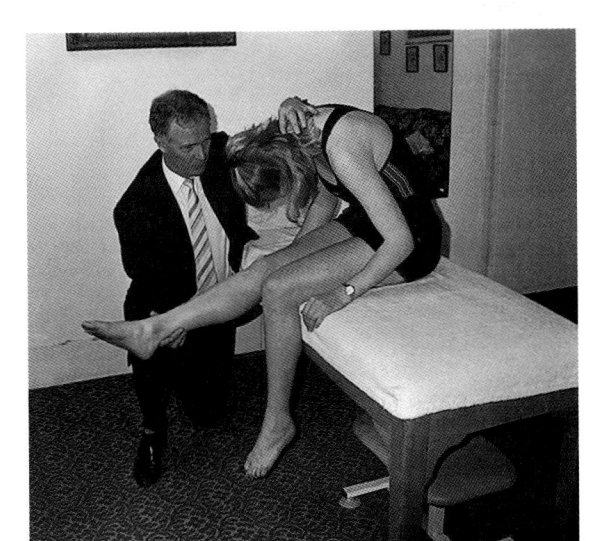

Figure 22.25 The slump test. If thought to be positive then extension of the neck in this position should relieve the symptoms.

SPECT

Single photon emission computed tomography. Extremely sensitive bone scan. See *Computed tomography*.

Speed's test

For **bicipital** impingement and tendonitis. Resisted flexion, adduction and supination of the humerus with the elbow extended produces pain at the shoulder. See *Yergason's test*.

Spurling's manoeuvre

For **cervical root entrapment**, where extension and rotation pinches the nerve in the lateral canal of the neck producing nerve root symptoms.

Steinmann test

Similar to McMurray but the object is to record pain rather than clunks over the joint line. Pain that moves posteriorly with increasing degrees of flexion suggests **meniscal** pathology. See *McMurray's test*.

Stieda process

Posterior protrusion from the back of the **talus** that may be impinged in a similar way as an os trigonum. See *Os trigonum*.

Stork test

For the **pelvis**, when the pelvis is X-rayed with the weight standing on one leg and then the other. A shift in the pubic symphysis of over 2 mm is significant.

Straight leg raise (SLR)

A **dural stress test** for the lumbar disc and sciatic nerve but by itself represents tensioning of the nerve roots or sciatic nerve. See *Adverse neural tensioning*.

Sudek's dystrophy

A **reflex sympathetic response** usually following trauma such as a Colles fracture, but it may be represented in an early stage as the shoulder/ hand syndrome. See *Reflex sympathetic dystrophy*.

Sulcus sign

For **shoulder instability** where a sulcus shows between the humeral head and the acromion with downward traction of the humerus if **inferior subluxation** is present.

Supination/pronation

At **foot** strike the foot needs to be firm to meet the impact – the weight being on the outside of the heel and the mid foot is lifted upwards to produce a high arch (supination). During mid stance the foot has to adapt to the ground, and to do this it rolls inwards and becomes soft so that it can seek the ground (pronation). To push forwards, the foot, at the lift off, must go hard to give a solid base and once again supinates, although the centre of the load is through the first and second toes. This is normal. Failure to resupinate at lift off, referred to as overpronation, produces a soft foot (like running off jelly), and tracking and overload problems at the knee.

Surgery for the spine

Loss of bowel and bladder control or altered peri-neal sensation indicates a S3/4/5 root compression and must be relieved surgically as an emergency. Surgery for the spine is becoming more definitive to the problem, i.e. discectomy for the disc, lami-nectomy for spinal or lateral canal stenosis, fusion for spondylolisthesis, etc. When should a back have surgery? Most backs get better with conser-vative management and repeat scans show either the reduction in size of a prolapsed disc over time or reduction in symptoms despite the ongoing disc. Probably the best guide is failure to progress, either with pain or mechanical signs, over 1 month in spite of the correct conservative therapy. The unstable back with repeat episodes of severe to moderately severe problems may earn their surgery on the recurrent history alone.

Syndesmal stress test

For syndesmal disruption between the tibia and fibula at the **ankle**. One hand prevents the tibia and fibula from rotating whilst the other forces dorsiflexion of the foot and then external and internal rotation.

Tarsal coalition

Calcaneo-navicular and talo-navicular joints can have a congenital fibro-cartilaginous or osseous union of the **two tarsal bones**. See Chapter 14.

Tennis elbow

Lateral epicondylitis of the elbow.

TENS

Transcutaneous electrical nerve stimulation.

This uses the 'gate principle' of spinal nerve con-duction to stimulate a new area thus interrupting the noci stimulus from the painful area. It may be used to provide a gentle faredic twitch to a damaged muscle.

Terry Thomas sign

The wrist with widening of the **scaphoid lunate gap** on X-ray showing disassociation from liga-mentous damage.

Thomas test

For **hip contraction**. Flex the hip until lumbar lordosis reduces and the back is flat on the couch. If the contralateral hip is tight it will have lifted off the couch.

Thomas test, modified

This extends the contralateral hip with a straight knee to test psoas contracture (Fig. 22.26). Then, with the hip extended, the knee is flexed as far as it will go to assess **rectus femoris** tightness (Fig. 22.27). If both have a full range but the knee moves laterally it is because the **tensor fascia lata** is tight (Figs 22.28 and 22.29).

Thomson's test

For **ruptured Achilles**. First described by Sim-monds. With the patient lying prone, squeezing the calf muscle produces a plantar flexion of the foot if the Achilles tendon is intact and no move-ment with an Achilles rupture. Note, however, that a too wide a grip of the calf muscle may squeeze the posterior tibialis and produce some plantar flexion movement.

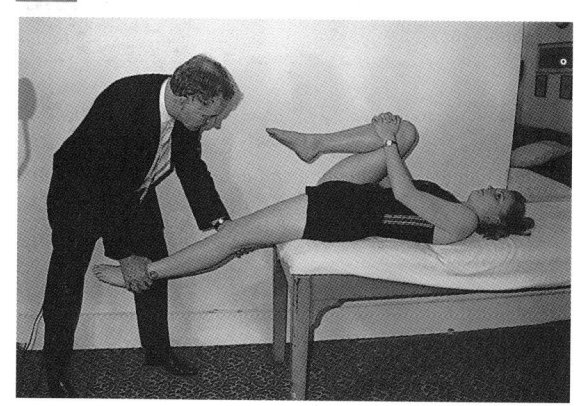

Figure 22.26   Modified Thomas test for psoas tightness.

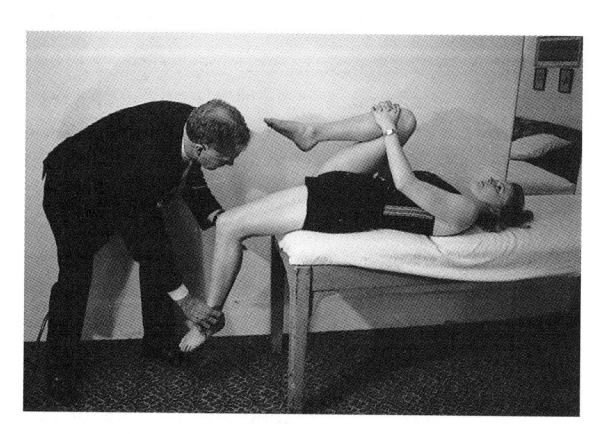

Figure 22.27   Modified Thomas test for rectus femoris tightness.

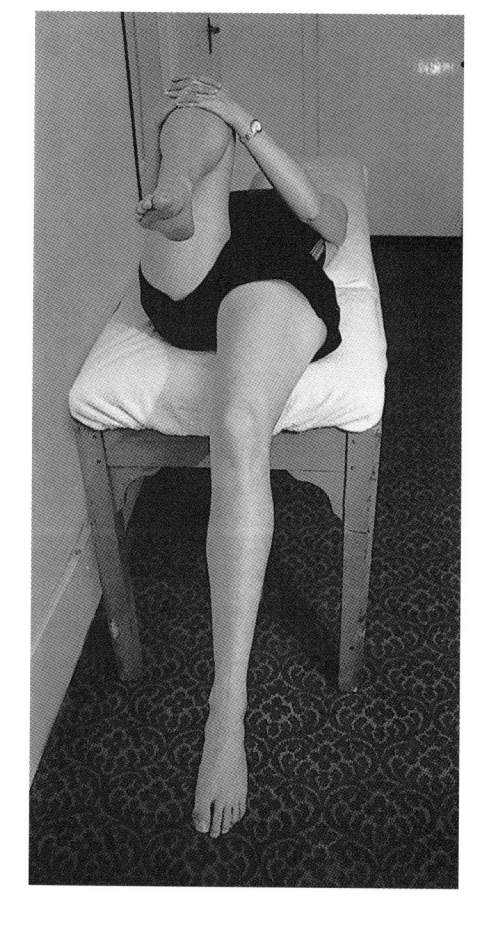

Figure 22.28   Modified Thomas test with a normal tensor fascia lata.

Three-phase bone scan

See *Bone scan*.

Tinel test

Tapping over a nerve produces pain and tingling or paraesthesia distal to the point of pressure. A test used particularly for the median nerve at the wrist (carpal tunnel) and the posterior tibial nerve (tarsal tunnel).

Tip toe stand

Nerve weakness. To test for weakness from the calf muscle and if no muscular or tendinous damage usually the cause is from a S1 root palsy.

Traction

The idea is to pull the vertebrae apart so that a negative pressure effect is exerted on the disc trying to reduce disc herniation, especially useful when an 'arc' of pain exists with SLR and this may be done in:

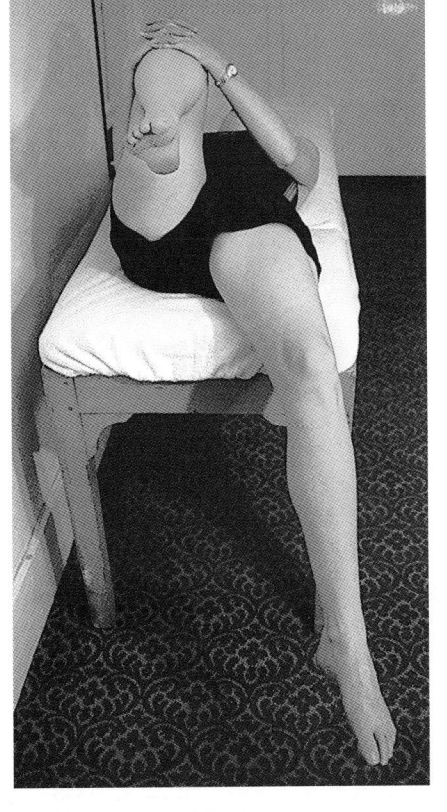

Figure 22.29   Modified Thomas test with a tight tensor fascia lata.

(a) Fowler's position, hips bent calves up on a stool. Good for L5 S1 collar stud disc, the early stage of L2/3.3/4 discs.

(b) Supine or prone. Good for discs improved with extension or worse with flexion. L4/5 later L5 S1 when extension does not make worse. L2/3.3/4 discs which no longer irritate the dura (can straighten and do extension manoeuvres without pain). Traction can be given daily or every other day, the kilo-pull will be increased as required by the therapist. Beware of a history of shooting pains and/or sudden stabs of pain into the leg, because the patient is wonderful on traction but may need an epidural to get them off traction. See Chapters 2 and 5.

Trendelenburg gait

Whilst standing the abductors of the **hip** tighten to support the pelvis. When the contralateral leg is raised, the pelvis should remain parallel or rise on the contralateral side. Lowering or excessive side flexion to the ipsi-lateral side is positive. The sign occurs with an osteoarthritic hip, stress fracture of the hip and trauma to the abductors.

Ultrasound

(a) **Diagnostic**. Ultrasound is very useful for soft tissue injuries, and particularly so for displaying haematomas and intratendinous cysts. In experienced hands tendinous tears, scar tissue and abnormal muscular contraction can be displayed.

(b) **Therapeutic**. Ultrasound appears of value to treat scar tissue as an adjunct to mobilization and stretching regimens. In particular, it has been shown to advance the migration of mast cells to, and their action at, the site of tissue damage. This is often degradative during the first 24–48 hours, which indicates that ultrasound should be applied around but not on the site of an acute lesion but after this time the reparative function of mast cells is enhanced and serial observations of tissue fractions show an advance in healing by about 4 days. The problems of penetration depth, standing waves and cavitation should be understood by practitioners using therapeutic ultrasound [10].

Valsalva

A dural stress test. Exhalation against a closed glottis or 'popping an ear' increases intraspinal pressure. See *Dural stress tests*.

Vastus medialis obliquus (VMO)

Part of the quadriceps muscle that attaches to the medial aspect of the patella and can therefore help to pull the patella medially and control maltracking. See Chapter 11.

Ward's triangle

Area of weakness noted in the trabecular lines in the inferior neck of the femur that may be the site of a stress fracture – the compression stress fracture.

Watson Jones

Operation for **unstable ankle**, using peroneals to strengthen the lateral complex.

Weiberg score

Defined from 1 to 4 with a Jagerhutt variety and is a classification of patella shapes relating to the femoral sulcus. The higher the score, the more likely the tracking problem causing anterior knee pain.

Wright's manoeuvre

The pulse of the abducted and externally rotated arm disappears when the neck rotates to the opposite side, and the shoulders are depressed and a deep breath taken. This may be positive for **thoracic outlet syndrome**. False positives occur.

Yergason's test

For bicipital tendinitis where resisted flexion and supination in the neutral position of the arm are painful. See *Speed's test*.

Further reading

1. O'Brien, S. J., Pagnani, M. J., *et al.* (1998) The active compression test: a new and effective test for diagnosing labral tears and acromio clavicular joint abnormality. *Am. J. Sports Med.* **26**, 610–613.
2. Butler, D. and Gifford, L. (1989) The concept of adverse mechanical tension in the nervous system. *Physiotherapy* **75**, 622–636.
3. Adler, G. G., Hoekman, R. A. and Beach, D. M. (1995) Drop leg Lachman test. A new test for anterior knee laxity. *Am. J. Sports Med.* **23**, 320–323.
4. Coates, G. C. and Keir, K. A. I. (1991) Connective tissue massage. *Br. J. Sports Med.* **25**, 131–133.
5. Coates, G. C. (1994) Massage – the scientific basis of an ancient art: part 2. Physiological and therapeutic effects. *Br. J. Sports Med.* **28**, 153–156.
6. Noyes, F. R., Grood, E. S., Cummings, J. F. and Wroble, R. R. (1991) An analysis of the pivot shift phenomenon. The knee motions and subluxations produced by different examiners. *Am. J. Sports Med.* **19**, 148–155.
7. Bobbert, M. F., Huijing, P. A. and Schenau, G. J. van I. (1987) Drop jumping. 1. The influence of jumping technique on the biomechanics of jumping. *Med. Sci. Sports Exercise* **19**, 332–338.
8. Bobbert, M. F., Huijing, P. A. and Schenau, G. J. van I. (1994) Drop jumping 2. The influence of dropping height on the biomechanics of drop jumping. *Med. Sci. Sports Exercise* **19**, 339–346.
9. Ho, S. S. W., Illgen, R. L., *et al.* (1995) Comparison of various icing times in decreasing bone metabolism and blood flow in the knee. *Am. J. Sports Med.* **23**, 74–76.
10. Dyson, M. (1987) Mechanisms involved in therapeutic ultra sound. *Physiotherapy* **73**, 116–120; and lecture series and personal communication, Mary Dyson, Guy's Hospital, London.

Index